Allergy Relief
& Prevention
THIRD EDITION

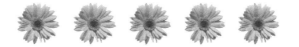

Allergy Relief
& Prevention

THIRD EDITION

Jacqueline Krohn MD

Frances Taylor MA

Erla Mae Larson RN

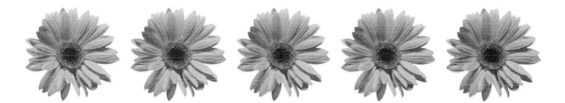

Hartley
&Marks
PUBLISHERS

Published by
HARTLEY & MARKS PUBLISHERS INC.
PO Box 147   3661 West Broadway
Point Roberts, WA   Vancouver, BC
98281   V6R 2B8

LIBRARY OF CONGRESS CATALOGING-IN-PUBLICATION DATA
Krohn, Jacqueline, 1950–
    The whole way to allergy relief and prevention : a doctor's
complete guide to treatment & self-care / Jacqueline Krohn,
Frances Taylor, Erla Mae Larson. — Rev. ed.
        p.   cm.
    Includes bibliographical references and index.
    ISBN 0-88179-194-6
        1. Allergy—Popular works.   i. Taylor, Frances A., 1938– .
ii. Larson,   Erla Mae, 1925– .   iii. Title.
    RC584.K76   1996
    616.97—dc20   96-29185
                                                    CIP

Design and composition by The Typeworks

Set in Scala

U.S. portion of the pollen map on page 222 courtesy of: Alk-Abelló,
Inc., 1700 Royston Lane, Round Rock, Texas 78664.

NOTE TO THE READER

This book is meant to be a source of information for those who are
not enjoying the best of health because of their allergies or sensitivities. Everyone has different problems and different needs based on
age, sex, lifestyle, health status, genetics, diet, psychological state,
and spiritual maturity. Our intent is to share our experience and
offer guidelines to help you become more informed about your
health. In cooperation with your physician, you can then take the
necessary steps to enjoy optimum health.

This book is not intended to be a substitute for consultation with
a physician. Neither the authors nor the publisher take medical or
legal responsibility for the reader who uses the contents of this book
as a prescription.

IN MEMORIAM

A special tribute to Dr. Theron Randolph, a pioneer in environmental medicine, whose genius forever changed the philosophy and practice of medicine.

TO OUR PATIENTS

who have taught us as we have attempted to teach and help them; who have presented innumerable challenges that have forced us to sharpen our skills; who have given us love beyond the love we have given them; and who have made all of our labors rewarding and worthwhile.

Contents

Foreword

EVERYTHING YOU ever wanted to know about allergies is in this book.

All pediatricians have to become allergists. At least 25 percent of their phone calls and office visits are related to allergy or sensitivity problems of some sort. Even infections are frequently triggered by allergies; we know that allergic people seem to be sick more frequently. The freckle-faced, ginger-haired youth is more susceptible to strep and rheumatic fever, probably because he has milk allergies. It is well known by most children's doctors, for instance, that ear infections (*otitis media*) begin as an allergic reaction to cow's milk that closes up the eustachian tube. Germs love to grow in that walled-off phlegm. Fever, pain, and a call to the doctor soon follow.

Decades ago, colic due to cow's milk sensitivity was estimated to upset only five to 10 percent of babies. By about 1970, workers at free clinics in large cities realized they were giving soy-based milk to at least half their clients because of sensitivities to cow's milk. Pediatricians have become adept at prescribing the usual control substances-antibiotics, antihistimines, sedatives, ointments, and gas dispersers-but little attention has been paid to the causes of allergies/sensitivities and their removal.

These infants grow up, of course, and they become allergic/sensitive children and then carry their problems into adulthood. School stressors, pollutants, sugar-laced foods, accidents, divorce, or death in the family are the stressors that seem to hit almost all of our children or patients. An overlooked fact is that about 80 percent of people in North America are too alkaline to some degree. This metabolism imbalance prevents minerals from being soluble and usable by the enzymes that allow the body to function optimally.

I have formulated a rule that works for me: If you do not understand something, it is probably due to an allergy. Everywhere I go in the US and Canada, and it has also happened in Australia and New Zealand, the natives say, 'This is allergy valley,' or 'This is hayfever hill.' It seems that only a few people do not have allergies/sensitivities of some sort or another. This book by Dr. Jacqueline Krohn will help the reader sort them out. There are many positive answers in this well-researched book, so don't give up!

Lendon H. Smith
Portland, Oregon

To the Reader

THE INFORMATION contained in this book is based on personal experience, as well as on knowledge gained through study and clinical experience. All of the authors have experienced, in varying degrees, allergies and sensitivities to foods, chemicals and inhalants; chronic fatigue syndrome; candidiasis; subclinical parasitic infections; mercury toxicity; and electrical imbalances. By using the treatment methods presented in this book, we have all recovered sufficiently to be able to conduct a full-time medical practice in environmental medicine.

From the beginning of our practice, we felt that an informed patient would be a more cooperative patient. We soon learned that a well-educated patient was more likely to comply with treatment, and to have a better chance of recovery. To aid in this educational process we wrote our *Allergy Patient Manual*, the nucleus from which *Allergy Relief and Prevention* grew. It is our intention that this book be useful to people with only a few allergies and sensitivities as well as those with environmental illness. Our primary goal, both in our practice and in this book, is to help people improve the quality of their lives.

We have used the most current, up-to-date information available. Although information and theories have been accumulating for many years, only recently have studies provided evidence that these theories are true. Environmental medicine is developing at a rapid pace, and this is not without controversy. It remains for health practitioners to interpret and implement this information, in innovative ways, for the care of their patients.

Controversy centers around nomenclature. In some instances we have tried to avoid this conflict by using the terms "sensitivity" or "intolerance" rather than allergy. The debate will continue for many years to come but will not solve the more important problem—the sufferer's distress. Our aim is to provide proper treatment and education to alleviate that suffering, whether symptoms are due to so-called "true" allergy or hypersensitivity syndromes.

Jacqueline A. Krohn, MD
Frances A. Taylor, MA
Erla Mae Larson, RN
Los Alamos, New Mexico
2000

Acknowledgments

Our sincere thanks to:

- Our predecessors and colleagues in the field of science and medicine, particularly in environmental medicine, for the work, research and publications that enabled us to write portions of this book.
- Colleagues who encouraged us and provided information and guidance.
- Our office staff for doing extra work to help us maintain our regular schedules while writing this book.
- Cheryl Sedlacek for the many hours she spent at the computer.
- Alice Kernodle, Susan Deininger, and Melissa Schneider for the many fact-finding exercises they performed on our behalf.
- Deborah Brandt for her contributions.
- Our families, who cheerfully endured the hours we spent writing this book.
- Elizabeth McLean, our editor for this third edition, whose knowledge, patience, enthusiasm, and talent enables our books to be organized and easy for readers to understand.
- The very capable staff of Hartley & Marks, particularly Susan Juby who puts everything together.

Introduction

A LARGE PART of the population of North America suffers from some type of allergy. Over 13 percent have pollen allergies. When the number of individuals who have food and chemical sensitivities is factored in, the total of those affected is over 25 percent of the population. In the United States, as many as 35 million people are affected by allergies, 6 million of whom are children. Allergies run in families, and if one parent is allergic, the children have a one-in-four chance of developing an allergy. If both parents have allergies, two of three children will be allergic.

Some physicians believe that the figures for allergy sufferers are low because, in addition to not including chemical and food sensitivities, they also do not include the many people who do not seek medical attention. Pollen allergies alone are responsible for 10 million physician office visits, 28 million days of restricted activity, 10 million missed workdays, and 2 million missed school days.

Some people are unaware of their allergies, many view their allergies simply as a nuisance, while others have symptoms severe enough to interfere with their chosen lifestyles. There are many clinical portraits of the person with allergies. The five main clinical descriptions are:

- those who have essentially only pollen allergies. They sniff, sneeze, cough and wheeze during pollen season, yet for the rest of the year feel reasonably well.
- those who have predominantly food allergies. They have no seasonal symptoms, but experience varying symptoms whenever they eat a food to which they are sensitive.
- those who have predominantly chemical sensitivities. They will suffer from exposure to perfume, gasoline, fabric softener, tobacco smoke, and other chemicals, but may not have symptoms from pollen or foods.
- those with a combination of pollen, food, and chemical allergies and sensitivities. There are infinite numbers of allergy combinations, varying in severity, and from person to person.
- those with such severe allergies and sensitivities, overlaid with other health prob-

I

Health is More Than Luck

Good health and a strong immune system are our most precious possessions. Allergies are not just a nuisance to be ignored until they can no longer be denied—they constitute a health problem that must be treated. Untreated allergies can lead to more serious difficulties as we get older. Blood pressure problems, diabetes, cardiovascular disorders, arthritis, and other degenerative diseases can develop as a result of untreated allergies.

If we do not take the time to treat our allergies and to get well now, we will have to take the time to be sick later. Good health does not depend on luck; it depends on having a healthy lifestyle.

into use each year, hazardous exposure is rapidly increasing. Our immune systems are often so overloaded that unless prevention and treatment are practiced, dysfunction and illness may result.

In this book, we present a complete look at allergy relief and prevention. Anyone with allergy problems, ranging from a minor sensitivity to environmental illness, will find information pertinent to his or her condition. Our practice evolved from and is based on the principles of clinical ecology and environmental medicine.

Clinical ecology is the study of our relationship with and adaptation to our environment (food, water, chemicals, air, inhalants, and medications) and the diseases and adverse reactions resulting from environmental sources. Environmental medicine is the practice of directly correcting or improving such environmentally caused problems with a minimal use of drugs. Its main goal is to reduce or eliminate the reactions a sensitive person experiences by using a combination of approaches, including environmental control, detoxification procedures, immunotherapy, nutritional supplementation, and rotation diet. In many cases, this comprehensive treatment enables the immune system to repair itself.

lems, that they are considered to be "universal reactors" and are described as ecologically or environmentally ill.

Environmental illness is the result of adverse reactions to substances in the air, water, food, home and work environments, and to medications. It can cause many varied, chronic symptoms, and it can involve many systems of the body, including the nervous, endocrine, immune, digestive, upper respiratory, muscular, and skeletal systems. Environmental illness frequently masquerades as other types of diseases and is often undiagnosed or misdiagnosed.

Unfortunately, environmental illness is becoming more and more prevalent. With over 5,000 new chemicals being brought

The "Tacks" of Illness

Dr. Doris Rapp of Scottsdale, Arizona says that having health problems is like having tacks in your shoe. People enjoying optimum health have shoes free of tacks; they experience no symptoms and enjoy life to its fullest. The rest of us have varying numbers of tacks in our shoes, depending on how many allergies and other health problems we may have. The environmentally ill person will possess the largest number of tacks.

We are born with some of our tacks, because we all possess hereditary factors, both positive and negative, that predispose us to some disease processes. To minimize the effect of these genetic traits, we can choose to alter our personal environment and lifestyle in order to maximize our strengths and minimize our weaknesses. We receive other tacks in our shoes as we journey through life and as our environment affects us. Infections give us one tack; the development of pollen allergy adds another. Chemicals in our environment, food sensitivities, nutritional deficiencies, electrical imbalances, dental problems—and even unresolved emotional issues—contribute still more tacks.

In order to improve our health and to eliminate the pain from these tacks, we must remove them. If we remove only a few, our pain level will be changed very little. In order to free ourselves entirely of pain, we must remove all of the tacks—we must travel the whole way to allergy relief.

Many treatment approaches are used to remove our "tacks" of ill health, and are discussed in detail throughout the book. Some people may require the use of only one approach to return to health. Others may need to use several to restore their health and well-being. In addition to our concern with allergy relief—with the removal of those tacks from our shoes—we are also interested in preventing and avoiding the accumulation of tacks. Prevention can be accomplished by reducing exposure in the immediate envi-

ronment and taking appropriate detoxification and nutritional measures before problems occur. Just as lifestyle management is the key to recovery from allergies, it is also the key to prevention.

Considering the Whole Person

Providing an in-depth history and evaluating all facets of your life helps your healthcare practitioner to guide you in removing the obstacles to healthy functioning. In such a lifestyle review, diet, habits, environmental exposure, psychoemotional functioning, and your particular experiences are essential pieces of data that determine the course of care. Looking at the whole person in this way allows the healthcare practitioner to individualize a program that will optimize your health.

▮ DIET ESSENTIALS

- *Healthy, high-quality diet:* Any junk food in the diet should be replaced with quality whole food that is organically grown, if possible. Fresh food devoid of pesticides and chemical fertilizers will promote and improve health.
- *Elimination diet:* Common allergenic foods and those suspected of causing allergic symptoms are temporarily eliminated. This helps both to identify allergens and to detoxify the body.
- *Rotation and allergen avoidance:* Improving your diet and using rotation of foods on a four- to seven-day basis helps to control food sensitivities, and prevents new sensitivities from developing. The complete avoidance of some foods may also be necessary.

■ LIFESTYLE ESSENTIALS

- *Proper exercise and rest:* Although exercise is a well-known stress reducer, most people who are not feeling well believe they should not exercise. Even mild exercise benefits the body by increasing the excretion of chemicals and toxins. Muscular activity acts as a pump for the proper flow of body fluids; nutrients and oxygen are carried to the cells for energy and repair; and waste products are carried to the proper organs for excretion. Then, during periods of rest, the repair processes are intensified.
- *Relaxation and meditation:* Stress, regardless of its origin, adversely affects the immune system. Relaxation and meditation reduce stress and calm both the mind and the body. Your attitude improves and problems can be approached with renewed vigor when your body, mind, and spirit are refreshed.

■ ENVIRONMENT AND DETOXIFICATION

- *Exposure reduction:* Reducing exposure to toxins, both internal and external, decreases the body's toxic load and allows it to heal. Diet alterations reduce internal exposures.
- *Environmental cleanup:* Unwanted or xenobiotic (foreign to the body) chemicals and cleaning supplies must be removed from your home and work environments in order to reduce your body's toxic load. Air or water filtration may also benefit your health. Natural methods of pest and fungus control must be used, rather than pesticides and fungicides. If you use natural gas, substituting alternative methods of home heating and cooking may be necessary.
- *Body cleansing:* Ridding the body of the unwanted chemicals it has absorbed is essential for recovery from health problems. Body functions improve when the toxic overload is treated by such techniques as detoxification saunas or baths, exercise, and massage. True healing begins only once the body's toxic burden has been reduced. Rest and appropriate support speed healing.

■ INDIVIDUALIZED EVALUATION AND TREATMENT

- *Allergy testing and desensitization with immunotherapy:* Identifying your major allergens and treating them with desensitizing extracts helps to control allergic reactions to foods, chemicals, and pollens. Hands-on allergy treatment will also desensitize people to foods, chemicals, and pollens.
- *Nutritional therapy:* Some infections and disease processes increase the demand for specific nutrients to amounts much greater than can be obtained from food. Nutritional deficiencies resulting from poor eating habits also contribute to the development of allergies and poor health. Vitamin and mineral supplementation will give your body additional nutrients to aid in the repair process.
- *Treatment for infection:* Allergies or sensitivities can follow a severe infection, and latent infections intensify allergies. Any ongoing viral, bacterial, fungal, or parasitic infection should be treated along with your allergies or sensitivities in order to reduce the total burden on your immune system.

The Right Doctor

It is vital to choose a healthcare practitioner with whom you feel comfortable enough to discuss all aspects of yourself and your health. A physician who is a true healer will be willing to listen and consider your ideas when developing a treatment plan. Your physician brings the benefit of experience with these complex health problems to the partnership. (See Choosing Your Physician in chapter 22.)

- *Evaluation and treatment of digestive function:* Poor digestive function can exacerbate allergies. By determining the level of acid in the stomach and the alkaline level in the small intestine, deficiencies can be corrected through supplementation.
- *Hormonal therapy:* Appraisal of the endocrine system for hormone imbalance can be important. Premenstrual syndrome, low thyroid function, thyroiditis, adrenal insufficiency, and other imbalances must be evaluated and addressed.
- *Identifying electrical imbalances:* The human body is electrical as well as chemical in nature. Electrical imbalances due to genetic predisposition, a diet poor in essential minerals, and environmental factors can adversely affect healing.
- *Evaluating dental health:* For some people, amalgam (silver-colored) fillings in the teeth lead to health problems. The mercury leaking from these fillings is a toxin responsible for a variety of adverse symptoms. Root canals can also be a hidden source of problems as toxins are released from minute remaining pockets of infection. Cavitations (necrotic areas in the jaw bones) are also a hidden source of toxins.
- *Emotional and spiritual health:* There is a crucial relationship between good health and your emotional, mental, and spiritual condition. Working to resolve emotional and psychological problems, trauma, or conflicts enhances and supports your recovery. Self-acceptance and self-expression enhance your healing.

Partnership with Your Physician

Dr. Marshall Mandell of the New England Foundation for Allergic and Environmental Disease in Norwalk, Connecticut has said that in order to treat our illnesses, we "look for magic, but must in the long run settle for hard work." Many people look for a "magic pill" that will cure their health problems without any effort on their part. There is no such pill. However, the hard work can be shared in partnership with your physician. He or she can help to diagnose your health problems and suggest ways for you to proceed.

An environmental medicine physician is the most knowledgeable ally to guide your recovery from allergies and sensitivities. Your adherence to the recommended treatment will determine your success. Your active participation keeps you motivated and moving toward health.

As you and your physician work through your particular "tacks" or problems, an individualized treatment program will be developed. Ideally, your body will respond to your patience, consistency, and commitment to your recovery with a lessening of and then an end to the symptoms. For some people, treatment will be very simple, requiring only a few changes, while for others their allergy symptoms may be only a small part of the whole picture and other factors will have to be considered.

Becoming an Active Patient

An active, informed patient is at the center of a health restoration program. The better you understand your body, its functions, and its problems, the more helpful and efficient you can be in implementing beneficial changes. Your dedication to the process immeasurably increases your health and quality of life.

The length of your recovery period depends on several factors: the number of your allergies or sensitivities; the length of time you have been ill; uncovering and resolving hidden infections; your nutritional state; your level of exposure to environmental elements; your compliance with treatment; and your desire to get well. The whole person needs to be considered: body, mind, emotions, and spirit. This approach to good health may seem slow at times, but given the right support your body can repair itself.

As you progress in your treatment, you will gradually learn to "read" your body and become more aware of subtle changes indicating problems or improvements. If you listen to its messages, your body gives much information about how well you are functioning. Most of us have been taught to ignore symptoms, to "grit our teeth" or numb ourselves. We continue routines that get us through the day, but damage the body and exhaust our energy. We have learned to ac-

cept less than optimum health. You can emerge from this state of "half health" as you learn to read your body, and you will be amazed at the volume of information that surfaces.

True healing is brought about through an internal process of self-knowledge and self-renewal. Choosing daily to take the small steps to move toward health replaces the "magic pill" approach. Optimal health is within your reach, as long as you are willing to work for it. As Dr. Lendon Smith, author and retired pediatrician from Portland, Oregon, remarks, "Not everyone needs to do all this: just those of us who want to stay well."

The holistic way of healing is a rebalancing process. There is a period of adjustment as you change your living habits to effect permanent benefits. You need to be supported through this time of learning and growth with the help of caring, experienced healthcare professionals. Gaining the skills that enable you to restore and maintain an optimal level of health may prove to be the adventure of a lifetime.

Natural Allergy Programs Work!

In our practice, we frequently tell our patients that their health and treatment can be compared to a flower bulb, its many layers representing the different health problems they may have. These problems can be treated and corrected, layer by layer. When the center of the bulb is reached, we discover the "flower of good health."

Some people have few health problems, and thus have small flower bulbs with few layers. Others have large flower bulbs with many layers that must be peeled back, using several different facets of treatment, in order to reach the flower. Regardless of the number of layers needing treatment, we all have the capacity to heal.

▮▮ SUE'S STORY OF RECOVERY

One of our patients with a very large "flower bulb" healed dramatically because of her diligent adherence to her treatment program. Sue was a 38-year-old woman who came to us complaining of severe headaches, extreme weakness, fatigue, hives and frequent rashes, colitis, intestinal cramps, nausea and vomiting, low energy, dizzy spells, arthritic symptoms, "heart cramps," sleep disturbances, bronchitis, and edema (swelling). She also experienced frequent sinus, bladder, and kidney infections.

Sue's history indicated severe allergies to pollen, dust, mold, and animal dander; acute chemical and food sensitivity; and evidence of Candida overgrowth. She had previously been given allergy shots containing formaldehyde as a preservative and, as a result, had acquired blood vessel damage both because she was allergic to formaldehyde and because of its toxic nature.

Her daily medications, prescribed by her previous physician, included:
- Lanoxin—0.25 mg, one per day
- Thyrolar—1 grain per day
- Entracin—5 grams, eight per day
- Tetracycline—250 mg, two per day
- Maxibolin—2 mg (half a tablet), three per week

Sue also had on hand, with instructions to take as needed:
- Lasix—40 mg, one every other day
- Ethaquin—100 mg, one per week
- Stelazine—1 mg, once per day
- Empirin #2—three per day
- Hydergine—1 mg, one or two per day
- Bentonite liquid, as needed
- Natural vegetable laxative, as needed

Other medications Sue had taken included cortisone, hormones, phenobarbital, sleeping pills, birth control pills, Inderal, Isuprel, and numerous antibiotics; nose drops; and antihistamines. She had a history of allergic reactions to drugs, including penicillin, sulfa drugs, and scopolamine, as well as reactions to bee stings.

Because Sue was suffering from numerous severe symptoms, we suggested that she leave her job as a substitute teacher to concentrate on her health care. Fortunately, she was financially able to do so, and she devoted her attention to taking care of her own health and that of her family. (Sue's two sons also had severe allergies.)

Sue's treatment began with allergy testing for pollens, dust, dust mite, mold, and animal danders. She tested positive to 9 trees, 6 grasses, 14 weeds, dust, dust mite, *Alternaria, Aspergillus, Hormodendrum (Cladosporium), Penicillium, Pullularia (Aureobasidium), Fusarium, Helminthosporium, Mucor, Rhizopus*, orris root, tobacco, histamine, cat, dog, and horse dander, and sheep's wool. Allergy extracts were made for her, based on these test results. The extracts were to be taken approximately once each week, after she determined her optimal dose.

We then tested Sue for chemicals, and found her to be sensitive to phenol, ethanol, benzyl alcohol, chlorine, glycerine, formaldehyde, and hydrocarbons (emitted by automobiles). Extracts for these chemicals were prepared, to be taken three times per day. Once Sue knew how it felt to be clear of symptoms, she began taking them once daily, repeating them as needed. Environmental cleanup was also recommended, and she followed the instructions to the last detail. Sue removed all harmful substances from her home, began using only safe products, and purchased an air cleaner and a water filter.

Testing Sue for food sensitivities both intradermally and sublingually, we found that she was sensitive to bananas, lemons, oranges, carrots, corn, garlic, onions, peanuts, pinto beans, potatoes, rice, soy, spinach, tomatoes, cow's milk, goat's milk, eggs, cane sugar, chocolate, barley, wheat, and yeast. This particular food grouping was consistent with the fact that Sue was an ovalacto vegetarian and these were the foods she ate most often. She was given food extracts for all of these foods, to be taken before her exposure to them.

Sue also began rotating her foods, following a four-day rotation diet. Day 1 was Italian day, Day 2 was Oriental, Day 3 was American, and Day 4 was Mexican; Sue prepared recipes that reflected the "national flavor" of each day while avoiding eating the same foods on successive days.

Sue's Candida questionnaire, symptoms, and culture were positive, indicating Candida overgrowth. Acidophilus and Nystatin powder were prescribed, and we recommended that she omit refined sugar from her diet. She was tested and given an extract for Candida and T.O.E. (*Trichophyton, Oidiomycetes*, and *Epidermophyton*).

At one time, Sue's pollen allergies were so severe she could not go outdoors for any length of time during pollen season. Grass mowing anywhere in the neighborhood caused her to react severely. Within a short time, the pollen extracts were giving Sue enough relief for her to be able to leave her home whenever she desired. Her tolerance to molds increased, and animal danders no longer caused her problems.

Chemical extracts allowed Sue to drive her car without developing acute symptoms, and she gradually was able to shop without experiencing a reaction. Exposures to personal care products worn by other people had limited her social activities; after treatment had begun, she was able to gradually resume her social life. The "heart cramps" Sue had experienced when bathing and washing her hair also disappeared.

Sue's creative rotation diet and her food extracts allowed her to eat without discomfort. Her colitis, alternating diarrhea and constipation, and headaches gradually subsided, and her rashes became a thing of the past.

One grain of thyroid was prescribed for daily use (based on basal temperature readings) to control her symptoms of hypothyroidism. Sue also used buffered Vitamin C and a heparin extract in addition to her extracts to control any allergic reactions she experienced, and she took a high-quality multiple vitamin and mineral supplement.

It was difficult for Sue to relinquish her many medications, but she gradually weaned herself from them as she began to feel better. She put the rather large sack of her medication bottles in her back storeroom, "just in case she needed them." She confessed that many times she was tempted to take some of them, because they provided what she felt was an easy "fix." We knew Sue was truly on the path to recovery when, after nine months on her program, she brought the sack of medications to us to throw away.

Sue experienced both ups and downs during her treatment program, but she persevered, faithfully following the prescribed treatment. Her cooperation, understanding, attention to detail, and creative spirit also contributed much to her recovery. After 18 months, she was back at work full-time, in a secretarial position where she was exposed to numerous chemicals with no ill effects. She was also able to use carefully selected makeup and hair care products.

As treatment progressed, Sue's family was able to get an outside dog, and Sue was able to gradually relax her rotation diet. Over a period of time, Sue was able to phase out her extracts, but she continued to use the air cleaner and water filter. When she occasionally became overloaded, she would increase her vitamin C intake and pay more attention to her exposures and diet. By exercising common sense, Sue was able to live a busy and healthy life. Her "flower of good health" flourished once she was able to peel away the many layers of her illness.

Sue's sons were both treated for their allergies also and did extremely well. Both boys had missed many days of school each year because of the symptoms caused by their allergies. The year after their allergy treatment, one of them had a perfect attendance record, and the other missed only two days of school with the flu.

PART I

Our Body Systems and Allergies

SCIENCE AND MEDICINE have categorized our body by systems that include the cardiovascular, musculoskeletal, immune, nervous, digestive, endocrine, respiratory, genitourinary, and other systems. These systems enable study of the body in great detail, and scientists and physicians have fully examined and defined each system. However, while this method of categorizing the body has some advantages, it also has disadvantages. Looking at individual body systems fosters the idea that these are separate, independent systems. The body is not considered as a whole and interdependently functioning unit.

In reality, the body systems are all interrelated, each affecting the other. There is a complex communication between the body systems, and more is discovered each year about the extensive nature of this communication. The body maintains a homeostasis or balance between the systems, so that any change or problem in one system affects all of the others. The body then has to establish a new balance. The more seriously one system is affected, the more difficulty the body has in re-establishing the balance.

Many of the body systems play a major role in, or are particularly affected by allergies. It is important to understand their role in the allergic phenomenon, as well as understanding the effects of allergies on these systems. Only those body systems that are most affected by allergies, and those playing a direct role in allergic reactions, are discussed in this section. Treatment possibilities for problems caused by allergies affecting these body systems are also presented.

CHAPTER I

Our Immune System

THE IMMUNE SYSTEM is our first line of defense against substances that would otherwise harm or destroy our bodies. So important is the immune system to our survival that it is distributed throughout our bodies and functions on a 24-hour basis. It is genetically programmed to fight off diseases from colds to cancer. The cells of the immune system communicate with each other, while acting with the endocrine and nervous systems to maintain body homeostasis or balance. Immune system functions are extremely intricate and complex—we still do not fully understand how an organism triggers, regulates, completes, or stops an immune response.

The immune system is affected more than other body systems when an allergic reaction occurs. This chapter describes the events that take place.

Organs and Lines of Defense of the Immune System

The immune system is a composite of cells and organs that extends throughout the body. The various organ components are listed below.

- *The skin:* The largest organ of the body, the skin protects the body against the invasion of harmful organisms.
- *The mucous membranes:* A thin sheet of tissue that lines parts of the body, the mucous membranes contain mast and basophil cells, T-cells, and IgA. These cells produce the chemicals that are released during an allergic reaction. They also secrete mucus that engulfs microorganisms and propels them for excretion.
- *The thymus gland:* Located at the base of the neck under the sternum at the level of the second rib, the thymus gland is the principal activator of the immune system. Known as the master gland of immunity, this gland was thought for many years to be useless after the age of puberty.

The primary function of the thymus gland is to produce T-cells, which are one type of lymphocyte (white blood cell). It also produces hormones that help initiate, mature, and regulate the function of the immune system. The thymus initiates the differentiation of the one trillion white blood cells of the body into several different types. These include neutrophils; macrophages; two kinds of lymphocytes, known as T-cells and B-cells; and eosinophils.

- *The lymphatic system:* A complex network of vessels that move fluid (lymph) from body tissues to the bloodstream. It is a pathway for the exchange of toxins, electrolytes, proteins, water, cell debris, and chemicals.

Lymph nodes are small protuberances along the lymphatic network that filter lymph and prevent foreign substances from entering the bloodstream. These nodes are found in the groin, the armpits, the covering of the intestinal tract (mesentery), the neck, between the ribs, along the spinal column, and in soft tissue in the knees and elbows. These nodes contain aggregations of lymphocytes (white blood cells) and antigen-producing cells, and become enlarged when they are actively fighting off an infection or increased numbers of allergens.

- *The tonsils and adenoids:* Composed of lymphoid tissues, the tonsils and adenoids act as a barrier to infectious organisms. The tonsils are a paired mass of lymphoid tissue at the back of the mouth while the adenoids are in the back of the nasal passage, on the wall of the nasopharynx.
- *The spleen:* Largest of the lymphoid organs, the spleen is in the left side of body between the diaphragm and the stomach. It produces some of the white blood cells that ingest foreign proteins and debris, and helps resist infections of encapsulated organisms, such as pneumococcus.

- *The appendix:* Also composed of lymphoid tissue and considered a part of the immune system, the appendix is attached to the cecum, which is the first part of the large intestine.
- *The small intestine:* The small intestine is the largest part of the digestive tract and contains collections of lymphocytes (both T- and B-cells) on the mucosal wall, known as Peyer's patches. Secretory IgA (an antibody) is produced by local plasma cells.
- *The liver:* During an immune response, the liver is stimulated to release a large number of protein molecules known as acute phase proteins. They exert an important influence on tissue repair, immune cell functions, and the inflammatory process. Located in the upper right part of the abdominal cavity, the liver is involved in ongoing body detoxification and takes some of the burden off the immune system by breaking down immune complexes.
- *The bone marrow:* The specialized soft tissue found inside the bones, the bone marrow is the production site for two types of white blood cells: B-cells, which secrete antibodies; and neutrophils, which consume foreign cells.

▮▮ CELLULAR COMPONENTS OF THE IMMUNE SYSTEM

The immune system functions through the action of highly specialized cells.

▮ T-CELLS

T-cells receive their name from the fact that they are produced in the thymus. Mature T-cells have a number of functions and are divided into three categories. Killer T-cells recognize and destroy foreign protein, such as bacteria, viruses, cancer cells, fungi, and protozoa. When a killer T-cell encounters an antigen, it attaches itself to the invader and "injects" it. These T-cells also activate phagocytes cells that engulf foreign substances to destroy the pathogens they have absorbed. Helper T-cells activate B-cells to make antibody molecules. Suppressor T-cells signal B-cells to turn off their production of antibodies.

▌ B-CELLS

B-cells are produced in the bone marrow and spleen, and in the lymphoid tissue of the immune system, not in the thymus gland. B-cells have the ability to multiply rapidly when they encounter antigens. Their function is to secrete chemicals known as antibodies or immunoglobulins, which circulate freely in all body fluids. These cells inactivate or eliminate offending organisms or antigens.

For each antigen present in the body there is a specific antibody produced by an individual B-cell, which remains committed to the production of that particular antibody. However, a shortage of T-cells will prevent the activation of the B-cells.

▌ LEUKOCYTES

Five types of cells make up the leukocytes, or white blood cells. There are three types of granulocytes that contain granules in the cell cytoplasm, including neutrophils, basophils, and eosinophils. Lymphocytes and monocytes have no granules in their cytoplasm. Leukocytes engulf and digest bacteria and fungi, and also function during allergic reactions and responses to cellular injury.

▌ MAST CELLS

Mast cells are large connective tissue cells that contain histamine, heparin, serotonin, and bradykinin. These chemicals are released by the mast cells in response to injury, inflammation, or allergic reaction, further adding to the inflammation.

▌▌ COMPLEMENT SYSTEM

The complement system, in partnership with antibodies, contributes to the destruction of pathogenic organisms. Complement is present in fluid of the blood and consists of over 20 proteins, each having a specific function. At least 9 of these complex serum protein units (C_1 to C_9) circulate in the body in inactive form. Once activated—usually by antigen-antibody binding (immune complexes)—they join and split one another sequentially, thus producing active, but short-lived, enzymes that bind to and rupture the antigen surface. This sequential activation is known as the complement cascade.

Additionally, fragments of the complement enzymes attach to the antigen itself, labeling it an enemy, or move into the bloodstream to attract phagocytic cells. Some antibodies activate complement enzymes in a way that produces agglutination (or clumping) of cells. The sources of these proteins are not fully known, but C_1 is thought to be produced in the colon, C_2 is made by macrophages, and C_3 is found in the liver. The purpose of the complement system is the destruction of "foreign" cells by lysis, or dissolution.

In the step-by-step progression and activation of the "complement cascade," histamine and other chemicals are released from

Exposure Routes

Allergens can enter our body in many ways. We can breathe them in through our respiratory tract; they can enter the digestive tract with our food and drink; we can be exposed to them on the skin and mucous membrane, or by sexual contact; they can be inserted into the body by injection or by insect bite; and we can even manufacture them in our bodies.

mast cells and basophils and are increasingly recognized as contributors to hypersensitivity responses.

Complement enzymes can also destroy the body's own blood cells in some types of autoimmune disease syndromes, which can lead to anemia (subnormal levels of red blood cells) and to leukopenia (subnormal levels of white blood cells).

Allergens and Antigens

Antigens are any molecules that are recognized by the immune system as foreign and that induce an immune reaction. For example, microbial antigens prompt the production of antibodies that aid in the destruction of organisms, and prevent reinfection with the same organism in future. Antigens are often composed of protein, but non-proteins can also be antigens.

Antigens that produce a different type of immune response, known as an allergic inflammatory response, are called allergens. Allergens can be inhalants (pollen from weeds, grasses, and trees; terpenes; molds;

dust; dust mites; cat and dog dander; foods of all types; chemicals (either internal or external); microorganisms; or insects.

Some allergens, called haptens, are too small to elicit a reaction from the body. However, when these allergens couple themselves with proteins in the body, the body sets up an allergic response to this form of antigen. The ability of the immune system to remember the substance it has previously encountered can actually work against the body during an allergic response.

■ CHEMICALS RELEASED DURING AN ALLERGIC REACTION

Mast cells, basophils, and other cells release chemicals during an allergic reaction. These chemicals may account for varying degrees of sensitivity, various symptoms associated with sensitivity, and varying time lapses between exposure to an allergen and the response.

- *Acetylcholine (AC):* AC is a neurotransmitter, as well as a chemical mediator released by cells and known to produce allergic symptoms along with histamine.
- *Bradykinin:* One of several kinins released during an inflammatory process when mast cells and basophils split open. Kinins tend to act synergistically with other chemicals to add to inflammation. Bradykinin causes pain by stimulating nerve endings and causes blood pressure to drop by widening peripheral arteries.
- *Heparin:* Inhibits the action of thrombin, an enzyme essential to blood coagulation. This may lead to increased blood flow to the inflamed site. Heparin and histamine are released at the same time.

- *Histamine:* Responsible for two main effects in an inflammatory response. It causes the blood capillaries to widen and increases their permeability so more fluid passes from the blood into the tissues. This causes local swelling, as well as generalized edema and redness. Histamine also causes contraction of the smooth (involuntary) muscles in the lungs, blood vessels, heart, stomach, intestines, and bladder.
- *Interleukins:* Antigens involved in activating and differentiating lymphocytes. They irritate tissues and can set up inflammatory responses.
- *Interferons:* Produced mainly by certain stimulated lymphocytes, they act to regulate the extent and speed of other immune responses, and enhance viral immunity.
- *Leukotrienes:* Leukotrienes are found in cell membranes, and act more slowly than histamine. A higher level of leukotrienes is present in the skin in atopic dermatitis (skin inflammation) and psoriasis; in the colon in inflammatory bowel diseases; in tears resulting from uveitis (iris inflammation); and in the nasal passages in allergic rhinitis (mucous membrane inflammation). Leukotrienes cause the bronchospasms of an asthma attack by causing the bronchial muscles in the lungs to contract, which allows the adequate inhalation of air, but prevents adequate exhalation.
- *Lymphokines:* A group of molecules, produced by lymphocytes, that are involved in signaling between the cells of the immune system.
- *Prostaglandins:* Hormone-like substances that regulate cell functions in every part of the body. There are a number of prostaglandins and many have antagonistic roles (roles that have opposing functions). Prostaglandins act to dilate blood vessels, affect smooth muscle contraction, enhance the effect of other chemicals, heat inflamed tissue, and increase pain in affected areas.
- *Serotonin:* Plays a role in allergic responses, especially to foods. Ninety percent of the body's serotonin is found in the mucous membrane cells of the gastrointestinal tract. It acts differently from histamine, even though the end result of inflammation is the same. A chemical (5-hydroxyindoleacetic acid) is released with the breakdown of serotonin in mucous membrane, and this is thought to cause irritation of surrounding cells.

■ IMMUNE RESPONSE IN ALLERGY

The immune response is a stimulus-response sequence of events. The immune system protects us in two ways: one occurs through cell-mediated immunity, the other through antibody-mediated immunity. The work of the cell-mediated immune response is done by phagocytes, neutrophils, and macrophages (types of white blood cells). Phagocytes engulf and destroy a wide variety of nonspecific molecules, particles, and organisms. These scavengers are found in the blood and lymphatic systems and in most other tissues in the body. They are very efficient and engulf not only foreign materials but also "self" materials such as damaged or dead cells, causing localized or systemic inflammation. After these specialized white cells have destroyed the invader, they present it to the T- and B-cells.

The T- and B-cells prepare to destroy antigens. First the T-cells become sensitized and are released into the lymph system, the bloodstream, and eventually to all parts of the body. When the sensitized T-cells find the antigen, they attach in a "lock and key position" and inject them with "poison." The T-cells send out chemicals that sensitize other nearby T-cells and attract macrophages, which consume dead neutrophils and antigens.

While the T-cells are combating antigens, the B-cells, having "studied" the antigen, begin to grow and divide into daughter cells called plasma cells. These plasma cells act like factories, manufacturing antibodies. The antibodies then seek out and destroy any antigens resembling the one for which they have been programmed. It takes time for the B-cells to produce plasma cells, and for the plasma cells to produce antibodies. The T-cells and macrophages must continue the battle until the antibodies can come to their aid.

B-cells become long-lived memory cells that retain the original specific antigen-binding information. Later re-exposure to the same antigens stimulates these memory cells to divide and produce more cloned plasma cells, and to speed up the body's immune functions. This quick response accounts for sensitive people's instantaneous reaction to chemical, food, or inhalant antigens.

▌ IMMUNOGLOBULINS

There are five types of immunoglobulins (antibodies): IgA, IgD, IgE, IgG, and IgM, which are made by B-cells. (Tests to identify and measure immunoglobulins are discussed in chapter 8, Allergy Testing and Treatment.) Each has a different "weapon" for attack. Some neutralize antigens by covering up their active or toxic sites, while some render antigens harmless by binding or clumping them together. Some immunoglobulins "rip" open antigens, and still others prevent viruses from entering cells.

- *IgA:* Found mainly in the mucous membranes of the gastrointestinal and respiratory tracts and body secretions (tears, saliva), it protects mucous membranes from invasion by microorganisms.
- *IgD:* Found in cell membranes, and involved in cell activation, it is believed to play a part in recognizing "self" and "foreign" antigens.
- *IgE:* Frequently involved in allergic reactions to pollen and food, it is found both in blood and within the organs. It attaches to basophils (white blood cells) and other mast cells that are similar to basophils. Contact with an allergen causes these cells to burst, which in turn releases histamine or enzymes into the surrounding fluid to inactivate the allergen. The release of histamine causes either local inflammation and/or systemic (whole body) flushing and other adverse symptoms.
- *IgG:* Found in both blood and tissue fluid, it is the most abundant antibody in the body and is also involved in attacking bacteria and other antigens, such as food. IgG coats microorganisms, and high levels indicate a past infection.
- *IgM:* Found mainly in the bloodstream, and most often involved in attacking bacteria and other antigens, IgM is the first antibody that the body produces against a

foreign antigen. IgM also coats microorganisms, and high levels indicate a current or recent infection.

▋▋ ANTIBODIES AT WORK

Antibodies, which are the immunoglobulins, can rip open cell membranes and kill an antigen or can neutralize it by covering up its toxic site. Multiple antibodies can bind themselves to several antigens, rendering them harmless. About 75 percent of total immunoglobulins are IgG, which together with IgM attack bacteria and viruses.

Wherever there is antibody-antigen action in the body, there will also be an inflammatory response, accompanied by swelling (edema), redness, heat, tenderness, and impaired function. This response is the body's attempt to heal itself. The inflammation is caused by release of prostaglandins, serotonin, leukotrienes, kinins, and histamine, and by an increased blood supply carrying more white blood cells to the area.

For anyone with allergies, the most important portion of the immune response takes place after the antibodies have attached to the invaders. At this point, they carry the antigen to the mast cells and basophils found in the blood, skin, and mucous membranes, causing the cells to release histamine and other chemicals. Histamine increases capillary permeability, allowing the white cells to flow freely out of the capillaries and into the tissues, where they can fight invaders. This triggers water retention and swelling.

Because the histamine and other released substances irritate normal cells, the body turns off their release when the invader

has been repelled. When histamine levels around a mast cell reach a certain concentration, the mast cell releases a chemical that turns off histamine production in the releasing cells and all surrounding mast cells. In some people, however, this mechanism does not function properly and the reaction "cascades." The T-suppressor cells then work to prevent the formation of any more antibodies.

Immune System Stressors

Unfortunately, in the severely allergic person, the immune system is continually at work, much like a car with its engine left running. In his book *Type 1/Type 2 Allergy Relief,* Dr. Alan Levin from Nevada compares the B-cells to the car's engine and the T-cells to the brakes. Allergic individuals have high-powered engines and weak brakes, so their car—or immune system—often goes out of control. An overstimulated immune system follows the same general law that applies to other overstimulated tissues: overstimulation eventually leads to inhibition of function. This continuous assault can lead to recurrent infection and inflammatory diseases such as sinusitis, arthritis, asthma, bronchitis, colitis, myositis, migraine headaches, and ulcers. Undiagnosed or untreated allergic responses can, over a period of years, lead to degenerative diseases.

Each of us has a different level of immune competence. This level varies with hereditary factors; the number and degree of our exposures to infections, chemicals, and drugs; age; nutritional status; stress level; and amount of exercise. In some cases, the allergic person is genetically endowed with

Stress and Lowered Immune Function

Stress in any form has a negative effect on our immune system. Studies have shown that surviving spouses have lowered numbers of T-cells for several months after the deaths of their partners. Hormones produced by the adrenal glands in response to stress can interfere with T-cell functions. Even positive stress, such as winning a million-dollar sweepstakes, can adversely affect the immune system, which can be damaged by constant stress just as it can be impaired by chronic disease or infection.

Maintaining regular sleeping habits and healthy eating routines, exercising, and pursuing gratifying work or hobbies help to support mental and physical well-being during and after stressful periods.

too few T-cells or overactive B-cells, resulting in improper immune response and producing "allergic" symptoms. Others may have more sensitive mast cells and basophils and so may release excess histamine during reactions.

Dysfunction of the endocrine system can alter the immune system's ability to respond. Recent research has shown that the brain and nervous system play a role in regulating our immune response. Lack of adequate nutrients can also have debilitating effects on all parts and functions of the immune system. Repeated or chronic infections have long been known to lower immu-

nity, but the body's ability to fight back can also be compromised when we are "overloaded" and assaulted repeatedly by food, chemical, or pollen antigens.

Clinicians have found that the immune system can be improved and strengthened, even though it may be heavily damaged. Improving diet, getting adequate rest, modifying responses to stress, exercising, eliminating infections, and reducing environmental exposures all help to repair the immune system. In addition, immunotherapy, therapeutic levels of nutrients, detoxification, herbal and homeopathic preparations, and supplements of enzymes that quench free radicals, support and accelerate healing. (Free radicals are chemicals—atoms, ions, or molecules—that have an unpaired electron, are highly reactive, and can cause tissue and cell membrane damage. When produced in normal small amounts by the body, free radicals are helpful. However, tissue damage occurs when they are produced in larger amounts, triggered by external stimuli.)

▮ AUTOIMMUNITY

An extremely complex syndrome takes place when the body no longer tolerates "self" molecules, producing an immune response to the self that interferes with normal cell function. Diseases such as diabetes, rheumatoid arthritis, multiple sclerosis, lupus erythematosus, myasthenia gravis, and Grave's disease (hyperthyroidism) are thought to be related to autoimmunity. Although we do not yet understand the exact mechanisms, it seems that a combination of genetic susceptibility and unknown environmental agents may trigger this malfunction.

Many researchers believe that immune complexes may be involved in some of these diseases. Immune complexes are formed when antibodies and antigens bond; under normal conditions, these complexes are destroyed and eliminated shortly after their development. However, sometimes they are stored in body tissues, causing inflammatory reactions, formation of fibrin, and tissue lesions. These immune complexes are evident in all diseased tissues. As long as these tissue-bound immune complexes remain, the immune system will be overstimulated and overloaded. When additional antigen loads are placed on the immune system, it is unable to respond adequately and the person becomes increasingly immune deficient.

Total Load/Overload

In day-to-day living, our bodies are subjected to many stresses: physical, emotional, spiritual, and environmental.

- *Physical stresses:* These include infections (viral, bacterial, parasitic, and fungal); chronic disease; poor nutrition; food allergies; chemical allergies; allergies to pollens and other inhalants; pregnancy; inadequate or excessive exercise levels; insufficient fatty acids; vitamin, mineral, and amino acid imbalances; hormonal imbalance and/or sensitivity; yeast overgrowth; acid/alkaline imbalance; a toxic body burden, lowered immune system function; poor digestion, hampered by insufficient hydrochloric acid and/or pancreatic enzyme production; and insufficient sleep.
- *Emotional stresses:* Each of us has a unique response to our emotions regarding our work, family, and personal lives. Our ability to allow and express these emotions is a factor in our overall stress load. Our outlook and emotions can contribute to or be a burden on our health. Abuse of any kind (past or present), whether it be sexual, physical, or verbal, causes emotional stress, often with a high toll in body symptoms, obsessive behavior, and alcohol and drug dependencies that can require extended recovery.
- *Spiritual stresses:* Many people today have a spiritual injury that contributes to their emotional stress. Their sense of spirituality and connection with their own soul may never have had a chance to develop or may have been damaged by their life experiences. This spiritual injury manifests as physical symptoms that impair their health.
- *Environmental stresses:* These may be extremes of heat, cold, or altitude; air and water pollution; or food pollution. Other stresses include high-intensity electricity sources; radiation; excess lead or heavy metal exposures; pesticides; fungicides; toxic cleaning and laundry products; scented personal care products; tobacco and wood smoke; car and diesel exhaust; natural and propane gas; and new building materials.

Our body can usually adjust to a few stressors, but when there is an accumulation or repetition of stressors, our metabolism loses its adaptability. Any one of these stresses can upset the normal control mechanisms of the immune, nervous, or endocrine systems. At this point we develop symptoms because our total body burden is

Popcorn Overflow

An allergic response to a given substance can depend on the total load/overload of the person at the time. One of our patients who was exquisitely sensitive to corn clearly demonstrated this phenomenon. If her allergic load was low, she was able to attend a movie with no symptoms. If her total load was high, the smell of the popcorn caused her to develop a migraine headache long before the movie was over. Her "rain barrel" overflowed from the smell of the popcorn if it was full or nearly full before she went to the theater.

too high. The collective response exceeds a "threshold" level that the body metabolism can tolerate. The body can then no longer maintain health and balance.

However, we can learn to systematically reduce the overloading stressors so that the energy that the body produces can be rerouted to adequately perform all of its normal functions.

▮ OUR IMMUNE SYSTEM "RAIN BARREL"

Dr. William Rea of the Environmental Health Center in Dallas, Texas, describes our immune system as a rain barrel. Any combination of stresses "fills" our rain barrel. If we can keep our rain barrels emptied by controlling our allergies, cleaning up our environment, improving our nutrition, exercising

regularly, detoxifying our bodies, and reducing other controllable stress, we can tolerate moderate life stresses without overflowing our rain barrel. If, however, our rain barrel remains full, the slightest additional stress factor will cause it to overflow, resulting in distressing symptoms.

The rain barrel concept explains why sometimes we develop symptoms from an allergen, while at other times we do not. This depends on how full our rain barrel is at the time of the additional stress. In addition, some people have large rain barrels, while others have small ones—heredity plays a role in determining their size.

We need to drain our rain barrels and keep them as empty as possible, so that our immune system will not be pushed to exceed its adaptive capacity and will begin to heal.

▮ PREVENTING THE RAIN BARREL EFFECT

Evaluating the causes of each sensitive person's overload is important in planning an effective treatment plan. There are many paths to recovery that prevent the rain barrel effect:

• treating sensitivities through immunotherapy, hands-on allergy treatment, rotation of foods in the diet, and selective food elimination
• cleaning up the environment
• avoiding exposures to allergens
• treating infections
• alleviating stress
• nutritional therapy
• hormonal therapy

- detoxification procedures
- adequate rest/sleep
- exercise
- relaxation and meditation exercises
- counselling

As you begin to identify the stresses that are causing your overload, an individualized program can be implemented to help reduce your total load. Diligently reducing total load will help you tolerate those substances to which you are sensitive and put you on the path toward optimum health.

CHAPTER 2

Our Endocrine System

PEOPLE WITH environmental illness often show evidence of endocrine dysfunction. It is difficult to assess whether this is caused by hereditary factors, stress from environmental illness, or both. Endocrine dysfunction can be corrected by assessing and treating hormonal imbalance, testing for and treating allergies, detoxifying the body, taking nutritional supplements, and reducing stress.

Our thyroid, parathyroid, pituitary, hypothalamus, pancreas, adrenal glands, pineal glands, and gonads (ovaries and testes) are all ductless glands that make up our endocrine system. These glands produce hormones and secrete them either directly into the bloodstream or into extracellular fluids, allowing them to reach virtually all cells of the body. The gastrointestinal tract, kidneys, liver, and placenta are part of the endocrine system because they too produce hormones that are released into the bloodstream. The immune system and the central nervous system work together with the endocrine system.

It is the body's second most important communications system, after the nervous system. Many of the glands secrete more than one hormone, and some of the endocrine glands, such as the pancreas, also have exocrine functions, which include the release of digestive enzymes and the bicarbonate that neutralizes the acidic food from the stomach.

Our endocrine system:
- controls the rate of chemical reactions
- regulates cell membrane permeability
- activates specific functions of cells
- regulates the slower metabolic reactions
- regulates circulation
- maintains water and electrolyte (e.g., sodium, potassium, magnesium) balance
- regulates digestion and absorption of food
- balances energy and metabolism
- regulates the reproductive cycle
- responds to stress stimuli

Hormones

Specialized cells in the endocrine glands produce hormones that act as chemical messengers, to speed up or slow down our body's chemical reactions. There is a feedback mechanism between the hormones and the glands so that the hormones from one gland can stimulate the production of hormones from other glands. Hormones produced in one area of our body can have an effect elsewhere in the body. Hormone production can also be stimulated by the central nervous system, and by the concentration of available nutrients and minerals.

A specific hormone may be produced by more than one type of endocrine gland. For example, somatostatin is secreted by endocrine cells in the intestinal tract as well as in the pancreas and in the hypothalamus of the brain. Some of the molecules classed as hormones can also be produced by other body tissues and may act as neurotransmitters by transmitting nerve impulses.

Hormones are not secreted at constant rates but rather in short bursts, depending on the amount and duration of regulatory stimuli. Some glands, such as the pineal, follow circadian rhythms (based on daily alternations of darkness and light) in their hormone secretion. Others, such as the adrenals, produce more hormones in response to external stimulation at irregular intervals, while glands such as the ovaries release hormones at regular intervals in response to levels of other hormones in the blood.

Hormones would not function if there were not specific matching receptor sites on our cells for attachment of the hormones, similar to the lock and key mechanism of antigen/antibody binding (see chapter 1,

Our Immune System). This binding of hormone to target cell initiates a response from the target cell. Hormones are highly specific in that each one will affect only one organ or one group of target cells.

Our hormone levels depend not only on the amounts secreted, but also on our body's ability to remove the excess. This is accomplished by direct excretion through the liver and kidneys, and also through metabolic transformation and degradation by enzymes. If these functions are not performed adequately, excesses of specific hormones or metabolites (products of metabolism) can continue to circulate in the body, causing hypersensitivity reactions and/or autoimmune responses, such as thyroiditis or the production of anti-ovarian antibodies. It has also been suggested that incomplete unexcreted fragments of a hormone may mediate new and different effects of that hormone. These effects may be undesirable, as well as unpredictable.

There are three types of hormones:

- *Amines:* Derived from the amino acid known as tyrosine. It has three subtypes of hormones: thyroid hormone (produced in the thyroid); protein hormones (such as prolactin, produced in the pituitary); and epinephrine, dopamine, and norepinephrine (produced in the adrenal gland and other tissue, and which also have neurotransmitter action).

- *Peptides:* Range in size from a group of three amino acids to large groups of amino acids, such as insulin (produced in the pancreas). The majority of hormones are peptide hormones.

• *Steroids:* All steroid hormones are produced by the adrenal cortex, testes, ovaries, and the placenta, and require cholesterol for their production.

After secretion by a specific endocrine gland, a hormone may undergo further metabolic steps in order to be fully effective. Some enzymes are required to activate and bond certain hormones with receptor sites on cells. Other enzymes act to transform a stored hormone into its active state, to synthesize hormones in an endocrine gland, and to convert one hormone into another. The concentration of these key enzymes can be low or nonfunctioning because of hereditary or genetic factors, lack of proper nutrients, or damage from circulating toxins, either exogenous (originating outside the body) or endogenous (originating within the body). When this occurs, malfunction and disease processes can be set in motion, causing such ailments as hypothyroidism, hypoadrenal function, or hypersensitivity to one's own hormones.

Additional problems can arise if receptor sites for hormones are nonfunctional, damaged, overloaded, unable to uncouple or transform the attached hormone, or improperly stimulated or prepared by another hormone. Such malfunctions result in decreased hormone production, an excess of circulating hormones that can damage other tissues, or an inability of the receptor site to accept a hormone. These malfunctions can also lead to diseases. It is possible to adjust malfunctions by using varying dosages of specific hormones, such as thyroid, cortisol, DHEA, estrogen, pregnenolone, progesterone, and testosterone.

Pituitary Gland

The pituitary is a small gland that lies in a pocket of bone at the base of the brain. It is integrally connected to the hypothalamus (part of the brain that controls the endocrine system, autonomic nervous system, and many other body functions), which collects neural information about the status of body functions and conditions, including hunger, thirst, stress, emotional state, body position, internal and external temperature, talking and walking, and sleep. After the information is collected and processed, the hypothalamus stimulates specific cells of the pituitary to produce and secrete hormones.

The pituitary gland is made up of two lobes—the posterior and the anterior. The posterior lobe is actually an outgrowth of the hypothalamus and is composed of neural tissue. It secretes two hormones (vasopressin and oxytocin), which are synthesized in the neural tissue and picked up by surrounding capillaries. These hormones are also produced by nerve tissue elsewhere in the body, where they act as neurotransmitters. This is another example of the close interrelationship between the endocrine and nervous systems.

Vasopressin is known as an antidiuretic hormone. It regulates fluid levels in the body by directing the kidneys to reabsorb sodium ions but not water. The water is then excreted. Increased amounts of vasopressin are also released during stress situations. Oxytocin, the other hormone secreted by the posterior lobe, has an influence over uterine contractility and causes the contractions of the nipple in the "milk letdown" response of nursing mothers.

The anterior pituitary lobe is also regulated by the hypothalamus. While there is no important neural connection between the anterior lobe and the hypothalamus, the hormones produced by the anterior pituitary lobe act to stimulate the secretion of other hormones in a chain fashion.

Some of these hormones influence more than one type of hormone, and can inhibit as well as stimulate. Our bodies contain many such complex check-and-balance mechanisms.

If there is any malfunction of the interconnected endocrine glands, the feedback mechanism between the glands and the nervous system can ultimately affect the pituitary gland and the hypothalamus. The problem will then be compounded because incorrect messages are received, and then improper stimuli are sent back to the glands within the system.

Thyroid Gland

The first gland to be discovered, the thyroid, is located behind and below the larynx. The pituitary stimulates the thyroid to produce

> ## Hypothalamus Dysfunction
>
> *Damage or a nutritional deficit in the hypothalamus leads to a disruption of signals, and the wrong messages are sent to the endocrine glands. Excess sugar and alcohol disrupt hypothalamus function. Disruption over a long period of time will result in pituitary insufficiency and inhibited function of many of the endocrine glands, with long-lasting effects. Some examples of these effects are hypothyroidism, obesity, muscular weakness, edema, PMS, infertility, fatigue, stress syndromes, depression, irregular menses, and hypoadrenalism.*

three hormones: thyroxine (T_4 – containing four iodine), triiodothyronine (T_3 – containing three iodine), and calcitonin. Both thyroxine and triiodithyronine are produced from elemental iodine and tyrosine (an amino acid). The thyroid gland can store several weeks' supply of thyroxine bound to a large protein known as thyroglobulin. The

Pituitary Hormones	Stimulates Secretion Of
Thyroid stimulating hormone (TSH)	Thyroid hormones (thyroxine, triiodothyronine, and calcitonin)
Adrenocorticotrophic hormone (ACTH)	Cortisol from adrenal cortex
Follicular stimulating hormone (FSH)	Estrogen, progesterone, and testosterone
Luteinizing hormone (LH)	Regulates the growth of sperm and ova
Growth hormone	Somatomedin (growth-promoting peptide) has direct effect on carbohydrate, lipid, and protein metabolism
Prolactin	Stimulates the breasts to produce milk

Hypothyroidism

Hypothyroidism is frequently found in those with allergic symptoms, and it may also be associated with fatigue, weakness, constipation, loss of hair, coldness of extremities, menstrual problems, depression, headaches, dry, coarse skin and hair, brittle nails, hoarseness, and pale skin.

thyroid secretes more T_4 than T_3, but a variety of tissues, including the liver and kidneys, enzymatically split off an iodine atom, converting most of the T_4 to T_3, which is the more active hormone.

Calcitonin is released from separate cells in the thyroid. Calcitonin lowers plasma calcium by inhibiting its release from bone. It acts in opposition to the parathyroid hormone. Magnesium, zinc, copper, iodine, and cobalt are minerals essential for the function of the thyroid gland.

The thyroid gland:

- regulates our metabolic rate
- stimulates protein metabolism in cells
- stimulates chemical reactions in cells
- stimulates glucose absorption
- increases the rate of absorption of nutrients in the intestinal tract
- increases the intestinal tract's motility
- controls children's growth rate
- affects the rate of adult metabolic repair
- increases heat and energy production in cells
- increases oxygen consumption
- affects our heart rate and strength, the central nervous system, muscle function,

sleep quality, hormone production, and respiration rate

Thyroid dysfunction symptoms are caused by either an acceleration of these functions (hyperthyroidism) or a slowdown (hypothyroidism). The classic symptoms of thyroid dysfunction are:

- increased allergic responses (hyper- and hypothyroidism)
- poor thinking processes (hyper- and hypothyroidism)
- digestive disorders (hyper- and hypothyroidism)
- memory loss, especially short-term memory (hypothyroidism)
- fatigue and waking up as tired in the morning as you were at bedtime (hypothyroidism)
- lowered sex drive (hypothyroidism)
- low basal temperature reading (hypothyroidism)
- insomnia (hyperthyroidism)
- palpitations and heartbeat irregularities (hyperthyroidism)
- nervousness, ranging from mild anxiety to full-blown panic attacks and suicidal tendencies (hyperthyroidism)

Thyroid dysfunction can be caused by malfunction of the hypothalamus; infectious diseases (parasitic, viral, bacterial, or fungal); nutritional deficiencies; hereditary factors; prolonged stress; damage from toxic materials; or tumor growths. A person may manufacture anti-thyroid antibodies as a result of immune system malfunctions following prolonged stress, as in chronic allergic states or following infections. Some people may have an overfunctioning thyroid that is inflamed or enlarged and produces excess thyroid hormones, causing them to be hyperthyroid. The function then reverses. The gland remains tender, but slows down the production of hormones, resulting in hypothyroidism. This fluctuation between hypothyroidism and hyperthyroidism is known as Hashimoto's disease.

▮▮ TESTING THYROID FUNCTION

The following tests are used to determine thyroid function:

- Anti-thyroid Antibody Panel (includes determination of antithyroglobulin and antimicrosomal antibodies)
- serum levels of T_3 and T_4 (thyroid hormones), and TSH (pituitary hormone)
- radioactive iodine uptake
- basal metabolic temperature readings

The thyroid gland can function in a borderline way, creating symptoms that complicate the diagnostic picture. The problem may not be severe enough to show up in blood tests, but lowered body temperature readings indicate low function. Even with borderline thyroid function, the symptoms may be severe enough to cause distress and create changes in metabolism that mimic allergic reactions. Low-dose thyroid supplementation significantly improves the person's health in these cases.

▮▮ BASAL TEMPERATURE STUDY FOR THYROID FUNCTIONS

In spite of the highly sensitive tests available today, the true status of the thyroid gland is elusive. Laboratory tests for thyroid evaluation are relatively inaccurate for near borderline hypothyroid function. Most of these tests indicate the levels of thyroid hormone circulating in the blood, but they do not accurately represent the amount of thyroid hormone available and being used at the cellular level.

Functional tests tell us more about a person's thyroid. Body surface temperature, measured under the arm, is an indication of thyroid function. If the temperature is consistently low, an underfunction of the thyroid is suspected. Normal values for underarm temperature are 97.4 to 98.2°F. If the temperature is over 98.2°F, hyperthyroidism is considered a possibility. A temperature below 97.4°F is suggestive of hypothyroidism.

This basal temperature method is quite useful and accurate when done properly. Other conditions in which basal temperature may be low include starvation, adrenal or pituitary gland deficiency, and toxicity from microorganisms. Thyroid supplementation is useful in some deficiencies of the adrenal and pituitary glands.

▮ HOW TO TAKE YOUR BASAL TEMPERATURE

- Before retiring at night, shake down a mercury thermometer and lay it on your bedside table or nearby chair. Be sure it is shaken down to at least 96°F.
- The next morning, before getting out of bed, place the thermometer in the armpit of your bare arm. Press your arm against your body so the thermometer will not slip, making sure there is no clothing between your skin and the thermometer. An electric blanket or excess bed covers will cause the thermometer reading to be high.
- Leave the thermometer in place for 10 minutes. Stay in bed. Remove the thermome-

ter, and read and record the temperature.

- Record your temperature for 14 days. Note any symptoms of illness and/or menstrual cycle next to the temperature.
- For premenopausal women, begin the temperature readings on the second day of your period.

After recording your temperatures for two weeks, average the values. If your basal temperature average is below 97.4°F, you may want to discuss the possibility of trial thyroid supplementation with your physician. You should also consider the methods of thyroid support discussed below.

■ TREATING THYROID DYSFUNCTION

Thyroid support can be accomplished in a number of ways: using nutritional supplements that include iodine and tyrosine, initiating thyroid replacement with either desiccated thyroid preparations or synthetic single hormones, reducing infectious disease processes, improving diet, reducing stress, surgically removing tumors when indicated, and by using homeopathic and herbal preparations designed for thyroid support.

Several types of thyroid preparations are available for supplementation. Synthetic thyroid preparations are formulated in the laboratory and contain T_3 or T_4, two of the thyroid hormones. While the dose is standardized and controlled, T_4 is not the most active thyroid hormone. Also, some people are unable to convert T_4 to T_3, which is the more potent thyroid hormone required by the body, and must take T_3.

Natural desiccated thyroid contains both T_3 and T_4, and is easily assimilated by most people. Newer processing methods, enforced by strict government regulations, now provide a standardized dose. Natural thyroid is processed from either beef or pork thyroid glands. Good results are achieved with both of these, but the balance of the pork thyroid hormones is closer to that of our own. People who are sensitive to beef or pork may have difficulty taking these thyroid preparations.

Thyroid supplementation is the treatment of choice for those who manufacture anti-thyroid antibodies, which attack their own thyroid glands. Among those with allergies to other substances, a significant number of people also have anti-thyroid antibodies.

■ WILSON'S SYNDROME

Some people suffer from Wilson's Syndrome, which is slow metabolism resulting from an impairment in the ability to convert T_4 to the active thyroid hormone, T_3. The symptoms of this syndrome often occur after significant physical, mental, or emotional stress. Routine thyroid blood tests will be normal, but body temperature will be below normal.

Symptoms of this syndrome include waking up tired, fatigue, dry hair and hair loss, decreased memory and concentration, insomnia, intolerance to heat and cold, depression, fluid retention, inappropriate weight gain, dry skin, constipation and irritable bowel syndrome, decreased motivation/ambition, decreased sex drive, menstrual problems, infertility, decreased wound healing, increased skin infections, allergies, and other symptoms.

To help determine whether you have Wilson's syndrome, take your temperature by mouth, using a mercury thermometer. Take it every three hours, three times a day, beginning three hours after you wake up. Average the three temperatures for each day. Check your temperatures for a week. Women should not use the three days prior to the onset of their period because the temperature is always higher then.

If the temperatures consistently run low during the day, when temperatures are normally higher, the average body temperature will be low. Combined with symptoms, this is an indicator for Wilson's syndrome. Temperatures will run below 98.6°F, with 97.8°F being typical. Some people may be slightly higher, in the 98.0° to 98.4°F range, while others may have a temperature of less than 97°F. If you are presently taking a T_4 preparation, you must gradually stop taking it and take no thyroid preparation for 10 days prior to taking the temperature test for Wilson's syndrome.

Treatment for Wilson's Syndrome includes resetting the thyroid gland using proper T_3 therapy. T_3 therapy is useful both as a symptomatic and/or therapeutic intervention. Specially formulated T_3, Liothyronine, is used for this therapy, as Cytomel, the more common form of T_3, is not long-acting enough to give a smooth, continuous level of T_3.

Adrenal Glands

The adrenals are the "fight or flight" glands, located above the kidneys. They are composed of the medulla, which is the inner core, and the cortex, which is the outer covering.

The medulla secretes two amine hormones, epinephrine and norepinephrine, which are released directly into the bloodstream. Under extreme stress, the adrenal glands prepare the "fight or flight" response, increasing blood to the heart, brain, and the long muscles, while decreasing blood to the skin and intestinal tract. The skin becomes white, the hands get cold, and the mouth becomes dry.

Epinephrine, also known as adrenalin, is a dilator for the vascular (circulatory) system, and for the airways in the lungs. Epinephrine is a hormone and neurotransmitter, and regulates organic metabolic processes. It inhibits insulin secretion and stimulates the release of glucagon (a protein hormone), which causes increased plasma concentrations of glucose, glycerol, and fatty acids. By these functions, epinephrine is involved in the body's "fight or flight" response to real or perceived stress.

Norepinephrine is epinephrine without an attached methyl group (CH_3). It narrows the blood vessels and constricts peripheral circulation in the skin, eyes, and the body's mucous linings. It functions as an inhibitory neurotransmitter between the nerve fiber and the cells responsible for changes in organs. It is thought to decrease distracting background electrical activity in the brain so that sensory input from the body is made more clear. This results in improved information processing during directed attention or learning situations.

Enkephalin and endorphins (peptide neurotransmitters with inhibitory properties) are also released by the adrenal medulla, as well as by the pituitary. They in-

Stress, Cortisol, and Adrenal Symptoms

The chronic stress state produced by overproduction of cortisol, followed by underfunctioning of the adrenal gland, can cause such symptoms as chronic fatigue, hypotension (low blood pressure), dizziness, hair loss, weight loss, inability to exercise, inappropriate response to temperature changes, lack of perspiration, and depression.

terrupt memory formation, especially if a painful sensation is involved.

The cortex or outer layer of the adrenal gland is composed of three separate layers that have opposing enzyme functions. These enzymes interrelate to produce the adrenal cortex hormones. Cortisol and aldosterone are the most important of the hormones produced.

Cortisol release is stimulated in response to stress, activated by the secretion of ACTH (adrenocorticotrophic hormone) from the hypothalamus/pituitary axis. Cortisol causes the release of glycogen, which is broken down to glucose, providing instant energy. It also affects the breakdown (catabolism) of proteins that provide more energy and glucose, which is of major importance to brain function. With these physiological changes, the body is prepared for fight or flight in any stress situation.

In today's world, a large variety of psychological events occur that our bodies perceive as stress, and respond by releasing cor-

tisol. When the body is unable to appropriately utilize the excess cortisol through either fight or flight, the increased levels of cortisol circulate and damage body tissues. As a result, there is a profound reduction in the immune system's inflammatory response, which in turn decreases resistance to infection or effective response to allergens. A chronically high cortisol level also triggers the retention of sodium ions that can lead to hypertension. Increased cortisol reduces the stomach's ability to handle normal levels of acid, which can lead to gastritis and/or ulcers. It also inhibits secretion of growth hormones (and contributes to the breakdown of body protein during chronic illness).

Aldosterone, the other important hormone produced by the adrenal cortex, stimulates the reabsorption of sodium from the kidney in order to regulate the electrolyte balance in the body when plasma volume is decreased. Extracellular potassium concentration also works directly on the adrenal glands to stimulate aldosterone production. This helps to control arterial blood pressure and aids the body in acclimatizing to heat.

Adrenal androgens are similar to but much less potent than testosterone and are produced in small amounts. They have some effect on growth by stimulating protein synthesis, especially during puberty, and are thought to contribute to sex drive in women.

The adrenal glands also produce dehydroepiandrosterone (DHEA) and its sulphonated metabolite DHEA-S. The precise function of these hormones is uncertain, but they may be involved in the maturing and aging process, and their levels do decrease with age. Supplementation of DHEA in people with low levels of this hormone has resulted in improvements in sleep, relaxation, energy, handling stress, and joint pain.

■ TESTING ADRENAL FUNCTION

Adrenal function can be tested with a 24-hour urine collection that measures overall hormone production of the adrenal cortex. Adrenal reserve can be tested by an ACTH stimulation test, in which intravenous or intramuscular injections of synthetic ACTH (Cortrosyn) are administered and blood cortisol levels are obtained before and after stimulation.

Adrenal function and hormone levels can also be checked with a saliva test. Hormone levels that can be determined include DHEA, prednisone, aldosterone and cortisol. Two saliva specimens (taken at noon and between 4 and 5 p.m.) are usually required and are collected by saturating a cotton roll that is then sealed in a tube and returned to the lab for analysis. There are eating and drinking restrictions before taking the sample. Other hormone levels can also be determined from a saliva test, including estrone, estradiol, estriol, progesterone, and testosterone.

■ TREATING ADRENAL
DYSFUNCTION

Avoiding stress is the most important factor in supporting the adrenal gland. For hypersensitive people, any method aimed at relieving environmental, food, or inhalant stressors is encouraged. Immunotherapy helps to relieve the chronic stress of repeated reactivity. Suitable exercise will help to reduce and eliminate excess circulating cortisol before it can damage and alter cell function. The adrenal gland needs vitamin C, potassium, and pantothenic acid (B_5) to function properly.

Many people who have repeated allergic reactions have exhausted adrenals. Fatigue and deep internal back pain above the waist may be a signal of this condition. This pain is frequently mistaken for kidney pain. People with exhausted adrenal glands should never undertake strenuous exercise. Supplementation with a dessicated adrenal glandular supports the adrenal gland and allows it to recover. The supplement supplies some of the hormones the adrenal gland is unable to make, and helps to relieve the fatigue and back pain.

Thymus Gland

The thymus gland, considered the master gland of immunity, is a small gland under the breast bone by the second rib, surrounded by ropes of nerves. At one time the thymus was thought to be useless because it shrinks and becomes fibrous at puberty. The adrenal glands swell under stress, whereas the thymus shrinks. It secretes thymosin, which stimulates T-cell function. Up to age seven, it regulates, through the T-cells, the amount of immunity you will have for the rest of your life. B-cells migrate from the bone marrow and undergo a differentiation process to become T-cells as they move from the outer shell of the thymus to its center.

After this differentiation, the T-cells leave the thymus and make their home in other lymph tissues throughout the body. The thymus continues to influence the T-cells and their clones by means of a hormone (thymosin) that is excreted by the cells on the inner lining of the gland. The T-cells produce interleukins and interferon, which stimulate cell division and further differentiation during an infectious or inflammatory process.

For a time, researchers used thymosin injections (obtained from calves after slaughter) to enhance the function of the immune system, but it was an extremely expensive material to use. Although thymosin has been successfully synthesized, its availability in North America has been restricted by health regulatory boards.

Inadequate nutrition stresses the thymus. Vitamin A, a powerful immune stimulant, will increase the function of the thymus gland and reduce the shrinking process in the thymus during infection or inflammation. Zinc deficiency has also been found to shrink the thymus. Any of the following antioxidant vitamins and minerals are helpful for thymus gland function: vitamins A, C, and E; sulfur-based compounds (methionine, cysteine, glutathione, or taurine); selenium and zinc. Desiccated glandular substance (usually obtained from cow's or pig's thyroid, or sometimes from sheep's or lamb's thyroid) may also help to boost some people's immune function. People who are sensitive to these meats may have difficulty taking these preparations.

Parathyroid

The parathyroid is composed of four lobes on either side of and behind the thyroid. It regulates blood calcium and phosphate metabolism.

Parathyroid hormone is controlled by the calcium concentration in the extracellular fluid surrounding the parathyroid glands. Lower levels of calcium stimulate the production of the hormone and higher levels have the opposite effect. The parathyroid hormone:

• stimulates the kidney to synthesize vitamin D (also a hormone). An increase in the level of vitamin D heightens intestinal absorption of calcium and phosphate.
• increases reabsorption of calcium in the kidneys.
• reduces reabsorption of phosphate and thus increases phosphate excretion, which in turn increases calcium deposits on bone. This is one step in maintaining a homeostasis of extracellular calcium and phosphate.
• increases the movement of calcium and phosphate from bone into extracellular fluids so there is an available source of extra calcium when needed throughout the body.
• increases the excretion of phosphate in the kidneys for protein balance in the body.

Pineal Gland

The pineal gland is located near the midbrain. It regulates growth and is very active until the age of seven, after which it tends to become more fibrous and begins to atrophy. Until recently, it was thought that the gland had no further function after this age; however, it is now felt that light passing the retina of the eye stimulates the pineal gland and the hypothalamus to create a sense of well-being. For this to happen, the light must be from a natural ultraviolet source, as some artificial forms of light can actually disrupt the pineal gland's function. The pineal gland is also stimulated by adrenalin.

Production of sex hormones, growth hormones, and some liver enzymes are all influenced by the pineal gland. It produces the hormone melatonin, a metabolite of tryptophan, which is responsible for regulating circadian rhythms in the body and sleep-wake cycles. Melatonin production responds to light stimulation, even in some totally blind people. Winter months, with their shorter days and less natural light, can lead to depression and lethargy. Called Seasonal Affective Disorder Syndrome (SADS), it is thought to be caused by a disruption in melatonin production. During prolonged periods of stress, melatonin production is suppressed.

Melatonin level abnormalities are found in many low-tryptophan diseases. Low levels of melatonin are found nocturnally in the depressive state of manic-depressive disease, in people with anorexia, schizophrenia, psoriasis, Cushing's disease, and hypopituitarism. High levels of melatonin are found in people with narcolepsy, obesity, spina bifida, sarcoidosis, and delayed puberty.

Pancreas

The pancreas, which is below and behind the stomach, has both endocrine and exocrine functions. The endocrine portion of the pancreas produces three protein hormones: insulin, glucagon, and somatostatin. They are produced by clusters of en-

Pancreas Dysfunction

If it is overstimulated, the pancreas eventually functions poorly. Addictions of all types (alcohol, food, chemical, or tobacco) lead to overstimulation, followed by pancreatic insufficiency of both exocrine and endocrine functions. This process is often seen in hypersensitive people.

Early signs of insufficiency are associated with hypoglycemic symptoms: loss of stamina one hour after meals, dizziness, cravings for sugar, sweating or chills, blurred vision, and headache. If untreated, further damage can result and may lead to diabetes mellitus.

docrine cells in the pancreas, called islets of Langerhans.

The hormone insulin acts on most of the body's tissues. Its secretion is stimulated by eating, which increases glucose, and is inhibited by fasting, which reduces glucose. Insulin stimulates the diffusion of glucose into the cells of muscles and adipose tissue. It also stimulates the active transport of amino acids into most cells, making them available for protein synthesis. Insulin inhibits almost all the liver enzymes that release glucose from the liver and increases the activity of the enzyme that catalyses the first step in glucose metabolism.

Glucagon, a second hormone produced by the pancreas, acts in opposition to insulin, increasing the:

• breakdown of glycogen in the liver.

• production of glucose and ketone bodies in the liver. Ketone is a byproduct of fat metabolism.
• breakdown of fat tissue.
• plasma concentration of glucose and fatty acids.

Somatostatin is the least well understood of the pancreatic hormones. It is an intercellular chemical messenger produced by cells in several locations in the body. It is released from the pancreas during the absorption of a meal. Somatostatin helps prevent excessive levels of nutrients in the plasma by slowing and restraining the rates of food digestion and absorption.

Preventing damage to the pancreas is most important for hypersensitive people. Avoidance of any addictive syndrome is foremost. Following a diversified rotation diet, taking nutritional supplements, reducing sugar intake, obtaining immunotherapy for allergies to reduce stress load, making hormone adjustments by taking exogenous hormones or allergy extracts, and reducing other stressors that trigger a glucose/insulin roller-coaster effect all help prevent damage to the pancreas.

Hyperinsulinemia (too much insulin circulating in the blood) is a primary cause of obesity and cardiovascular disease. It is caused from the production of too much insulin, as well as by the inability of insulin to bind to the cellular insulin receptors. This condition is known as insulin resistance.

When glucose enters the cells, a drop in insulin takes place, and serotonin is released by the brain. The serotonin release produces the "full" feeling, or satiety. In people with hyperinsulinemia, the level of insulin does not fall, serotonin does not rise, and the person does not feel full.

The elevated insulin levels prevent the release of glucagon, which signals the liver to stop making cholesterol. Without glucagon release, cholesterol levels will continue to rise. In cardiovascular disease, insulin resistance also causes glucose intolerance, a resistance to insulin-stimulated glucose uptake, increased very-low density lipoprotein cholesterol and triglycerides, decreased high-density lipoprotein cholesterol, and hypertension.

Most obese people are insulin resistant. Their glucose is converted to glycogen and triglycerides in the liver. Insulin stimulates fat synthesis, causing obesity. Exercise decreases insulin resistance.

The main causes of hyperinsulinemia are carbohydrate, fructose, fat, and alcohol ingestion. Hyperinsulinemic people release too much insulin in response to the carbohydrates they eat. These elevated insulin levels create an appetite for more carbohydrates and the person becomes a carbohydrate addict.

Kidneys

The major function of the kidneys is to excrete waste products and water, and to regulate the homeostasis between sodium, potassium, calcium, hydrogen, and bicarbonate ions. The kidneys also produce the hormones known as erythropoietin, renin, and 1,25 dihydroxyvitamin D.

Erythropoietin acts on bone marrow to stimulate the proliferation and maturation of one type of red blood cell (erythrocytes). Its secretion is stimulated by a decrease in the level of oxygen delivered to the kidneys. Testosterone, the major male sex hormone, also stimulates the release of this hormone.

Renin is involved in fluid balance. The parathyroid hormone acts on 1,25 dihydroxyvitamin D. Vitamin D plays a role in calcium absorption from the intestinal tract.

Gastrointestinal Tract

Five hormones are secreted by cells throughout the gastrointestinal tract.

- *Gastrin:* A peptide hormone secreted in the stomach lining that stimulates gastric secretions and some gastric contractions.
- *Secretin:* A peptide hormone produced in the small intestine. The presence of acid in the small intestine stimulates its release, and secretin in turn prompts bicarbonate release from the pancreas and the liver. Acid secretions and stomach motility are inhibited by the action of secretin.
- *Cholecystokinin:* Also produced in the small intestine in response to acid material. It enhances the action of secretin, stimulates pancreatic enzyme secretion, stimulates gallbladder contraction, and stimulates the bicarbonate secretion of the liver.
- *Somatostatin:* Decreases the rate at which food is digested and absorbed. It inhibits production of growth hormone and thyroid-stimulating hormone from the pituitary, and the release of gastrin from the stomach and insulin from the pancreas. It is also thought to act as a neurotransmitter. Somatostatin is secreted by the pancreas, hypothalamus, and the stomach.

- *Gastric inhibitory peptide hormone:* Secreted by the stomach, this hormone inhibits the secretion of acids and pepsin, and stimulates the release of insulin as part of the digestive process.

Gonads

Gonads (the testes in the male and the ovaries in the female) are our main reproductive organs. The gonads produce sex hormones that are stimulated by two gonadotrophic hormones from the pituitary: follicular stimulating hormone (FSH) and luteinizing hormone (LH). These are steroid hormones, synthesized from cholesterol, that induce development of the sex organs and many of the sex characteristics and changes that occur throughout life. Sex hormone secretion begins around the age of eight to ten and reaches a plateau within five to ten years.

▌▌ MALE HORMONES

In men, the testes produce the hormone testosterone and reproductive cells (sperm) at a constant rate. The effects of testosterone are to:

- maintain the function of male reproductive organs.
- stimulate male secondary sex characteristics (hair growth).
- stimulate growth and bone growth.
- maintain sex drive.
- inhibit LH production.
- aid sperm production.

Testosterone, which can also be produced by the adrenals, has a mild effect on the thymus. The testes also produce a small amount of estrogen, less than one-fifth of the amount produced in women.

■ ANDROPAUSE

In men, the climacteric or "menopause" occurs when there is a gradual slowing of testosterone production. This condition is called andropause. The pituitary attempts to stimulate the production of testosterone, but because the testes are no longer able to produce it, there is an excess of follicular stimulating hormone. This excess causes changes in mood and perception—effects that can be more emotional than physical. However, many men experience weakness, impotence, pain, stiffness, drooping muscles, depression, irritability, and excessive sweating with intolerance to heat.

Symptoms of andropause can be helped with the following methods:

• *Diet:* Eliminate sugar, caffeine, and alcohol. Cut back on red meat and fat, and foods containing nitrites, such as luncheon meats. Eat a diet high in soy, fiber, and organic vegetables, particularly those that are red-orange in color. Also eat seafood, lean meat, and grain products. Drink 1/2 ounce of pure tolerated water per pound of body weight each day.

• *Exercise:* Exercise regularly to increase fitness levels.

• *Nutrients:* The following nutrients, including vitamin E, copper, zinc, DHEA, essential fatty acids, octocosanol, a multivitamin and mineral, and raw orchic glandular can improve andropause symptoms.

• *Herbal and homeopathic remedies:* Specific remedies selected for the man's symptoms can alleviate problems.

• *Hormonal treatment:* Extracts or hand-on allergy treatments for testosterone sensitivity may be indicated. In some cases, supplementation with natural testosterone from a compounding pharmacy is necessary.

■■ FEMALE HORMONES

The female gonads, the ovaries, have three functions:

• producing ova (eggs)
• preparing the body for conception and gestation
• determining the length of pregnancy

The ovaries are stimulated by luteinizing hormone (LH) and follicular stimulating hormone (FSH) to produce the two steroid hormones, estrogen and progesterone. The ovaries also produce a small amount of testosterone. Their rate of production is cyclic, not steady, as is testosterone production in men. Estrogen creates a negative and positive feedback on the pituitary to regulate the production of LH and FSH.

Estrogen actually refers to a group of steroid hormones that have an effect on the female reproductive system similar to estradiol, which is the major estrogen secreted by the ovaries. Estriol is also produced in small amounts by the ovaries and is the major hormone secreted by the placenta, along with progesterone and chorionic gonadotropin, during pregnancy. Estrone is the third form of estrogen, and is produced from estradiol and other hormone precursors.

Estradiol, estrone, and estriol are commonly referred to as estrogen. Estrone and estradiol have been found to be carcinogenic under some circumstances. Estriol is considered not only to be noncarcinogenic but anticarcinogenic.

Estrogen causes secondary sex characteristics. There are six different stages of estrogen production and utilization. In the liver, excess estrogen is changed to estriol, which is less active and is excreted. The effects of estrogen are to:

- stimulate growth of the ovaries, follicles, and external genitalia.
- initiate breast development.
- cause females to have shorter bones.
- increase protein synthesis in pregnancy.
- increase fat deposits in the breasts, hips, and thighs.
- soften the skin because of fat and increased vascular supply.
- stimulate the growth and maintenance of smooth muscle and lining of the reproductive tract.
- cause fluid retention.

Recent evidence points to excess estrogen as being the cause of endometriosis, a condition in which the uterine lining proliferates outside the uterus. The liver is unable to convert other forms of estrogen to estriol for excretion, causing excess estrogen in the body.

Progesterone prepares the uterus for pregnancy and develops the breasts for lactation. It also provides a negative feedback control over LH and FSH, and regulates secretions in the reproductive tract.

▌ PREMENSTRUAL SYNDROME

Many hypersensitive women develop other problems as a result of prolonged allergic reactions. Because the endocrine, immune,

> ## Symptoms of PMS
>
> - *Psychological and neurological symptoms: Depression, irritability, memory loss, sleep disorders, anxiety, hostility, crying spells, lethargy, paranoia, tension, dizziness, headaches (migraines), fainting, seizures*
> - *Glandular symptoms: Swelling and tenderness of breasts and the vaginal mucosa, increased sex drive*
> - *Gastrointestinal symptoms: Abdominal bloating, constipation, abdominal cramping, craving for sweets, lowered tolerance for alcohol*
> - *Dermatological symptoms: Facial acne*
> - *Other physical symptoms: Fatigue, swelling of extremities, weight fluctuation, thirst, pelvic pain*

and nervous systems are so closely interrelated, a stress on one system eventually overflows to place stress on another system. A common complaint from such women is known as premenstrual syndrome.

Premenstrual syndrome (PMS) refers to the complex of symptoms from which over 20 million North American women suffer. Most women with PMS experience several of these symptoms with each period. We hope that no woman suffers from all of them. Some women's symptoms begin at mid-cycle, and others have them immediately before menstruation begins. The beginning of menstruation usually relieves the symptoms, although they may last as long as four days after the onset of the menses.

■ TREATMENT OF PMS

There is no single "magic pill" to relieve or cure the symptoms of premenstrual syndrome. PMS involves a dysfunction of the immune and endocrine systems of the body. The best approach is to address the whole body. Some ways to do this are by diagnosing and treating abnormal levels of estrogen, progesterone, FSH or LH; diagnosing and treating endometriosis (dysfunction of the uterine membrane); reducing and treating allergies and infections; and cleaning up the immediate environment to reduce allergens and other toxic exposures. This will enable the endocrine and immune systems to function more efficiently.

Because many factors are involved in PMS, treating it involves a variety of therapies:

■ *Treating Hormonal "Sensitivities"*

PMS symptoms are relieved through treatment with the proper hormonal extract or hands-on allergy treatment for hormones. Most PMS patients have normal hormone levels, but when they are tested for progesterone, estrone, or LH, they show acute sensitivities to these hormones. A neutralizing dose of these hormones helps to relieve the symptoms of PMS. Hands-on allergy treatments for hormones will also help. Both types of treatment are also useful in relieving morning sickness and menopause symptoms.

■ *Treating Candidiasis*

Treatment of candidiasis to relieve the symptoms associated with yeast overgrowth also helps relieve PMS symptoms. This involves the use of antifungal agents, diet control, mold control, and the use of extracts or hands-on treatment to stimulate the immune system. Progesterone release in the body may aggravate Candida overgrowth and may cause or increase some premenstrual symptoms. (See *Candida albicans/ Yeast Infection* in chapter 17, Fungi, Yeast, and Mold.)

■ *Treating Food and Chemical Allergies*

Food addiction plays an important role in PMS. People tend to be addicted to the foods to which they are allergic. Control of food allergies by testing and treatment with extracts or hands-on treatment for offending foods will significantly reduce the body's total load. Cleaning up the environment, avoiding chemical exposures, and treatment with chemical extracts or hands-on treatment for chemical sensitivity will also help.

■ *Controlling Diet*

Many studies have been done linking diet to PMS. Eliminating caffeine, sugars, salt, alcoholic beverages, and highly refined carbohydrates will reduce PMS symptoms. Caffeine prolongs the action of adrenalin, which affects the stimulation of other hormones. Adrenalin stimulates gastric secretion and adversely affects blood pressure, fat metabolism, and insulin requirements. Caffeine also acts as a stimulant to the central nervous system and cardiac muscle.

Sugar and highly refined carbohydrates rapidly raise blood sugar levels, forcing the hormonal system to be overworked. This may lead to shakiness, dizziness, and headaches.

Salt contains sodium and chloride, which are essential for maintaining the body's water (and acid) balance. They also affect the nerve cell excitability and muscle contraction. Women will experience monthly water retention when sodium excretion is inhibited by pituitary hormones that are released in response to excess estrogen. Excess sodium may create an imbalance with potassium, causing erratic contractions of the uterus resulting in cramping.

Alcoholic beverages affect both the absorption of many nutrients and carbohydrate metabolism. An interim product in alcohol metabolism is acetaldehyde, which is toxic to the body, causing dizziness, disorientation, headache, cloudy vision, poor concentration, and poor memory. Acetaldehyde is also one of the many toxins released by the Candida organism during its metabolic processes.

I *Nutritional Supplements*

Vitamin A helps maintain healthy epithelial tissue, which is a barrier to bacteria and infection, and it is essential for a normal estrus (fertility) cycle. It also helps prevent excessive bleeding during periods.

B complex vitamins, known as the antistress vitamins, are necessary for carbohydrate, protein, and fat metabolism, and assist in proper functioning of the nervous system. Vitamin B_6 helps to regulate the female cycle and balance sodium.

Vitamin C strengthens blood vessels, increases iron absorption and aids in the conversion of tryptophan to serotonin, which has a calming effect on metabolism. Vitamin C is necessary for maintenance and proper functioning of collagen fibers in the uterus, which provide the elastic qualities of the uterine wall.

Vitamin E helps maintain cell membrane integrity and aids in converting estrogen to estriol in the liver. It is vital to the proper functioning of the reproductive organs and helps reduce premenstrual edema. Vitamin E strengthens capillary walls, thereby improving the vascularity of the uterus.

Calcium and magnesium are important to muscle and nerve function, and are involved in transmitting hormonal messages. Magnesium is known as nature's tranquilizer and muscle relaxant. It will relieve uterine and vaginal cramping and will help to moderate PMS mood changes.

Potassium is required for proper functioning of the smooth muscle tissue of the uterus. It is also used by the adrenal glands during periods of stress.

Prostaglandins produced by the body play a role in PMS. One type of prostaglandin induces the kidney to retain salt, leading to water retention, and also causes inflammation. Both of these conditions contribute to menstrual cramping and the symptoms of PMS. Another type of prostaglandin causes relaxation of the uterine muscle. Evening primrose oil is a precursor to the beneficial prostaglandins and helps to relieve bloating, breast pain, irritability, and depression.

Nutritional programs work slowly to alleviate PMS and must be continued over a period of time before results are achieved. However, consistently using nutrient therapy will gradually decrease symptoms and prevent their recurrence.

I *Exercise*

Regular exercise helps to control PMS. It tones the muscles, relieves tension, aids in food metabolism, provides extra oxygen for improved cell metabolism, and leads to improved self-image and increased well-being.

❙ *Water*

Increasing water intake several days prior to the start of menses will help to flush out degraded hormones, as well as circulating nutrients more quickly to all cells. It will also keep electrolytes balanced in the tissues, which will reduce edema.

❙ *Stress Reduction Techniques*

Management and reduction of stress help in controlling PMS. Biofeedback, relaxation therapy, and changes in lifestyle are very helpful for some people.

❙ *Detoxification Procedures*

Procedures that increase the efficiency of the liver, such as liver cleanses, detox baths or saunas, exercise, and nutrients, enable the liver to more efficiently detoxify excess hormones produced by the body. Balanced hormones decrease the symptoms of PMS.

Some women have severe symptoms just before and during menopause. Many of the treatment methods discussed above that are helpful for PMS will also relieve menopausal symptoms, as well as painful menstrual periods. See Natural Remedies for Common Complaints in chapter 21, Solving Everyday Problems, for treatment of menstrual cramps.

CHAPTER 3

Our Nervous System

COMPOSED OF THE BRAIN, spinal cord, peripheral nerves, and special sense organs, our nervous system is our body's primary communication, regulation, and coordination network. (The other system used for communication is the endocrine system.) Our nervous system is also responsible for our behavior, learning, states of consciousness, emotional responses, motivation, memory, thoughts, and reasoning.

Our nervous system is directly affected by external toxins and allergens, as well as by toxins and substances produced within our body as a result of the malfunction of other systems. Recent studies indicate that the nervous system may play a major role in reactions to chemicals.

Nutritional factors required for proper support of the nervous system include B vitamins, calcium, copper, magnesium, manganese, potassium, sodium, zinc, coenzyme Q_{10}, glucose, choline, amino acids, and oxygen.

The Neuron

The basic unit of our nervous system is a cell called a neuron. Neurons come in many sizes and shapes, but they all have the same parts: cell body, dendrites, axon, and axon terminals. The dendrites are extensions (of varying complexity, length, and number) of the cell body that increase the surface areas of the nerve cell, where signals are received from other neurons. The axon or nerve fiber extends out from the cell body. Its length can vary from microscopic to as much as 30 to 40 inches. The longer axons connect with peripheral organs and limbs, while the shorter ones are found predominantly in the brain. Many axons are covered with a fatty membrane (myelin sheath) that protects and insulates. The end of the axon branches out into filament projections known as axon terminals. These extensions transmit chemical signals to the receptor sites on glands, muscles, and organs.

Receptors on the surface of cells detect

Common Neurotransmitters

NEUROTRANSMITTER	PRECURSOR	ACTION
Acetylcholine	Choline and Phosphatidyl choline	Excitatory
Amino Acids		
Glycine	Serine, Threonine	Inhibitory
Glutamic Acid	Aspartic Acid	Excitatory
GABA	Glutamic Acid	Inhibitory
Aspartate	Aspartic Acid	Excitatory
Glutamate	Glutamine and Glutamic acid	Excitatory
Taurine	Cysteine	Inhibitory
Biogenic Amines		
Serotonin	Tryptophan	Inhibitory
Dopamine	Tyrosine	Inhibitory
Epinephrine	Tyrosine	Excitatory
Norepinephrine	Tyrosine	Excitatory
Histamine	Histidine	Excitatory
Melatonin	Tryptophan	Inhibitory
Neuropeptides		
Enkephalins	Proenkephalins	Modulatory
Substance P	Protochykinin	Modulatory
Cholecystokinin	Procholecystokinin	Modulatory
ß-Endorphin	Pro-opiomelanocortin	Modulatory
Miscellaneous Gases		
Nitric oxide	Arginine	Regulatory
Miscellaneous Purines		
Adenosine	AMP	Regulatory
Adenosine triphosphate	ADP	Regulatory

environmental and/or chemical changes; as a result, some researchers use the term detector rather than receptor. These neural receptor sites are distinct from hormonal or chemical receptor sites elsewhere in the body. Each responds more readily to one type of energy than to another. For every type of sensation or stimulus there is a specific type of receptor. Candace Pert, former chief of brain biochemistry at the National Institute of Mental Health in Maryland, describes the receptors as "buttons." Depending on the button that is "pushed," different reactions occur in our brain or body—an emotion, the release of gastric acid, a constriction of blood vessels. Even changes in our thoughts, attitudes, and perceptions of the world around us can "push the buttons" by causing the release of various neurochemicals.

Neurotransmitters

The neuron's axon terminals and dendrites are not joined together but are separated by a narrow, extracellular gap known as a synapse. The axon terminals produce and store chemical substances called neurotransmitters that are released, on signal, into the synapse.

The chemical synapses operate in only one direction, so a signal or message is transmitted along a neural pathway only in that specified direction. The amount of time required for this is less than one-thousandth of a second.

After the release of the neurotransmitter and acceptance by the receptor site, the excess is removed from the synapse in one of three ways:

Chemical Messengers

Neurotransmitters are chemical messengers that trigger a response built into the target or receptor cell. They are picked up and bound by the receptor sites on the membranes of dendrites and nerve cell bodies, muscle cells, secretory cells, and skin cells.

This information transfer allows us to perceive, interpret, respond to, and interact with our internal and external environment. The neurotransmitters link our metabolic, chemical, muscular, behavioral, and hormonal functions.

- a chemical transformation of the neurotransmitter, by enzyme action, into an ineffective substance
- diffusion into extracellular spaces away from the receptor site
- transport of the neurotransmitter back into the specific releasing axon terminal

The release of a neurotransmitter from the axon terminals depends primarily on the concentration and movement of ions (atoms that have lost or gained an electron) such as calcium, magnesium, sodium, potassium, and chloride. Sometimes more than one neurotransmitter can be released from an axon terminal. One usually enhances the effectiveness of the other.

Some of the neurotransmitters are inhibitory (they depress function) and some are excitatory (they stimulate function). These opposing functions produce a check-and-balance mechanism in the nervous system to regulate body processes.

Neurotransmitters are formed within the nerve cell body from precursors, which include nutrients (proteins, fats, minerals, and vitamins) that circulate in the bloodstream and the cerebrospinal fluid. Over 50 compounds have been indentified and classified as neurotransmitters, grouped into five main chemical types. These include acetylcholine, amino acids, biogenic amines, neuropeptides, and miscellaneous neurotransmitters that include nitric oxide and purines. Twenty amino acids function as neurotransmitters, and the biogenic amines are synthesized from amino acids.

Many neuropeptides have a neuromodulatory action and have a biochemical effect in the nervous system. Neuromodulators either amplify or dampen the electrochemical activity of the neurotransmitters by causing chemical changes in the neurons. While the neurotransmitter function takes place in milliseconds, the neuromodulators tend to create long-term effects that can be measured in minutes, hours, or even days.

Some 85 neuropeptides have been identified as having neurotransmitter or neuromodulator action. Some of the modulators on the following list also have hormone function:

- adrenocorticotropic hormone
- aldosterone
- bombesin
- estrogen
- neurotensin
- oxytocin
- prostaglandins
- somatostatin
- testosterone
- thyrotropin-releasing hormone
- vasoactive intestinal peptide
- vasopressin (an antidiuretic hormone)

Neurotransmitters are heavily affected during debilitating, toxic physical states. The following factors can all affect neurotransmitter levels:

- age
- allergies
- chemical toxicity
- drugs
- electromagnetic impulses
- hereditary factors
- hypersensitivity
- infections (viral, bacterial, fungal, and parasitic)
- internal production of free radicals (see Immune System Stressors in chapter 2, our Immune System)
- nutritional deficiencies
- oxygen supply
- stress
- temperature variations

Some of these factors will cause changes in the production of neurotransmitters; blockage of receptor sites; changes in receptor site; changes in numbers of receptor sites; or inhibition of enzymatic degradation of excess neurotransmitters.

Divisions of Our Nervous System

The nervous system is divided into the central nervous system, made up of the brain and the spinal cord, and the peripheral system, consisting of the nerves that link the central nervous system to organs or limbs.

■■ THE CENTRAL NERVOUS SYSTEM

The central nervous system is composed of the brain, which weighs less than three pounds, and the spinal cord. The spinal cord is a long, slender cylinder that extends from the brain to the sacrum in the pelvis. It is surrounded by the protective sheath of the vertebrae.

The portion of the brain and the center of the spinal cord that is composed of brownish-gray nerve tissue are called the gray matter. It is made up of cells that communicate with one another within the nervous system. The white portion of the brain and the outer portion of the cord are composed mainly of myelinated nerve fiber and are called the white matter. This portion of the spinal cord contains groups of axons referred to as pathways. These pathways run the length of the spinal cord, with sensory pathways ascending and motor pathways descending.

The brain and spinal cord float in a cushion of liquid known as cerebrospinal fluid, which protects the delicate tissues from sudden, jarring movements. Cerebrospinal fluid provides a medium of exchange for nutrients to enter the brain cells and for end products of brain metabolism to leave the cells.

The brain is the body's central command headquarters. Its different sections—the brainstem, the cerebellum, and the forebrain—regulate different functions of the brain and body. These portions are subdivided into areas which all communicate with each other. Communication within the brain occurs between neural cells called neurons, which account for about 99 percent of all nerve cells.

The brainstem connects the spinal cord with the higher brain centers. The nerve pathways that run up and down the spinal cord also run through the center of the brainstem. Ten of the cranial nerves branch out from the brainstem to innervate the muscles and glands of the head and neck and many organs in the chest and abdominal region. They also supply the sensory nerves of these areas.

The cerebellum is located at the base of the posterior skull and is involved with skeletal muscle function. It helps to maintain stability of balance and position, and to provide smooth, directed movements.

The forebrain (cerebrum), the largest part of the brain, is divided into two hemispheres and a central core that contains the thalamus and the hypothalamus. The cerebrum is coated with a heavily convoluted or folded shell, called the cortex, which is about three millimeters thick. The convolutions provide a large surface area for the interaction between neurons. This area is responsible for integrating information from the sensory nerve fibers, and for processing the information into meaningful images. The refined messages are then transferred to the motor nerve fibers to initiate muscle impulse and control.

The cortex is subdivided into the temporal, frontal, parietal (side), and occipital (back) lobes. The lobes have circuitous interconnecting pathways associated with learning, emotions, pain and pleasure, sight, language, and hearing. Sensory input from all of these is then translated into motor response. The center of the brain contributes to the coordination of muscle movements.

The thalamus is a control board and relay station that integrates sensory input on its way to the cortex. The information that is relayed does not always become part of conscious experience, but may stimulate automatic, subconscious responses.

The hypothalamus is a tiny area in the mid-brain that is responsible for unifying many homeostatic functions of our body. Homeostasis is a balanced state that all body functions work to achieve and maintain. The hypothalamus also contains endocrine cells that produce hormones to interact with the neural tissues in the hypothalamus. The hypothalamus is an important control center that regulates our body's internal environment as we respond to the external environment.

■■ THE PERIPHERAL NERVOUS SYSTEM

The second division of the nervous system, the peripheral system, is composed of nerve fibers that extend from the brain and the spinal cord. These nerve fibers are classified according to two distinct functions.

The afferent fibers handle sensory information traveling from our body's periphery to the central nervous system. The nerve cell bodies of these fibers are located outside of the brain or spinal cord in structures called ganglia. One long projection of the nerve cell extends from the ganglia out to the receptors. Another shorter projection extends into the central nervous system, where it branches and synapses with the interneurons, which are groups of neurons between the sensory and motor neurons that govern coordinated activity. The interneurons receive the bits of information sent to the brain or spinal cord via the afferent fibers, and then send out signals along efferent fibers of the peripheral nervous system.

The efferent division has two parts, the somatic branch and the autonomic branch. The somatic fibers run from the central nervous system to the skeletal muscles. The cell bodies of these neurons are located in groups within the brain or spinal column, and their axons extend directly to the muscle cells without joining with other neurons. The innervation signals sent along this pathway cause contraction of the skeletal muscles. This type of neuron is sometimes called a motor neuron. Somatic fibers have only an excitatory function, and play no inhibitory role. The neurotransmitter released by these fibers is acetylcholine.

The autonomic fibers lead from the central nervous system to smooth muscle (digestive tract and internal organs), cardiac muscle, and glands. Autonomic responses usually occur without conscious awareness or control and are also called involuntary responses. However, because mechanisms to control heart rate and other body functions can now be learned through biofeedback, the term involuntary is no longer entirely accurate.

The sympathetic division of the autonomic nervous system mobilizes our body's resources to respond to pain, strong emotion, or extreme temperatures. It is triggered by the "flight or fight" reaction. In contrast, the parasympathetic division restores and conserves body energy, overseeing digestion and absorption of nutrients.

Autonomic fibers lead to organs in the chest area (sympathetic fibers) or to the craniosacral area (parasympathetic fibers), and some organs are innervated by both types of fibers. This dual function is evident in the relaxation and contraction of the lungs, the heart muscle, and the stomach, resulting in a finer, more accurate degree of control over the organ.

Neurotransmitters released by the sympathetic and parasympathetic fibers at the junction with the receptor sites differ. The sympathetic axon terminals release epinephrine, while the parasympathetic fibers release norepinephrine.

Neurological Dysfunction

Dysfunction of any part of the nervous system can be initiated by the same factors affecting neurotransmitter levels (see Neurotransmitters, above). Some common neurological dysfunctions lead to disease, while, in other instances, diseases cause damage to the neurological system that result in neurological dysfunction.

- *Chronic inflammation:* Allergens (including foods, chemicals, inhalants, and organisms) can cause inflammation of neural tissue as a result of the immune cascade. After years of a chronic inflammatory state resulting from unrecognized, untreated allergies, the nerves can become permanently damaged.
- *Multiple sclerosis:* In this disease, the myelin sheath covering and insulating the nerve fiber incurs multiple scars. Some multiple sclerosis patients have improved dramatically when their allergies have been identified and treated, and when amalgam fillings have been removed from their teeth.
- *Alzheimer's disease:* This disease involves the destruction of nerve cells that synthesize acetylcholine, and the availability of oxygen to the brain cells is also reduced.

The person affected progressively loses memory and cognitive function, undergoes regression and personality changes, and may eventually need complete custodial care.

- *Schizophrenia:* An increase in dopamine receptors stimulates excessive release of dopamine at the synapses. This creates a fragmentation of mental functioning with symptoms of altered motor function, perceptual distortions, altered mood, abnormal interpersonal behavior, and disturbed thinking.
- *Parkinson's disease:* The dopamine neurons degenerate, leading to difficulty with voluntary movements, tremors, and rigidity of the arms, legs, and facial muscles. The amino acid L-dopa has been used with some success to stimulate the activity of dopamine in the brain.
- *Encephalitis:* This disease is caused by infectious diseases carried by ticks or mosquitoes, or it can result from diseases such as measles, mumps, or influenza. It causes inflammation of brain tissue that can lead to sleeplessness or coma, tremor, rigidity, compulsive movements, and states of immobility.
- *Chronic Fatigue Syndrome:* The cause of chronic fatigue syndrome is not known, but neuroendocrine dysfunction, viral infection, environmental toxins, genetic predisposition, or combinations of these factors are suspected. There is evidence of neurotoxicity in chronic fatigue, as many patients test positive on the Romberg test. To perform the Ronberg test the patient stands with eyes closed and will sway if there are neurological problems. Some

physicians believe that chronic fatigue is a neurosomatic disease in which the brain misperceives sensory information. Information processing occurs appropraitely, but the control of data input and output from processing centers is dysfunctional.

■ NEURALLY MEDIATED HYPOTENSION

Hypotension is the medical term for low blood pressure, and neurally mediated hypotension occurs when there is a "miscommunication" between the heart and the brain, even though both organs are structurally normal. When a normal individual stands up, blood pools in the legs because of gravity, decreasing the amount of blood returning to the heart. A reflex is triggered, increasing heart rate and the strength of the heart's contractions. The blood vessels constrict, and the proper amount of blood flow to vital organs is maintained.

In neurally mediated hypotension, the signal to the brain is incorrect, the heart rate slows and the blood vessels in the extremities dilate, resulting in a reduced blood flow to vital organs, including the central nervous system. This results in a feeling of lightheadedness or fainting. These symptoms occur in affected people after prolonged periods of standing or sitting. Diagnosis of NMH is done on a special tilt-table, which stimulates the effects that can trigger neurally mediated hypotension.

When hypotension is triggered, in addition to lightheadedness or fainting, the person suffers from prolonged fatigue, muscle aches, headaches, and mental confusion. The cause of NMH is not known, but is suspected to be genetic. This simple dysfunction of the nervous system has repercussions throughout the body.

Many of the affected individuals have a low salt intake in their diet. This contributes to even lower blood pressure in these people. Increasing salt and fluid intake is the first step in treatment. Some people also require increased nutrients, such as potassium, as well as the administration of medications.

Research done in 1995 at John's Hopkins by P.C. Rowe and others shows that the nervous system may play a role in chronic fatigue immune dysfunction syndrome (CFIDS). In the study, neurally mediated hypotension (NMH) was treated in CFIDS patients, resulting in resolution of the CFIDS symptoms in almost half of the patients. However, not all CFIDS patients have NMH.

Treatment of Nervous System Disorders

Research is proceeding rapidly to discover treatments for nervous system diseases and anomalies. Some of the following methods are in their infancy, but further research will no doubt uncover more applications.

- Nutritional manipulation of diet, as well as the use of vitamin and mineral cofactors, and amino acid precursors, is effective in treating neurotransmitter dysfunctions. Supplying precursors helps people whose bodies do not produce enough neurotransmitters.

- Immunotherapy, avoidance of allergens, and detoxification procedures are all essential in reducing recurrent immune inflammatory cascades that damage neural tissues.

- Peptide neuromodulators are being used to address some of the dysfunctions involving neurons. Neuropeptides are composed of two amino acids linked together with a special chemical bond called a peptide bond. These chemicals modulate neurotransmitter function in the body, either inhibiting or augmenting it.
- Biofeedback retraining mechanisms can control pain, reduce blood pressure, and change body temperature. This technique has the added benefit of freeing people from the feelings of helplessness that can accompany chronic illness.
- TENS units (transcutaneous electrical nerve stimulation) are successful in modulating some types of pain. The low-voltage electrical shock waves are thought to stimulate the release of serotonin, a neurotransmitter that blocks pain.
- Battery-operated pacemakers are very effective in regulating the nervous impulses to the heart.
- Drug therapy is used to treat the blockage of some synapses and enzymes, and to stimulate neurotransmitter precursor production. However, drug therapies have a number of potentially devastating side effects.

Many people have imbalances in and sensitivities to their own body chemicals, including neurotransmitters. Immunotherapy with highly diluted neurotransmitters helps people who are unable to utilize the neurotransmitters their body makes. This method has been successful in modulating behavioral problems in children, ADHD, rage attacks, and autism. Neurotransmitter extracts are also helpful for alleviating depression and emotional problems, sleep problems, and obsessive compulsive behavior in adults.

Testing for neurotransmitter imbalance or sensitivity may be done either by EAV or provocative neutralization. Extracts are prepared like other chemical extracts or homeopathically. Hands-on testing and treatment will also help neurotransmitter imbalance or sensitivity.

The following are a few of the neurotransmitters we have found to be helpful.

- *Acetylcholine:* A major neurotransmitter in the body, it is helpful in turning off allergic reactions regardless of the cause. It also helps with brain allergy, depression, headache, learning disabilities,mood swings, senility, and many other symptoms.
- *Choline:* Helps with bloating, bowel problems, constipation, memory impairment, senility, stomach discomfort, and sweating.
- *Dopamine:* Helpful for anxiety, depression, dyslexia, hyperactivity, learning disabilities, panic attacks, and tremors.
- *Histamine:* Neutralizing doses are helpful in turning off allergic reactions regardless of the cause. Also helps to relieve asthma, depression, food allergy, and hay fever.
- *Malvin:* Not a true neurotransmitter, since it is not made in the body. However, it is a neurogenic compound and occurs in 35 foods. It is in every red or blue food, but because the color of malvin depends on pH, it is in foods of other colors as well. Malvin helps with anxiety, arthritis, asthma, depression, enuresis, headaches, joint pain, CNS symptoms, epilepsy, noise sensitivity, rage attacks, and suicidal tendencies.
- *Melatonin:* Particularly effective for Sea-

Three Generations of Serotonin Disorders

Neurotransmitter problems can have genetic origins. One family in our practice has a serotonin problem, with all of its facets being demonstrated over three generations. The mother (generation 1) is hyperinsulinemic and has sleep difficulties. (Very little serotonin is released by the brain in hyperinsulinemia.)

Her two daughters (generation 2) suffer from migraine headaches that are triggered by serotonin release and both women are severely hyperinsulinemic. One daughter can experience severe depression accompanying a serotonin problem, but her sister is only mildly depressed from time to time. They both have trouble tolerating high-tryptophan foods such as pork and turkey, because tryptophan is converted to serotonin by the body.

The granddaughter (generation 3, and the daughter of the sister with severe depression) received a double dose because her father also has serotonin problems. She suffers from migraine headaches, severe depression, anxiety attacks, and hyperinsulinemia. She also has sleep difficulties, and trouble tolerating turkey and pork, as do her mother and aunt.

Treatment with serotonin extracts and the supplements Anxiety Control and Balanced Neurotransmitter Complex have helped the sisters and the granddaughter.

sonal Affective Disorder Syndrome (SADS) and sleep problems.

- *Norepinephrine:* Used for anxiety, autism, depression, flat emotional response, drug use, eczema, excessive fears, headaches, hyperactivity, obsessive behavior, panic attacks, and temper tantrums.
- *Octopamine:* Extremely useful for patients with neurological problems. Also helps with headaches, metal allergy, mental acuity, and feelings of heavy chest or suffocation.
- *Phenylalanine:* Helps brain allergies, depression, headaches, heartburn, hyperactivity, learning disabilities, generalized pain, sleep problems, and sugar craving. We have seen improvement in a cranky disposition with this extract.
- *Serotonin:* A universal "reaction stopper."

Reduces aggression, food allergy, headaches, hyperactivity, insomnia, and mood swings. Also related to appetite changes.
- *Tryptophan:* Helps anxiety, bowel problems, constipation, depression, fatigue, insomnia, lethargy, and sleep problems. Tryptophan is not made in the body, but is found in many foods and is converted to several other neurotransmitters by the body.

In addition to being manufactured in the body, many neurotransmitters also occur naturally in foods, both from animal and plant sources. The role of these chemicals is unknown in plants. Their presence adds to the dimension of food sensitivity for people who are sensitive to neurotransmitters. See chapter 9, Food Allergy for more information.

CHAPTER 4

Our Body Electric

THE PRESENCE of electrical and magnetic forces has been documented for thousands of years. Inscriptions on Egyptian tombs describe the effects of electricity generated by a species of fish. Later, the Greeks described the use of electric eels to control pain. The Chinese perfected the art of acupuncture for healing and anesthesia, based on stimulation of the body's electromagnetic pathways. In acupuncture, the internal energy of the body is influenced by external energy, and the insertion of metal needles is electrical, while the use of lodestones (naturally magnetic black iron ore) on the energy points is magnetic. Shamans in all cultures have used the magnetic forces in stones and crystals to treat unhealthy people.

The German physician Friedrick Anton Mesmer (1734–1815) treated a variety of ills with magnetic therapy, and French chemist and bacteriologist Louis Pasteur (1822–1895) observed that placing a magnet near fermenting fluids and wines speeded up fermentation. Physiologist Otto Lowei proved in 1921 that transmission of a nerve impulse across a synaptic gap is also chemical, adding to Julius Bernstein's 1871 work that proved nerve impulse is electrical. In 1941, Dr. Albert Szent-Gyorgyi (1893–1986) proposed that the newly discovered electrical conductivity, semi-conduction, played a role in living cell function.

Every organism regulates its metabolic cycles in response to the fluctuations of the earth, moon, and sun. Oysters, placed in a water tank at a great distance from the ocean, continue to open and close in rhythm with the rise and fall of the ocean tides, which are governed by the magnetic energy of the moon's gravitational force fields.

We have evolved and adapted in an environment containing a full spectrum of magnetic and electric pulsations. Our body rhythms also respond to and resonate with the regular rhythms of the earth, moon, sun, and major planets, whose gravitational, magnetic, and electrical variations affect tides, radio waves, electrical transmissions, plants, and animals.

Our bodies interact with the electrical

and magnetic forces of the earth. Sometimes these effects are harmful. Admissions to psychiatric clinics are higher during magnetic disruptions in the ionosphere. Major biological and genetic effects, such as immune system dysfunctions, may be related to exposures to abnormal electromagnetic fields. Our bodies also interact with electromagnetic pollution created by humans. The effects of this pollution are considerable, and are a very important issue in this century.

Electrochemical Cell Function

All chemical reactions in our body are electrical in nature, as they involve the exchange or sharing of electrons and the formation of positive and negative ions. In fact, our cells function as batteries for which electricity is the driving force. The charges inside the cell are different from those outside the cell, with the fatty cell membrane acting as an electrical barrier. When a nerve cell is stimulated, a wave of current travels down the nerve fiber. Potassium is released, and sodium moves into the cell. When the current passes, the cell wall re-establishes the charge difference, and potassium returns to the inside of the cell. This exchange of ions across the cell membrane initiates a series of complex electrical/chemical events that produces a measurable voltage charge.

For this system to work, the proper amounts of potassium, sodium, calcium, magnesium, fatty acids, and water must be present. Intracellular fluid contains more potassium and magnesium, while extracellular fluid contains more sodium and calcium ions.

Nerve and muscle cells can allow differences in the exchange between sodium, potassium, magnesium, and calcium. This allows "signals," as well as nutrients, to be more readily transferred between cells. Nerve and muscle cell membranes can change their electrical potential hundreds of times in a second. This capability is described as the cell's excitability.

The following examples illustrate the correlation between chemical and electrical influences on cell function.

- Lowering extracellular calcium concentrations temporarily increases the cell's excitability. Lowering the calcium concentration still further may cause a complete loss of membrane excitability.
- Magnesium deficiency produces electrical instability in the heart muscle and nerve cells. This can result in arrhythmia and coronary vasospasms (contraction of blood vessels), and electrocardiograph abnormalities.
- Many drugs, chemicals, and toxins are capable of changing the permeability and electrical potential of the cell membrane.

Electrical Functions

The nervous system functions are not only chemical but also electrical. Each of the neurotransmitters, as well as the calcium, magnesium, sodium, and potassium ions within the nerve cell, carry specific electrical charges—positive, negative, or neutral. As a neurotransmitter contacts a receptor site on the next cell, an electrical "firing" occurs. The cells then enter a resting phase when ions are returned to their original position to await the next "firing." This electrical activity can be seen with the use of sophisticated electrical equipment.

Electrical pulsing can be detected by placing electrodes on the surface of the skin at specific points on the body, known as acupressure points. Nerve pathways and endings are close enough to the skin's surface that the electrical activity of the nerves can be determined.

Until the development in the 1990s of the all-digital real time EEG machine by Margaret Ayers of Beverly Hills, California, it was not possible to see EEG changes in real time. Averages were used and gave different sets of data, and, in addition, the speed of the ink pen in the old EEG instruments was a limiting factor. With real time EEG readings, it becomes obvious that the brain is an extremely important organ in allergic reactions. At rest, the brain wave activity of the frontal lobe has a frequency of 15 to 18 cycles per second. During an allergic reaction, the brain wave activity changes, and the distinctive allergy pattern has a cycle of 22 to 24 cycles per second. With the real time EEG, it is possible to see the differences in the brain waves before and after allergy treatment.

Magnetic Functions

Physics tells us that any flowing electrical current produces a magnetic field in the space around it. This field, carrying energy and information, is capable of producing an action at a distance. Every chemical bond has a magnetic field or vibration associated with its electrical field. It is important to understand that our body has chemical, electrical, and magnetic properties.

Electrical Rhythms of the Brain

Brain electrical function can be demonstrated with an electroencephalogram (EEG), which shows several types of electrical impulse. Alpha rhythms are linked with lower levels of attention, relaxation, and happiness. The beta rhythm's faster oscillation rate is associated with attention to stimuli. During sleep, the alpha rhythm is replaced with even slower frequencies that change during the varying stages of sleep.

Our brain and spinal cord carry a positive magnetic pole orientation, and the peripheral tissues carry a negative orientation. Each cell in the body has both a positive and negative magnetic field in its DNA, and the force that activates the function and division of cells is magnetic energy. Individual cells are dependent on magnetic energy for their function, and the interaction of the organs and systems of the body is dependent on the presence and influence of magnetic energy.

For example, the pineal gland is sensitive to the daily cyclic patterns in the earth's geomagnetic field. The gland's level of secretion responds to light wave impulses and geomagnetic rhythms in its production of the hormone melatonin and other chemicals that it secretes. Trace amounts of magnetite are present in the soft tissues of the human brain, and mediate the response of the body to the geomagnetic field of the earth. Biophysical elements related to magnetivity probably govern biochemistry in our body, rather than biochemistry being in total control of the body.

Electromagnetism Applied

Dr. Robert Becker, a pioneering researcher in biological electricity from New York, in his book *The Body Electric*, shows that growth and development, metabolism, and communication between organs and between cells cannot be explained only on the biochemical level. He proved that, in the healing process, electrical currents play a role in cell communication and division. By applying this knowledge, Dr. Becker learned to heal bone fractures by applying minuscule electric currents on either side of the fractures.

Electrosleep, used as a method for anesthesia, also developed as a result of Dr. Becker's work. The front of the skull is negative in electrical potential, while the back of the skull is positive. When electrodes are placed on the head (negative in front and positive in back) and small voltages and currents are applied, a feeling of well-being is produced. If the electrical potential is reversed, unconsciousness results.

The production of electrical and magnetic currents in our body can be measured using highly sophisticated electronic and magnetic devices such as an electrocardiogram (ECG), an electroencephalogram (EEG), galvanic skin response electrodes, and electromyelography. The nuclear magnetic resonance instrument (MRI) is replacing the X-ray for internal body imaging.

In 1970, Brian D. Josephson of England completed the development of the SQUID (superconducting quantum interferometric device). Through the use of this instrument, it is now known that our body contains both AC (alternating) and DC (direct) electrical fields of current. This instrument also determines magnetic fields associated with these currents in living organisms. The brain produces a steady DC magnetic field, which is one-billionth the strength of the earth's geomagnetic field.

▊ ENERGY MEDICINE

In addition to electromagnetic procedures for imaging and diagnoses, techniques are now applied for beneficial treatments as well. The term energy medicine is used to describe this type of treatment. Examples of energy medicine include:

- *Short-wave diathermy:* The generation of heat in body tissues by electric current is used for both surface and deep heating to relieve muscle and joint pain.
- *Oscillators:* Used to disintegrate gallbladder and kidney stones so they can be excreted more readily.
- *Electrocautery and electrosurgery:* A fine wire probe is employed, which produces a high-frequency electric arc between the probe and the tissue to be treated.
- *TENS units (transcutaneous electrical nerve stimulation):* These units deliver an electrical pulse to an area of pain through electrodes attached to the skin. They are in widespread use for pain relief, particularly after surgery. They can also be helpful for chronic, nonresponsive pain. Their use reduces the amount of analgesics needed by the patient.
- *Electroacupuncture (also called Neuro Electric Therapy):* Originally used for pain re-

lief, it is used as a treatment for drug dependency by measurably increasing the amount of natural brain endorphins. Unfortunately, its use has not yet been approved in North America.

Environmental Sources of Electromagnetism

Our sun produces solar winds composed of high-energy atomic particles, which travel at enormous speeds and collide with the magnetic force exerted by the earth. Some of these high-energy particles are trapped in two areas, known as the Van Allen belts, encircling the earth. These belts shield the earth from solar wind, X-rays, and other ionizing, high-energy radiation. Without this protection, life on earth could not exist. The interaction between the sun's high energy and the earth's magnetic force produces extremely low frequency (ELF) electromagnetic waves (between 0 and 100 cycles per second) and very low frequency (VLF) waves (between 100 and 1,000 cycles per second).

In an 11-year cycle, solar storms erupt on the sun, thrusting energy particles of increased intensity out into space. This, in turn, affects the strength of the earth's magnetic field. These surges disrupt radio and electrical transmissions on earth, as well as the electrical function and behavior of biological organisms, including humans. Many people have observed human and animal behavioral disturbances during magnetic storms.

Telecommunications, electrical power plants, transmission lines, appliances, and microwave, radar, and radio transmissions have all increased at an dramatic rate during the past 50 years. We generate and manipulate electromagnetic forces, but since we are beneath the Van Allen belts, they can give us no protection from the effect of these forces.

Long-term exposure to ELF waves causes biological effects that include increased serum triglycerides (linked with high cholesterol); increased cancer cell growth; decreased production of dopamine, serotonin, and norepinephrine (neurotransmitters) in the brain; alterations in biological cycles; and increased chronic stress responses that lead to immune system deficiencies. Although we have a very adaptable biological system, when faced with overwhelming insults, our normal mechanisms begin to fail. These effects are magnified in people who already have impaired immune, endocrine, or nervous systems. Exposure to VLF waves has been associated with reproductive difficulties.

Symptoms of Electromagnetic Imbalance

The following may indicate an electromagnetic imbalance:

- symptoms of any type that worsen before a thunderstorm or wind storm
- symptoms that improve after a storm has begun
- an electrical discharge that occurs when touching any object after walking across a rug
- nervousness, anxiety, and headaches from telephone use
- malfunction of electrical equipment or appliances in the presence of a person
- watches that stop, lose or gain time, or cause sleepiness

Electrifying People

We first became aware of electromagnetic imbalances a number of years ago when a patient announced to us that she had worn her battery-operated watch for four years without a battery and that it kept perfect time. She popped the back off it to show us that it indeed had no battery. She further stated that she was not allowed in the computer laboratory where she worked because her presence made the computers malfunction. In discussing this incident with our staff, we were startled when one of them stated that her computer always turned on by itself when she walked past it!

Problems with watches are common in cases of electromagnetic imbalance, but in most cases they will not run or keep time at all. Difficulty wearing hearing aids and sleep problems are also common symptoms of an electromagnetic imbalance.

- fluorescent lighting causing hyperactivity, headaches, or blurred vision
- symptoms that worsen when near high-powered electric lines or transformers
- nervousness or headaches that occur when wearing hearing aids
- sleep disturbances or insomnia (may signal an electromagnetic imbalance, which can be caused by a toxic body burden of metals)
- taking a shower or bath, or standing bare-foot on damp grass, relieves many adverse symptoms

Air particles become positively charged before a storm or during periods of high, dry winds. Water droplets change the positive ion accumulation in their immediate surroundings to negative. Once a rain or snow storm has begun, the positive ions are shifted to a negative charge.

Many people do not feel well when the air has a high positive ion level. Teachers are well aware of discipline problems in children prior to a storm. Hospital staff see worsening of symptoms in their very ill or elderly patients during weather changes. Animals are also known to be very restless when positive ion levels are high.

Symptoms associated with electric or magnetic field sensitivity or imbalance vary according to one's state of health and the intensity of exposure. Symptoms can be as mild as dizziness or headache, occurring only when you are exposed to an electromagnetic field. Repeated exposure can cause neurological reactions of confusion, hyperactivity, memory loss, paresthesia (tingling skin), or convulsions; chronic stress syndromes; lowered immune responses to infection; aggravated immune responses resulting in increased hypersensitivity reactions; and general debility, as in chronic fatigue syndrome.

How to Reduce Electromagnetic Effects

Our society, with its many advantages, is not risk-free. We must continually weigh the benefits derived from new materials and products against their potential hazards. Many problems arising from external sources of electromagnetic force are beyond our control—but we can make evaluations, take precautions, and exercise control over our own use of electromagnetic devices. Consider the length of time that you use appliances each day. Although the electromagnetic field generated by an electric razor or hair dryer is greater than that of a television set or computer, exposure time to these appliances is much shorter. Hearing aids contain batteries that can create electrical imbalance, causing dizziness, sinus congestion, or headaches.

The potential danger of high levels of electromagnetic waves has been well documented. In the absence of appropriate regulation, protection against the long-term effects of exposure requires personal precaution measures.

There are a number of simple precautions we can take to protect against low-frequency waves.

- Keep as few electrical appliances in your bedroom as possible. This will lower electrical exposure for at least eight hours of the day.
- Position the head of your bed facing north to take advantage of the earth's magnetic force. If this is not possible, east is the next best choice.
- Do not use electric blankets or heating pads.
- Check microwave ovens for possible leaks that can occur if food or other particles are stuck in the rubber insulating gasket on the door. Inspect the gasket for cracks or nicks. Stay at least four feet away from an operating microwave.
- Use a screening shield to reduce the waves that emanate from your computer screen.
- Check all electrical cords to be sure that their insulation is intact.
- Choose a bedroom location in your home that is far removed from the entry of the main electrical source to the house.
- If possible, choose a home site that is over 200 yards from high-voltage wires or transformers.
- Have a satellite dish mounted away from your house rather than on top of it.
- Use the telephone as little as possible. Cellular telephones may cause symptoms for hypersensitive people.
- Have mercury amalgam fillings removed by a dentist with experience in amalgam removal. This can be advantageous for electrically sensitive people because opposing charges build up on the amalgam, causing an electrical field discharge between the fillings.
- Go barefoot as much as possible.
- When traveling by automobile, try to get out of the car and walk around every half-hour to have ground contact. Air travel for extended periods may pose a problem because of lack of grounding.
- Supplement both trace and macro minerals if your drinking water is filtered or distilled. These minerals are essential to proper electrical function in the body.
- Purchase an automobile that does not have computer-regulated systems.
- Avoid using free-standing or individual room electric heaters.

- Use a negative ion generator. Take care in choosing a generator because some types produce ozone. *Note:* Not all people tolerate negative ion generators.
- Use homeopathic imponderables (homeopathic remedies made from various types of energy sources) such as X-ray, electricity, radiation, cathode rays, negative magnetic, positive magnetic, and others. These remedies are helpful for some people.

There is new evidence that wearing specially prepared magnets may help balance your body's electromagnetic function and reduce the effect of external electromagnetic forces. The use of diodes, a copper-colored solid composite, helps to maintain energy levels along acupuncture meridians, maintaining energy patterns and polarity balance in the body, and to counteract harmful electromagnetic energies. The number of diodes needed varies from person to person. Tachyon beads are also helpful for electromagnetic imbalances. These beads are made from a photon-emitting material and help maintain proper cellular metbolism. They also allow increased oxygen flow and absorption of important nutrients through their effect on water molecules.

If you are electrically sensitive, you will find that being near moving water is helpful when the positive ion level of the air is high. You can find some relief if you can be near a stream, lake, or ocean. Since this is not possible for most people, an alternative is to stand in a running shower. Even running water over your lower arms and hands a number of times each day can provide relief.

Mobile homes can be problematic for people with electromagnetic imbalances because the electrical wiring runs the length of both sides of the structure. Also, the sides and roof are nearly always made of metal, and the home is frequently not sufficiently grounded for electrically sensitive people. For extra grounding, drive a copper pipe two feet into the ground and attach a copper wire from the pipe to the metal frame or siding of the mobile home. This should be done at two different places on the mobile home, preferably at both ends of the home.

The sensitivity of biosystems to electromagnetic fields has been known for a long time. With the increase in artificially made force fields, sensitivities are becoming more evident. Intricate cell structure and functions in biosystems are affected. More research into these effects is needed to find solutions to the associated problems. The time has also come for medical science to incorporate new knowledge from the discipline of bio-physics, and to apply a new dimension of electrical and magnetic components to clinical practice. Diagnosing and treating illness can no longer be confined strictly to biochemical functions, but must take into account bioelectrical and biomagnetic factors.

CHAPTER 5

Psychoneuroimmunology
Bringing Systems Together

A NEW FIELD in medicine has gradually emerged since the early 1980s. Developed as an outgrowth of studies by biologists and physiologists, the discipline formed by merging immunology, neurology, and psychology is now designated as psychoneuroimmunology. Some have suggested it should be called psychoneuroendocrinimmunology because the endocrine system is also a part of the interrelationship!

Because of the vast amount of knowledge available and applicable in each field of medicine, practitioners of medicine have investigated and specialized in separate organ or systems function. However, this exclusivity has created many gaps in the care of people who do not have classically defined symptoms. After all, our body functions not as separate parts but as a complete, integrated, interdependent whole.

Hippocrates, viewed as the father of medicine (460–377 B.C.), was well aware of this. He insisted that medical students view the emotions as an integral part of the cause of disease, as well as a factor in recovery. Aristotle (384–322 B.C.) too discussed the role of emotions in both health and disease. He felt that the soul was housed in, and inseparable from, the body, and that all parts of our body are functionally related to serve the whole. He considered the soul to be "ideas expressed in matter." Moses Maimonides, a 13th-century Jewish philosopher and surgeon, thought the emotion of happiness would complete a healing process. However, with the discovery of the microscope and emergence of the germ theory, the idea developed that organisms were the sole cause of illness. That theory is too simplistic to assign to today's multisystem image of disease.

In the past, the family doctor tried to treat illness in relation to the whole person, as well as considering the person's relationship to family and community. This attempt was limited, however, because precise biological information was missing. Then, for a period of time, the pendulum of thought

A New Understanding of Allergies

With this "new" approach to medicine, the experiences of allergic and hypersensitive individuals can be validated. Neurological, behavioral, immune, hormonal, and emotional changes do occur during a reactive state and contribute to the overall debilitation of their health. Perhaps now people with allergies will no longer be misunderstood, and their symptoms will no longer be classed as merely subjective, anecdotal, or psychological.

Sensitivity responses affecting the central nervous system were previously not considered allergic in origin because evidence of immune system involvement was lacking. Now these reactions are shown to stem from chemicals released and mediated from any one or all three systems: the nervous system, the endocrine system, and the immune system.

shifted to viewing psychological factors as the root cause for all unknown disease syndromes. When the cause could not be determined in the laboratory, or if the symptoms did not fall into classic disease patterns, the problem was deemed psychological in origin. Fortunately, many physicians tempered this trend with a broader approach to diagnosis and treatment. Biologists and physiologists had not yet proved that cellular level function is interdependent for all of the systems of the body. But as this knowledge be-

came available, physicians were once again able to view people in their entirety.

The cooperative effort between specialists in the field of endocrinology, neurology, biology, physiology, psychology, and immunology is to be applauded. Laboratory proof of the interdependence between the systems will have a tremendous impact on the maintenance of health and the treatment of illness. Physicians will be interested not only in disease, but also in wholeness and well-being; not only in methods of treating disease, but in ways of preventing it; not only in identifying harmful microorganisms, but in knowing something about the situations that lead to their development; and, finally, not only in treating patients, but in fostering self-confidence so they can gain knowledge for self-care.

Medicine will be based on improving the quality of life rather than on preventing death. Medical intervention will include helping to explore and maximize one's creative potential. Medical practitioners will be able to go beyond the limited tools of their profession and help the patient find rewards from an evaluation of self and lifestyle precipitated by illness.

The Interconnection of Body Systems

Dr. Blair Justice of Rice University in Houston, Texas, in his book *Who Gets Sick*, states that "most of medicine continues to pretend that mind and body are separate and that pathways by which attitudes and moods physically affect our organs and tissues are really imaginary and that simple physical explanations will be found to account for major disorders, as if mind and brain have no physical reality." Adverse prolonged physical symptoms do have a profound effect on the emotions and the psyche, but the reverse is also true. Drugs used to treat illness not only affect the disease but change brain, immune, and endocrine function, as well.

Below are some findings that support the interconnection and communication between the nervous, endocrine, and immune systems.

- Dr. Candace Pert, former chief of brain biochemistry at the National Institute of Mental Health in Maryland, and researcher Solomon Synder succeeded, in 1973, in locating and labeling receptors which the brain uses for communication between cells. The brain releases neurotransmitters and hormones to communicate with receptors throughout the body, including receptors on endocrine glands and cells of the immune system. In turn, chemicals and hormones from the immune and endocrine systems communicate with and modulate the brain and nerve cell function.
- During the 1960s, Dr. George Soloman, a psychiatrist at Mount Sinai School of Medicine in New York, discovered that by electrically stimulating certain parts of the brain of research animals, their ability to fight infection was improved. By damaging those same areas, the effectiveness of the immune system was impaired. It was then found that macrophages (a type of white blood cell) had specific binding sites on their cell membranes for neurochemicals, including the mood-altering endorphins.
- Lymphatic organs (parts of the immune system) such as the thymus, spleen, and lymph nodes are supplied with cholinergic (which release the neurotransmitter acetylcholine) and adrenergic (which release the neurotransmitter norepinephrine) nerve fibers. T-cells from the immune system have receptors for both of these neurotransmitters on their surfaces, which either stimulate or inhibit the proliferation of the T-cells.
- IgA (immunoglobulin) production in the intestinal tract is stimulated by the neuropeptide VIP (vasoactive intestinal peptide). The B-cell lymphocytes that produce IgA have specific receptor sites for VIP. It is thought that this interrelationship may play a role in food allergy responses. VIP has also been shown to influence immune responses in lymph glands and responses in the brain tissue.
- The autonomic nervous system influences the rate at which gastrointestinal hormones are secreted, as well as the speed of glucagon release from the pancreas. Some of the gastrointestinal hormones are also produced by neurons in the brain and function there as neurotransmitters.
- Nerve fibers from the sympathetic branch of the nervous system terminate in the adrenal glands. This explains why the adrenal glands rapidly release epinephrine in response to stress, which stimulates the responses we associate with "fight or flight."
- Endorphins and enkephalins (peptide neurotransmitters) produced during acute episodes of stress tend to stimulate the production of the immune system's natural killer cells and T-cells. However, the prolonged stress of grief has been shown to inhibit production of killer cells.

• Chemical irritants bind receptors on nerves and cause the release of substance P and other inflammatory substances. Substance P causes the release of histamine from mast cells. This is known as neurogenic inflammation.

■ PSYCHOLOGICAL AND EMOTIONAL FACTORS

In our clinical experience, we have observed that in addition to physical problems, emotional and psychological stress factors underlie some cases of environmental illness. Psychological traumas from the past that have been long suppressed and forgotten by the conscious mind can heavily influence the immune, nervous, and endocrine systems. Many people will make progress toward good health through good physical care, but then reach a plateau and are unable to improve further.

With very careful investigation, gentle searching, and time, buried issues surface so they can be addressed and put in proper perspective. Some of the most common unresolved problems are:
• early childhood feelings of fear, abandonment, and rejection
• emotional pain transferred or reflected by a parent through body language, words, and actions
• sexual, emotional, verbal, or physical abuse
• grief caused by the death of a loved one
• emotional upheaval caused by unemployment, divorce, rejection by a parent or loved one
• alcoholism, addiction, or family dysfunction
• repressed anger

• lack of forgiveness of a personal wrong (resentment)
• guilt or imagined guilt from a lack of proper response to a situation
• loss of one's dreams or goals

A solution for such problems cannot always be found, but the affected person usually feels profound relief when their existence is at least recognized. An assessment can then be made of the general impact of these problems on physical status and emotional well-being.

Another encouraging aspect of this investigation is that many researchers and practitioners are clinically studying and applying techniques of healing thought. A group of distinguished physicians, scientists, psychiatrists, writers, and faculty members recently joined together at UCLA to investigate and correlate laboratory evidence of the overlap between body systems, and to gather more evidence on the way emotions influence body function. Researchers such as Hans Selye, Karl Menninger, and George Engel had already provided a great deal of evidence that thought, attitude, stress, feelings, and experiences all affect the body's physiological functions.

Norman Cousins showed by his own experience, recorded in *Anatomy of An Illness*, that positive attitudes could affect the body's ability to repair. He also determined that his own sedimentation rate (a blood indicator of inflammation) decreased by five points when he engaged in laughter. The UCLA task force worked to gather irrefutable evidence that one's attitude toward illness can improve health and enhance treatment. The enlightening outcome of this cooperative effort was reported in Cousins' book *Head First—The Biology of Hope*. Ongoing related studies are being conducted in many universities and laboratories as a result of the task force's effort.

Norman Cousins, Bernie Siegel, Gerald Jampolsky, Oscar and Stephanie Simonton, Robert Schuller, Norman Vincent Peale, and Ron Del Bene have all paved the way with their lectures and writings for the application of positive thinking to the improvement of health, even in the presence of terminal diseases. (See also the discussion of hope in chapter 24 on Body, Mind, and Spirit.) They have proved that feeling love for others triggers lower levels of the stress hormone, nor-epinephrine, and a higher ratio of helper/suppressor T-cells in the immune function. David McClelland, a psychologist at Boston University, discovered that higher levels of IgA antibodies and lower levels of infection are found in people who receive high scores on intimacy questionnaires.

We know that areas in our brain and nervous system regulate and control most of our body's functions. Our brain in turn receives messages from our body and responds with appropriate signals to all systems. It seems to follow that our minds can also be conditioned and taught to control body functions during illness to enhance healing and recovery.

CHAPTER 6

Our Digestive System

OUR HEALTH, and indeed our existence, is dependent on our having a healthy, efficient digestive system. It is this system of the body that enables us to utilize the food we consume to build, repair, and maintain our bodies. The mouth, pharynx, esophagus, stomach, small intestine, large intestine, and rectum make up this system. In addition, glandular organs such as the salivary glands, liver, gallbladder, and pancreas secrete substances into the digestive tract that are esssential to digestion.

During the digestive process, food is broken down into its constituent parts. The body then extracts nutrients from these well-digested food molecules.

However, when digestion is abnormal, many food materials are not adequately broken down. This can lead to sensitivity to those foods. For example, if protein molecules are too large when they are absorbed into the bloodstream, the body treats them as invaders, just as it does bacteria or viruses. The immune response sends extra white blood cells to destroy the invaders and

histamine, serotonin, and kinins may be released—an allergic reaction is put into motion. Food allergy reactions are not confined to proteins, as originally thought, but can include all food categories and chemicals found in foods, especially those contacted most frequently.

The Process of Digestion

The process of digestion is a complex one, and each part of the digestive system plays a unique and important role. Improper functioning of any part can adversely affect the overall process. Proper digestion is a key factor in recovering from food sensitivity.

■■ MOUTH

Digestion begins in the mouth, where chewing physically breaks food apart into small particles, increasing the surface area available for the action of acid in the stomach and enzymes in the small intestine. Chewing also lubricates the food with saliva for ease in swallowing. Saliva is secreted by salivary and parotid glands, and contains the enzyme amylase, which initiates carbohydrate digestion.

■■ ESOPHAGUS

The next step in digestion is swallowing, which propels food through the esophagus, the tube connecting the mouth and stomach. The waves of contractions from swallowing further propel the food into the stomach. The swallowing process is complex, involving muscles in the tongue, larynx, pharynx, respiratory tract, and esophagus. All of these muscles work to prevent food from entering the nasal passages or lungs.

■■ STOMACH

While in the stomach, food is churned and mixed by the action of many muscle bands that alternately contract and relax. Hydrochloric acid is secreted into the stomach by parietal cells lining the stomach. The vagus nerve signals the parietal cells to begin acid production after it receives stimulus from the sight, smell, and taste of food and from the process of chewing. The higher the protein content in the meal, the greater the stimulation of gastric acid release. Caffeine also stimulates acid release. Hydrochloric acid is highly acidic and kills bacteria that entering the stomach along with food. This is not 100 percent effective, however, as a few bacteria survive to take up residence and multiply in the intestinal tract.

Optimum digestive function in the stomach occurs in an acid medium of pH 1.8 to 3. (pH is a measure of acidity or alkalinity; 7.0 is neutral, 1.0 is extremely acidic and 14.0 is extremely alkaline.) The acid mixture starts to work on the protein structure, disintegrating connective tissue and cells in the ingested food. Stomach acid has only a limited capacity to work on complex proteins or carbohydrates, and no capacity to digest fats. Cells lining the stomach produce an "intrinsic factor" that is essential for the absorption of vitamin B_{12} in the small intestine.

Hydrochloric acid activates the secretion of the enzyme pepsin, the hormone gastrin, and additional mucus. Mucus protects the stomach wall from the effects of hydrochloric acid. Pepsin works to break down protein, while gastrin helps to stimulate acid release and contractions of the stomach. Histamine, found in the mucosa of the stomach wall, also plays a role in the release of hydrochloric acid. Very little of what is eaten is absorbed through the stomach wall—only water, alcohol, and a few minerals.

Some people have excessive acid secretion, which can cause a burning sensation in the upper abdomen and in the esophagus, burping of sour-tasting liquid, and excessive gas. This condition is known as hyperchlorhydria. Anxiety, anger, stress and caffeine will all contribute to the overproduction of acid. Taking calcium supplements with meals will help to absorb excess acid.

In contrast, hypochlorhydria occurs when acid secretion is diminished, resulting in inadequate amounts of hydrochloric acid. Achlorhydria is the term used when hydrochloric acid is present in extremely low amounts in the stomach. This results in improperly digested food. Symptoms of low levels of stomach acid are often the same as those experienced by people with excess acid levels.

The usual over-the-counter treatment

for stomach symptoms is the wrong approach for treating low stomach acid because, as advertisements tell us, antacids "absorb up to 45 percent of their weight in stomach acid." The cause of indigestion or stomach pain should be investigated before antacids are prescribed or taken.

Symptoms accompanying hypochlorhydria can include poor nutrient absorption from either food or nutritional supplements, sensitivity to foods, longitudinal ridges on fingernails, nails that break easily, rosacea (small broken blood vessels on cheeks), belching or bloating soon after a meal, regurgitation of sour liquid, burning in the stomach area or esophagus, food "sitting in the stomach" for long periods, or hypoglycemia-like symptoms. Some people report having diarrhea, constipation, or undigested food particles in their stools.

Levels of gastric acid can be measured by radiotelemetry (Heidelberg gastrogram), discussed below.

▌ ALLERGIES AND STOMACH ACID

Food sensitivity is frequently associated with inadequate levels of stomach acid. Those with low stomach acid have poor nutrient absorption, and supplements are usually needed.

Hydrochloric acid supplementation returns acid secretion to normal levels in hypochlorhydric or achlorhydric individuals, but it must be used only when indicated and with careful supervision. The acid should never be used in conjunction with anti-inflammatory medications such as aspirin or ibuprofen or with corticosteroid preparations because of the risk of inducing bleeding or ulcers. Hydrochloric acid is

Low Stomach Acid and the Elderly

Clinical observation has shown that low stomach acid levels increase susceptibility to and severity of bacterial, fungal (including yeast), and parasitic bowel infections. Stomach acid levels are inadequate in 50 percent of people over the age of 60. This contributes to the poor nutritional status (especially low calcium levels) seen in many older people.

available in tablet, capsule, or liquid form. Capsules are the most convenient and effective form, since tablets do not readily dissolve and liquid hydrochloric acid can damage tooth enamel. People with low stomach acid may have difficulty dissolving capsules in the stomach. If this is a problem, small pinpricks may be made in the capsule before swallowing it.

Hydrochloric acid is also available with and without pepsin, and with betaine or glutamic acid as carriers. Taking gradually increased amounts of lemon juice, vinegar, and ascorbic acid (vitamin C) also provide small amounts of acid. Just before a meal, take 1 gram of vitamin C, 1 Tbsp. apple cider vinegar, or a quarter of a lemon. These amounts can gradually be increased to 4 grams of vitamin C, 2 Tbsp. vinegar, or half a lemon. Excess amounts of supplemental acid will cause stomach burning, which can be neutralized immediately with a form of bicarbonate. If burning occurs, the dosage of acid must be reduced.

SMALL INTESTINE

The final stage of digestion takes place in the small intestine, where most of the absorption occurs. From the stomach, the partially digested food mixed with acid (called chyme) enters the small intestine. Chyme is very liquid and highly acidic. This movement occurs about 45 minutes to an hour following a meal.

Here, enzymes work to convert proteins into amino acids, fats into glycerin and fatty acids, and carbohydrates into monosaccharides (sugars). These simple molecules are then small enough to pass through the mucosal lining of the intestine into the bloodstream to form "building blocks" for the body. Water, minerals, ions, and vitamins are also absorbed.

The small intestine is 9 feet long, but its absorptive surface is 600 times that length. Its inner surface is highly folded and covered with small fingerlike projections called villi, which, in turn, are covered with microscopic projections called microvilli. This surface is where absorption and the final stage of digestion occur. Villi cells function only for a few days and then disintegrate. The intestinal lining renews itself constantly if proper nutrients are available.

LARGE INTESTINE

Ingested food molecules are absorbed long before reaching the large intestine, which serves mainly as a storage and dehydrating organ. It takes 12 to 14 hours for materials to make the circuit of the large intestine, and by the end of this trip the indigestible material has been condensed into feces for elimination from the body. A large part of the feces is composed of bacteria. Over 400 species of bacteria live in the large intestine, some of which synthesize vitamins that are absorbed by the cells lining the large intestine. However, the amount of vitamins produced this way is far below the daily level needed for optimal body function.

Some yeast organisms also colonize areas of the large intestine, and help to disintegrate fibers in the waste material. The overgrowth of undesirable bacterial or fungal organisms will lead to production of toxins and gas. The gas (flatus) is composed of nitrogen, carbon dioxide, and small amounts of hydrogen, methane, and hydrogen sulfide. Many of the toxins that are released by the yeast are water-soluble and are absorbed into the bloodstream.

DIGESTIVE ENZYMES

Digestion involves the exocrine, or internal, functioning of the pancreas. Pancreatic enzymes specific for each of the three classes of foods—protein, carbohydrate, and fat—are manufactured and stored in the pancreas until the stomach signals for their secretion. These enzymes, which complete the work of digestion, enter the first part of the small intestine from the pancreas. The enzymes present in the pancreatic fluid are also essential to the processing of the fat-soluble vitamins A, D, E, and K.

The pancreatic enzymes function only in an alkaline medium provided by bicarbonate solutions secreted from the liver and the pancreas. The amount of bicarbonate that is secreted is normally equal to the amount of acid released by the stomach. An alkalinity of pH 8.0–9.0 is essential for proper pancreatic enzyme function. If the alkaline (bicarbonate) level is not adequate, the pancreatic enzymes are destroyed or inactivated. Generalized body acidosis can then occur after meals, and the intestinal mucosa can be damaged by the excess acid.

Bile, from the liver, is stored in the gallbladder and is dumped into the small intestine through the same duct as the pancreatic enzymes. Bile contains bile salts, cholesterol, lecithin, minerals, and bile pigments. The first three ingredients help to digest fats, while the minerals provide bicarbonate ions to neutralize stomach acid.

Bile insufficiency is easy to detect because of the color of the stool. Normal stool is a medium to dark brown color. Stool that is predominantly clay-colored (yellow), grayish, or very light brown usually indicates low bile content. Taking supplements of taurine, an amino acid, can help stimulate bile production and thin the consistency of the bile so it will flow more readily. Choline, inositol, methionine, or lecithin are also helpful in increasing bile production.

Bile salts are also available as a supplement. The correct dosage is indicated by a return to a normal stool color. Take care while increasing dosage because diarrhea can be easily triggered, causing greenish, unpleasant, and irritating stool. Bile salts are derived from animal sources, so you should also be aware of its allergenic potential.

Irritation of the tissues surrounding the bile duct opening into the small intestine can be caused by repeated exposure to allergenic foods, candidiasis, or parasitic infections. The local irritation causes a swelling of the duct, and backs up bile into the gall-bladder. This results in thickening of the bile and in gallbladder pain, which can be misdiagnosed as gallstones. Eliminating offending foods and/or treating organisms will often reduce this type of pain.

Low pancreatic enzyme and bicarbonate secretion frequently occur together with low stomach acid secretion because adequate stimulation from stomach acid is essential for the production and release of pancreatic enzymes. Insufficient pancreatic enzymes result in lowered fat digestion and a subsequent rise in blood phospholipid/cholesterol ratios. One sign of inadequate pancreatic enzyme and bile function may be floating stools.

■ MEASURING ENZYME LEVELS

The radiotelemetry method of diagnosis (see below) is helpful in determining the levels of available bicarbonate in the small intestine. If the levels are low, pancreatic enzyme function is also reduced, since pancreatic enzymes are activated only in an alkaline medium created by bicarbonate.

Blood, hair, and urine analyses can help determine your nutritional status (levels of minerals, vitamins, and amino acids). An assessment of intestinal digestion and absorption can also be made from these results. Stool examination can detect undigested protein and vegetable fibers, starch granules, and excess fat globules, all of which indicate impaired digestion.

Impaired Digestion

Improper secretion of enzymes and bicarbonate from the pancreas or liver—or impaired digestive and absorptive surfaces in the intestinal tract—can have a variety of consequences, the most important of which is poor nutrition. Since nutrients are the building blocks of our cells, a deficiency will mean lowered functioning of all body systems, including the immune system. Lack of adequate nutrients will cause frequent infections; disruption of hormone levels; poor memory and decreased mental acuity; lack of cell enzyme production, resulting in fatigue; inability to cope with stress; and increased allergic inflammatory reactions.

A major digestive problem is "leaky gut" (altered intestinal permeability), which occurs when the intestines absorb larger molecules than usual. This condition is initiated by repeated exposure to foods that cause inflammatory reactions, leading to abrasion of the microvilli. This leaves larger openings in the intestinal wall, allowing larger molecules of food to pass into the bloodstream, where further inflammatory processes develop.

This chain of events heightens food allergies. More antigen reaches the liver and the white cells, putting more stress on the immune system and increasing the person's sensitivity. In addition, the hepatic (liver) detoxification pathways are forced to work harder, and some of the amino acids are depleted.

The lining of the intestinal tract is designed to keep antigens, toxins, bacteria, yeasts, and parasites out of the body. People with yeast or bacterial infections, overgrowth of the intestine, inflammatory bowel disease, or food allergies have abnormal intestinal permeability. The ingestion of alcohol or anti-inflammatory drugs such as ibuprofen or naproxen can also cause a leaky gut.

Digestive Dysfunction Can Cause Allergies

When our digestive system is not functioning properly, it can have an adverse effect on our health. Our bodies will not be nourished properly, but more important, improper food digestion leads to food allergy. The body does not recognize improperly digested food as being nutritional and treats it as a harmful foreign substance. Food allergies, with their many and varied symptoms, quickly develop.

Undigested food in the stool can be a sign of improper digestion, but it may also indicate food allergy. Simple measures, such as supplementing with acid, if hydrochloric acid levels are low, and digestive enzymes, can help to correct poor digestive function. (See Allergies and Stomach Acid)

Other problems are associated with improper digestion and absorption. Excessive blood sugar fluctuations act as a stressor to the pancreas, liver, brain, and adrenals. Eating many times during the day (nibbling or snacking) puts an added burden on the pancreas, eventually reducing pancreatic enzyme production. Excessive eating of the same food also stresses the digestive enzyme systems so that they no longer produce adequate amounts of enzymes. Foods are then improperly digested, causing allergic reactions. This constant irritation can lead to irritable bowel syndrome. Reduced acid production in the stomach and less efficient nutrient absorption from the small intestine tend to accompany the aging process.

Infants up to six months of age do not have adequate levels of IgA in the cells lining the intestinal tract. These cells prevent the absorption of large particles that may be allergenic. Early exposure to solid foods (before the age of six months) can initiate food sensitivities. The infant's intestinal tract is unable to properly digest the food, and the protein or carbohydrate molecules are absorbed whole into the bloodstream. The body then mounts an immune response and produces antibodies to the food molecule. Thereafter, whenever that food is encountered, an immune reaction will occur.

■■ RADIOTELEMETRY—HEIDELBERG GASTROGRAM

The gastrogram test is an important aid to investigating digestive problems. In this test, a miniature high-frequency transmitter is encapsulated in an easy-to-swallow capsule. The transmitter is calibrated to receive the pH values (acidity and alkalinity) from the stomach and small intestine. These frequencies are picked up by a belt antenna, worn by the person being tested, and are transmitted to a receiver. The receiver displays the information on both a meter and a graph.

During the test, the following information can be gathered:
• acidity of the fasting stomach
• ability of the stomach to reacidify if challenged by sodium bicarbonate or food
• emptying time of the stomach into the small intestine

• bicarbonate levels in the small intestine (necessary to activate the pancreatic enzymes)
• transit time of food and waste in the gastrointestinal tract
• presence of a mucus mass in the stomach that would interfere with the action of hydrochloric acid
• presence of gastric or duodenal ulcerations

Treatment of Digestive Irregularities

Pancreatic enzyme supplements can reduce reactions, provide adequate enzymes for digestion, and allow the pancreas to repair and recover its function. Some of the available enzymes are bromelain (from pineapple), papain (from papaya), superoxide dismutase (SOD), and pancreatic enzymes (from lamb, beef or pork). The wide variety of enzyme sources is an aid to those who follow a rotation diet, as they can also be rotated to prevent developing a sensitivity to any one preparation. In addition, enzymes improve food digestion, making any diet more effective. (See chapter 10, Eating Safely, for a discussion of the rotation diet.) These enzymes are taken with meals as digestive aids and between meals for their anti-inflammatory function.

Since pancreatic enzymes do not function in an acid medium, bicarbonate supplements should accompany pancreatic enzyme therapy. The alkaline material should be taken 45 minutes to an hour following a meal, when the chyme (partly digested food) from the stomach begins to enter the small intestine.

The bicarbonate may be obtained from a variety of sources: buffered forms of vitamin

C; combinations of potassium, magnesium, and calcium bicarbonates; sodium and potassium bicarbonates; or ascorbates formed by combining ascorbic acid with either sodium, magnesium, or calcium. Bicarbonates also neutralize the stage of an allergic reaction when the body tends to become acidic.

All raw foods contain enzymes that will digest the food in which they are contained. These enzymes can help to body digest the food, but are removed during cooking and methods of food processing that extend the life of the food. Animal (pancreatic) enzymes work in a pH of 7.0 to 9.0. Plant enzymes work in a pH range of 3.0 to 9.0. Taking plant enzyme supplements greatly increases the digestive capabilities of the body, allowing some digestion to take place in the acid climate of the stomach. The digestive system does not have to assume the entire burden of digesting the food and there is no accumulation of food that it cannot assimilate.

Nutrient supplements that aid function

> ## Diet Repair
>
> *One of the most important ways to treat digestive malfunction is by eliminating the offending allergenic foods or with a diversified rotation diet. Elimination diets (diets in which the allergenic food is totally eliminated) or rotation diets remove the stress load on the pancreas and reduce the inflammatory reactions to allow repair of the pancreas and small intestine. (See The Rotation Diet in chapter 10, Eating Safely, and Recommended Books for more information.*

and repair of the pancreas and intestinal tract include vitamins A and C, calcium, magnesium, manganese, potassium, zinc, and amino acids.

Many supplements will help repair a leaky gut. Glutamine, an amino acid, is a growth factor for the intestine. Essential fatty acids, bioflavonoids, vitamin E, and glutathione will help heal the intestines.

CHAPTER 7

Allergy and Disease

DISEASE SELDOM has a single cause. In evaluating any set of symptoms, the role of allergy or sensitivity should be considered as a primary cause or at least a strong contributing factor. Allergy is the common denominator in many different diseases, including degenerative diseases.

Almost half the people in North America suffer from some form of degenerative disease, and the statistics worsen every year. The central factor of all degenerative disease is stress, which affects all biochemical and metabolic processes. Among the stress factors in degenerative disease are chronic addictive reactions, including sensitivities to foods, chemicals, and inhalants; heavy body levels of toxins; nutritional deficiencies; and infections.

These stress factors cause an imbalance at the cellular level, as the dysfunction of biochemical and bioelectric metabolic processes increases. As the imbalance continues, deficiencies and organ malfunctions set off a chain reaction that can affect the whole body. These increases in toxicity and dys-

function make it impossible for the body to maintain the biochemical balance necessary for health.

In his book *Brain Allergies*, Dr. William Philpott, a pioneer in environmental medicine and a researcher in magnetic therapy, of Choctaw, Oklahoma, describes the degenerative disease state: "The different diseases we all know are named according to the specific tissues inflamed, the particular metabolic symptoms interfered with, the secondary invading opportunistic organisms involved, the behavioral symptoms displayed, or the specific gland which is disordered; however, it is the underlying disease process and its related organic factors in the basic foundation from which all of these different reactions are built."

Allergic reactions to foods stress the metabolic process. Food, chemical, and inhalant reactions can disrupt the endocrine system function, and adversely affect the respiratory system. In addition, nutrient deficiencies in the diet produce organ and metabolic functional deficiencies in the

Tobacco, Alcohol, and Food Addiction

In 1980, the late Dr. Theron Randolph of Chicago defined obesity and alcoholism as "similar illnesses, one dealing with addicting foods in their edible form and the other in their potable form."

Also in 1980, Dr. William Philpott observed that after a two- to three-week abstinence from tobacco use, about 10 percent of his schizophrenia patients had psychotic episodes following reintroduction to tobacco smoke. Tobacco is a member of the nightshade food family, along with eggplant, potato, tomato, pimento, and peppers. Addictions are usually to the food component of the substances to which a person is allergic. (See chapter 9 for more information on food allergy and addiction.)

body. Maladaptive allergic and addictive food and chemical reactions usually bear a direct relationship to nutritional deficiencies. Whole organ systems are affected and a host of symptoms can result.

Disordered metabolism causes cells to react with more sensitivity to allergic foods and chemicals, and enzymes become depleted. This sets up a chain reaction of inflammatory reactions throughout the body that are a major contributor to the development and symptoms of many different disease processes. For example, any time there is an inflammatory edema, it causes a reduction in oxygen to the tissues involved in the reaction, resulting in a favorable biological state for a flareup of infection.

Several phenomenon occur during an infection. Organisms multiply and produce toxins that can be both toxic and allergenic. The body also responds allergically to the protein in the body of the organisms both during the infection, and to any debris left after the infection. Infections cause nutritional deficiencies that lower immune defenses, caausing allergies to become more severe. Many infections can produce reactions as specific as those produced by food, chemicals, and inhalants.

Dr. Philpott states that in diagnosing any diseases, the following factors must be considered as causes of the symptoms:

- nutritional deficiencies or exceses
- heavy metal toxicity
- reactions to foods, chemicals, inhalants, and microorganisms and their toxins
- learned psychological responses to life experiences and exposures

Common Diseases and Allergies

In a report on chemical sensitivity prepared for the New Jersey State Department of Health 1989, Dr. Nicholas Ashford and Dr. Claudia Miller document many correlations between the allergy/sensitivity/maladaption process and subsequent degenerative or autoimmune diseases.

■ BLOOD DYSFUNCTIONS

A type of eosinophilia (increase in a type of white blood cell) with accompanying muscle pain, insomnia, and fatigue is seen frequently in allergic people.

As early as 1962, anemia caused by allergy to cow's milk was reported in the *American Journal of Diseases in Children* by Dr. D. Heiner.

▌▌ CARDIOVASCULAR DISEASE

Higher histamine levels have been found in the coronary arteries of cardiac patients, as reported in *Science* by S. Kalsner and R. Richards in 1984.

In clinical practice, we have observed a number of patients with arrhythmias, palpitations, edema, and increased pulse rates after exposure to foods, chemicals, inhalants, or hormone fluctuations, or during testing sessions. These abnormalities dramatically subsided with neutralizing doses of the offending substance. One female patient experienced an increase of 40 to 50 points in her systolic blood pressure and 10 to 20 points on the diastolic reading when she ingested rice. (The systolic blood pressure is the maximum arterial blood pressure during the cardiac cycle, and the diastolic blood pressure is the mimimum arterial bood pressure during this cycle.)

Repeated exposures and resulting inflammatory reactions such as these will eventually lead to biochemical dysfunction of the cardiovascular tissue. This damage is also caused by unresolved kinin release and inflammation. (See chapter 1, Our Immune System, for more information on kinins.)

▌▌ CHRONIC FATIGUE SYNDROME

Dr. Jesse Stoff of Tucson, Arizona, in his book *Chronic Fatigue Syndrome*, implicates allergic responses as contributing factors in the baffling syndrome of chronic fatigue. In environmental medicine clinical practices, this debilitating syndrome is a predominant complaint.

Dr. Theron Randolph demonstrated, in 1944, many abnormal lymphocytes in the blood of chronic allergic patients, similar to white blood cells seen in mononucleosis patients.

Robert A. Buist reported in his book *Chemical Hypersensitivity* that a great majority of chronic fatigue syndrome (CFS) patients had been or are being exposed to environmental pollution, causing damage to the lipid (fat) component of red blood cells and lymphocytes. In 1988, in *the Journal of Allergy and Clinical Immunology*, S.E. Strauss and J.K. Dale reported that up to 75 percent of CFS patients had pre-existing inhalant, food, chemical, or drug allergies.

▌▌ DERMATOLOGIC DISORDERS

Food challenges (in which test foods in pure form are given under controlled conditions) on patients with atopic dermatitis (eczema) not only worsened the rash, but also triggered gastrointestinal and respiratory symptoms in a 1988 study done by A. Burks and colleagues and reported in the *Journal of Pediatrics*.

Dermatitis herpetiformis, a chronic skin disease in which there is eruption of blisters that itch and occur in symmetrical groups, is associated with gluten sensitivity.

A number of allergists recognize that urticaria (hives, which are raised, itchy skin patches) can be caused by foods and food additives, but are hesitant to accept that chemical contacts can also cause some forms of urticaria. Delayed-pressure urticaria (hives that appear after pressure is relieved on an area of skin) has been seen to occur with food challenges and to clear with fasting. Secondary skin rashes have also been noted in cases of sensitivity to molds and fungi.

In the August 1991 issue of *Annals of Allergy*, Nicholas Orfan and colleagues reported the case of a five-year-old boy who had systemic cold urticaria (hives). This child had elevated plasma histamine corresponding to the onset of hives.

Many people regard rosacea, a disorder in which there is marked flushing of the facial skin, as a skin problem or inherited skin disorder. Rosacea can be accompanied by acne vulgaris and seborrheic dermatitis, making diagnosis more difficult. Dr. Jonathan K. Wilkin, director of dermatology at Ohio State University in Columbus, Ohio, has been experiencing success in treating rosacea following the principles of allergy treatment. He has his patients follow an allergy elimination diet, eliminating foods and beverages, adding them back one at a time to determine what might provoke the rosacea. In addition, he recommends eliminating all chemicals that can cause redness, as well as avoiding extremes of sun, heat, or cold.

▮ EAR, EYE, NOSE, AND THROAT DISORDERS

Repeated inflammation of throat and eustachian tube tissues because of ingesting allergenic foods such as milk is known to predispose children to recurrent otitis media (middle ear infection). Natural gas exposure in the home or at school can also cause this disorder.

Chronic sinusitis with accompanying debilitating headaches can be caused by tissue reactivity to the presence of molds.

In a challenge study, F. LaMarte and colleagues demonstrated a sixfold increase in plasma histamine release and observed a swollen larynx in a patient exposed to the manufacture of carbonless paper. The report of their study in the July 1988 issue of the *Journal of the American Medical Association (JAMA)* reported symptoms of hoarseness, coughing, flushing, itching, and rash within 30 minutes of exposure.

Ear, nose, and throat specialists repeatedly see chronic inflammatory tissue damage in sinusitis, as well as vertigo, hearing loss, ringing in the ears, Meniere's syndrome, nasal obstruction, adenitis (lymph gland inflammation), and salivary gland enlargement as a result of untreated allergies.

▮ ENDOCRINE DYSFUNCTION

The late Dr. Phyllis Saifer of Berkeley, California, implicated untreated allergy in autoimmune thyroiditis.

The relationship between the stress of chronic allergy states and hypoadrenalism is well known. Traditional allergists commonly treat this disorder by administering cortisone to boost the function of already exhausted adrenal glands, often with severe side effects. Early, proper management of allergies would make this type of treatment unnecessary.

Doctors Donald Sprague and William Rea of the Environmental Health Center in Dallas, Texas, and Charles Mabray of Victoria, Texas, found that many premenstrual abnormalities improved following adequate allergy management.

In the November 1990 issue of *Immunology and Allergy Practice,* J. Scinto and colleagues reported the case of a woman who had had five documented episodes of life-threatening anaphylaxis during treatment with estradiol birth control pills. These episodes occurred within 10 hours after ingestion of the pills, and in a laboratory test leukocyte histamine release was demonstrated to progesterone and pregnanediol.

■ GASTROINTESTINAL DISORDERS

Food sensitivity has been clearly linked to disease of the intestinal tract, including gluten reactivity relating to celiac disease, and milk sensitivity causing small, white blisters in the mouth. In 1990, Dr. Ronald Finn and others implicated sensitivity to baker's and brewer's yeast in Crohn's disease in their report in the *International Archives of Allergy and Applied Immunology.*

In his study reported in the August 1981 issue of *Annals of Allergy,* Dr. J. Siegel found a higher incidence of accompanying hay fever, eczema, and asthma in patients with inflammatory bowel disease. For these patients, when the other systemic allergic responses were treated, their bowel disease was controlled. Cortisone injections reduced their symptoms, thus indicating further that an allergic response was active. Irritable bowel syndrome will often improve when common allergenic foods, such as milk, soy, wheat, corn, or sugar, are either eliminated or rotated in the diet, and when immunotherapy is utilized.

When the pancreas begins to function poorly, metabolic acidosis occurs in the small intestine. Lowered enzyme levels cause amino acid deficiencies and a rise in kinin inflammatory reactions in tissues and organs.

As early as 1949, allergy was also implicated in chronic ulcerative colitis by Dr. Albert Rowe in a report in the *Annals of Allergy.*

"Leaky gut" syndrome plays a large role in food allergy because the body does not recognize the undigested food as nourishment and this food becomes allergenic. Dr. Leo Galland, author of *The Four Pillars of Healing,* states that "Leaky gut syndrome isn't a disease itself, but is thought to play a part in other diseases. Allowing undigested food or bacteria into the bloodstream sets in motion a chain of events: the immune system reacts, the body thinks it's sick and expresses it in a number of ways, such as a rash, diarrhea, joint pain, migraines, even psychological symptoms such as depression. Those problems can add up to a disorder that has no obvious relation to the original cause."

■ GYNECOLOGICAL DISORDERS

The methyl xanthine contained in coffee, colas, tea, chocolate, and Theophylline (used to treat asthmatics) causes a common sensitivity response in some women, known as fibrocystic breast disease.

■ INFECTIOUS DISEASES

Recurrent viral, fungal, or bacterial illnesses occur more frequently in allergic people because the chronic stress imposed by the allergy state impairs and stresses the immune function that is designed to protect the body from the invasion of pathogenic organisms.

The hyperpermeable ("leaky") gut and respiratory tract, due to continual irritation from histamine, serotonin, and leukotriene production and release, allow easier entry for organisms. These body chemicals all participate in the inflammatory process of the allergic cascade. Damaged skin surfaces that occur with the inflammation response of allergic rashes and eczema also allow easier access for microorganisms.

▮▮ KIDNEY AND UROLOGICAL DISEASES

Cystitis and urinary bleeding often result from allergies to the more common foods, especially wheat and dairy products. Untreated wheat and milk allergies have led to irreversible glomerulonephritis (kidney disease). R. Finn, in *Clinical Nephrology* in 1980, reported renal (kidney) damage caused by occupational exposure to hydrocarbons.

▮▮ METABOLIC DISORDERS

Liver dysfunction is associated with allergy, sensitivity, and intolerance to drugs, alcohol, and chemicals.

Gallbladder disease (including stones) is usually aggravated by repeated exposure to allergenic foods.

Dr. William Philpott, in his book *Brain Allergies*, describes the progression from hypoglycemia to diabetes mellitus in the following way:

1. Acute allergic reaction involving the pancreas and/or liver
2. Several years of adaptive addictive adjustment with the consequences of episodic hypoglycemia
3. Metabolic failure by fatigue and/or exhaustion of the adaptive stage of the body resulting in a degeneration of the pancreas, and the logical onset of diabetes mellitus

Hypoglycemia and hyperglycemia are caused by allergy-evoked carbohydrate metabolism interference. Dr. Philpott states that both foods and chemicals can evoke these symptoms and that diabetes and hypoglycemia should be viewed as degenerative disease processes.

▮▮ NEUROLOGICAL DYSFUNCTIONS

In 1980, an article in *Lancet* by Jean Monro and others reported that two-thirds of migraine sufferers are allergic to certain foods. Often, the implicated food relieves a headache because of the addictive response described by Dr. Theron Randolph. (See chapter 9, Food Allergy, for more information.)

Some seizure disorders, including gait changes, slurred speech, tremors, and petit mal seizures are initiated by exposure to foods and chemicals even when minute amounts are administered during allergy testing. Dr. Marshall Mandell of the New England Foundation of Allergic and Environmental Disease in Norwalk, Connecticut, has videotaped these types of symptoms during allergy testing.

Symptoms of multiple sclerosis can subside after the removal of mercury amalgam fillings. Sensitivity to the amalgam stems from the mercury content as well as other metal components. Symptoms of multiple sclerosis also frequently improve after treatment of food, chemical, and inhalant allergies.

Nightshade Arthritis

Allergies to food can cause the joints to ache and deteriorate. We have several patients whose hip, knee, and ankle joints become excruciatingly painful if they eat wheat, sugar, or any member of the nightshade family, such as potatoes, tomatoes, eggplant, peppers, and pimentos. Some of them choose to eat these foods occasionally, particularly sugar, with the full knowledge that their painful joints are going to adversely affect their sleep and ability to move for several days.

▋▋ PSYCHOLOGICAL AND BEHAVIORAL DISORDERS

In his books *Human Ecology and Susceptibility to the Chemical Environment,* and *An Alternative Approach to Allergies,* Dr. Randolph clearly denotes the adaptive, stimulatory, and withdrawal effects of all allergens on psychiatric symptoms.

Dr. William Philpott, a psychiatrist, described maladaptive emotional reactions to allergens ranging from "mild central nervous system symptoms such as anxiety, dizziness, weakness, and depression to dissociation, paranoid delusions, and visual and auditory hallucination."

▋▋ RHEUMATOLOGIC DISORDERS

Arthritic symptoms are a common complaint of people as they grow older. Many physicians view it as a natural consequence of aging. However, allergy can play a role in this disease. In his book *Nutritional Therapy,*

Dr. Jonathan Wright of Kent, Washington includes allergy as a prominent, causative factor in rheumatoid arthritis. Some clinics have demonstrated relief of joint swelling, pain, and movement loss following carefully monitored fasts. Symptoms returned with deliberate food challenges.

Dr. Randolph also includes the inflammatory disease syndromes of ankylosing spondylitis (spinal stiffness), osteoarthritis, Reiter's syndrome, and other forms of arthritis in the same category as allergy-induced rheumatoid arthritis. Sensitivity to a variety of chemicals and foods has also been implicated in cases of lupus erythematosis.

The Goal of Treatment

The aim of this discussion is not to oversimplify complicated medical conditions, but rather to look beyond obvious symptoms and classifications, to ferret out the subtle nuances of early warning signs, and to uncover underlying causes that lead to degenerative diseases.

The goal of treatment should be diagnosing the basic biochemical and metabolic dysfunctions, and using all possible measures to restore the rhythm and balance of our body to achieve and maintain health. Dr. Philpott refers to lifestyle changes as "...giving promise of reducing or eliminating the disease process," rather than using only palliative measures to treat the symptoms. This approach does not diminish the science or art of healing disease, but enhances and augments our human capacity to grow, develop, and adapt to our environment in constructive and creative ways.

PART II

Understanding Allergies

M ANY PEOPLE ARE unaware that they have allergies. Unless they are sneezing, coughing, wheezing, or have watery eyes during pollen season, they feel that they are allergy free. They may boast that they have no allergies, even though they have health problems that are directly attributable to allergic reactions. The scope of allergies and their effect on health is far broader than most people realize. Many symptoms that people take for granted as a condition of life are actually symptoms of an allergic reaction.

Unless they undergo allergy testing, many people will be unaware of their sensitivities. Many different types of testing are available that allow a variety of treatments for any allergies found. Most people and many physicians are familiar only with the scratch test and do not realize that there are many other very accurate methods of testing. An overview of these tests is presented in chapter 8, along with treatment possibilities.

The most common substances to which people may be allergic or sensitive are presented in chapters 9, 11, and 13. Food, chemical, and inhalant are the main categories to which people may develop allergies or sensitivities. (Microorganisms are also a common cause of allergic reactions, and they are covered in Part III.) Symptoms from their allergies can significantly lower the health of the sensitive person. Untreated allergies can gradually damage the body and result in more serious problems later in life.

Once you understand the nature of your allergies, however, you will be able to use the information in chapters 10, 12, and 14 to minimize your exposures to allergens. The home survey in chapter 15 will help you to identify problem areas.

The task of implementing the measures recommended in this section may seem overwhelming at first, but changes can be done in stages. Keep in mind that any positive changes you make will significantly benefit your health. Knowing specific steps that you can take to improve the quality of your life gives you a sense of control that will increase your confidence in your ability to attain optimum health.

CHAPTER 8

Allergy Testing and Treatment

THERE ARE NUMEROUS methods of testing for food, chemical, pollen, mold, dust, dust mite, and animal dander allergy or sensitivity. The accuracy of any test depends on the skill and competence of the technician, laboratory, or physician. Because of their differences in background and training, all healthcare practitioners utilize the testing methods that are the most effective for their particular skills. In addition, practitioners attract different patient populations, depending on their particular expertise. For example, a physician who can offer the services of an environmental unit will have more seriously ill patients than a healthcare practitioner who is not a physician, but has expertise in some types of therapy. The testing methods used by a given practitioner will be those best suited to their skills and the needs of their patients. The testing methods that are more common or used more frequently are presented in this chapter.

There are also many different ways of treating allergy. Some methods are palliative, while others are curative. Each type of testing permits different treatment possibil-

ities, which are discussed in detail, in addition to immunotherapy and hands-on allergy treatments.

Avoidance and Challenge

This type of allergy testing involves a challenge in which the patient is exposed to the test substance under controlled conditions. Some protocols or exposures call for an avoidance period before the challenge. A symptomatic response to the test substances indicates allergenicity or sensitivity, and there are several types of challenge testing.

▮▮ FASTING AND DELIBERATE FOOD TESTING

This method involves four- to seven-day fasts and then reintroducing foods, one at a time, to observe any resulting symptoms. Although this can be done at home, fasts are not safe for everyone, and because of the allergy/addiction phenomenon (most people are addicted to the foods to which they are allergic), withdrawal symptoms from foods can be severe. (See chapter 9, Food Allergies, for more information.) This type of food test-

Pros and Cons of Fasting

Fasting detoxifies the body, unmasks sensitivities, and makes it easier to identify an offending food. However, fasting can be a painful experience for many, and reactions to the reintroduced foods may be severe.

ing is best done under medical supervision if a person has multiple or incapacitating symptoms.

The foods used in the test meals must be free of chemical contaminants and prepared with no seasonings, to avoid confusing results. Only one food must be given at a time unless you are testing for food combinations. People need to test for food combinations only when foods eaten together appear to give them symptoms, but when tested separately are not a problem. When testing for food combinations, test for only two foods commonly eaten together.

Meals should be spaced three hours apart, and testing must be completed in 10 days because cyclic food allergies may not be detectable after this avoidance time. Smoking is not allowed during the testing period, as it can cause symptoms and confuse the test results.

When done properly, this method gives very accurate results. The symptoms experienced when foods are reintroduced offer definite proof to the sensitive individual that a particular food is an offender.

Deliberate food testing can also be done without fasting, by eliminating only suspected foods. After four to seven days they are reintroduced one at a time, and symptoms will result if a food is an offender. However, testing foods without a fast is not as accurate, and will not identify any food combinations that are a problem. In addition, suspected foods must be eliminated completely, including possible hidden sources of a given food, to avoid inadvertently consuming it.

Fasting and deliberate food testing is sometimes supervised by a physician in a hospital setting, in special environmentally controlled units. This ensures that the fast is a true one, that the food tested is in pure form, and that there is no negative environmental exposure to confuse results. Medical help is available should symptoms become overwhelming.

▌▌ DELIBERATE CHEMICAL TESTING

A type of deliberate chemical testing, also called the Bronchial Inhalation Challenge, is performed in a chemical testing booth. Unlike fasting and deliberate food testing, this test cannot be done at home. It must be supervised by a physician in a specially constructed testing booth. The person's pulse, blood pressure, and symptoms are noted before the test, and mental ability is tested.

The person is then exposed, in the booth, to the specially prepared chemical. This is a double-blind test, so that neither the person nor the supervisor knows which chemical is being tested. Pulse, blood pressure, and symptoms are again noted, both immediately after the test and 30 minutes later. The tests for mental ability are also repeated at these intervals.

Changes in pulse, blood pressure, symptoms, and test performance will reveal which chemicals are causing problems. Since neither the supervisor nor the person being tested know the identities of the chemicals, personal bias cannot affect the test results.

■ PULSE TEST

The pulse test involves taking a resting pulse, eating a certain food or being exposed to a particular substance, and then taking the pulse again after 30 minutes. A significant increase or decrease in pulse rate indicates a sensitivity to the substance being tested. Smoking, snacking, and chewing gum must be avoided during testing. The pulse is taken several times a day for two to three days before the test in order to establish a baseline average pulse.

If you are taking the pulse test at home, before beginning testing obtain a resting pulse after sitting quietly for 10 minutes. For the pulse test, suspected foods should be eaten singly and in pure form. Frequently eaten and favorite foods should also be tested. Let the pulse return to normal for at least one hour before testing the next food.

The pulse test may also be used to identify sensitivities to chemicals. Problems with general chemical levels in large areas, buildings, rooms, and cars may be identified in this way. Discovering sensitivity to a single chemical is more difficult, since exposure must be limited to only that chemical.

General reactions to pollens and molds may also be tested by the pulse method, but isolating a specific pollen or mold is difficult in a home situation. It is hard to determine exactly which pollen or mold is causing the pulse change.

One advantage of the pulse test is that it can be done at home. Generally speaking, it is safe and, of course, it is free. However, one must take care that physical or emotional activities and responses do not affect the results. Inadvertent exposure to other allergens can also undermine its accuracy.

For some, however, the pulse test will not be helpful. Some people—those who are not "pulse changers"—will not experience significant pulse change even when exposed to substances to which they are quite sensitive. Also, those whose pulse is difficult to detect will not be able to use this test.

Avoidance is the main treatment method for all challenge tests. However, some homeopathic remedies, and allergy extracts prepared homeopathically are also treatment possibilities.

■ BLOOD TESTS

Several allergy testing methods utilize the person's blood. With one type of blood test, changes in the white blood cells (harvested from a blood sample) are noted after exposure to a test antigen. Another method involves using serum, the liquid remaining after the blood clots. This type of test allows the determination of the presence of specific antibodies that have been given a special identifying tag for detection either by a counting instrument or by color changes

■ ANTIGEN LEUKOCYTE CELLULAR ANTIBODY TESTING (ALCAT)

This method uses a Coulter Counter to count and size white blood cells (granulocytes and lymphocytes) and platelets in blood samples. The counting is done before and after a person's serum and white blood cells (red blood cells have been destroyed) are incubated with a food- or mold-impregnated disc. Changes in cell size and numbers are noted, and a certain percentage of change signals a problem reaction to the food or mold. Avoidance of the allergenic substance, or immunotherapy based on test results, are possible treatments.

∎ CYTOTOXIC TESTING

The cytotoxic test is a blood test for foods (and some chemicals) in which live white blood cells from the patient are mixed with a food antigen. The white cells will show various types of deterioration if the person is sensitive to the food being tested. If the person is not sensitive or allergic to the substance, there will be no change in the white blood cells.

The cytotoxic test gives immediate, objective results, and detects masked sensitivities. However, it is expensive and will sometimes show a false negative result if the food has not been eaten for several months. The skill of the person reading the slides also affects its accuracy. Cytotoxic testing has been found to be very accurate for some people, while less so for others. The treatment for this type of testing is avoidance of the allergens.

∎ ELISA

Enzyme-linked immunosorbent assay, often called the ELISA, can detect IgE antibodies in serum. A variation of this test, called the ELISA/ACT, can diagnose all delayed immune reactions which involve other types of antibodies. This technique uses the antigen binding properties of antibodies to detect specific antigens or antibodies in the serum from the patient.

For this test, antibodies are labeled with enzymes. The enzyme-antibody combination attaches to its specific antigen, and visualization is made possible by enzyme interaction with a substrate in which an indicator, usually a dye, changes color. Both the presence and amount of antibody or antigen can be measured by this sensitive method that can detect as little as 10^{-10} g/ml. Many substances, including antibodies to foods, pollens, molds, and microorganisms, can be detected by this method. Avoidance or immunotherapy based on test results are possible treatments for this method of testing.

∎ RAST

The Radioallergosorbent Test (RAST) is a blood test in which IgE and IgG antibodies are labeled with a radioactive substance. The amount of antibody found in the blood in response to a given food, pollen, mold, dust, dust mite, or dander can then be measured with a Geiger-counter type of instrument. For the RAST to be accurate for foods, both IgE and IgG must be measured. Sometimes this test will yield false negatives if a food has not been eaten recently.

The RAST can test for sensitivities to a large number of substances in a short period of time. It is objective, and the only trauma to the patient is the taking of the blood sample. However, the RAST is expensive and works only with immunological antibodies; it cannot identify problem substances for which there is no antigen-antibody response.

Avoidance of the allergens is the most common treatment used after RAST testing, although it is possible to prepare immunotherapy based on the test results.

Skin and Sublingual Testing

Skin testing involves several different methods, including the scratch or prick test, and intradermal testing, in which larger amounts of antigen are injected just beneath the skin. In both of these tests, the growth of a wheal (a raised red bump) indicate a positive reaction to the antigen.

Allergy testing can also be done sublingually (under the tongue). Any substance, including testing antigens, placed under the tongue will be absorbed by the blood vessels (sublingual vessels) under the tongue almost as rapidly as giving the substance intravenously. Symptoms and pulse changes are used as reaction indicators for sublingual testing, since there is no wheal.

▌▌ SCRATCH OR PRICK TEST

In this test, a drop of concentrated antigen is placed on the skin, which is then pricked or scratched so that a minute amount of antigen is absorbed. The growth of a wheal surrounded by erythema (redness) indicates a response to a problem substance. If a sensitive person has high IgE levels, the scratch or prick test will accurately determine allergy to pollens, molds, dust, dust mite, and animal dander. However, if IgE levels are low, a wheal may not develop even if the person tested is sensitive to these inhalants.

Immunotherapy based on these test results is determined by the personal judgment of the physician. This immunotherapy

is given by injection and, because of the danger of anaphylaxis, must be administered in the office of the physician.

When the scratch test is used for food testing, only food allergies for which the person has an extremely high IgE level will be uncovered. Since over 85 percent of food allergy is non-IgE mediated, this type of testing cannot give an accurate picture of a person's food problems. The scratch test also cannot be used for testing chemicals, since most chemical reactions are not IgE mediated. No immunotherapy is given for foods and chemicals tested by the scratch test, and these substances will have to be avoided.

▌▌ PATCH TEST

This test is used to diagnose contact allergies. A patch with an antigen on it is applied to the skin and is left in place for 24 to 48 hours. Lesions, a rash, erythema (redness), or hardness of the skin under the patch indicate sensitivity to the test substance. Avoiding problem substances and topical palliative treatment are considered the best treatment possibilities with this method of testing.

▌▌ PROVOCATIVE NEUTRALIZATION TESTING

This test may be performed either intradermally (under the skin) or sublingually (under the tongue) to identify problem foods, chemicals, and inhalants. Each involves the use of antigens serially diluted at a 1:5 ratio.

In intradermal provocative tests, baseline symptoms are noted, and an antigen is injected under the skin. The wheal is measured immediately after injection and again

Convincing Results

Provocative neutralization is a very useful test. Because there is usually more than one test factor—either a wheal and symptoms or the pulse and symptoms—the results are accurately determined. Vivid symptoms help to convince the more skeptical that the test substance is indeed a problem. While some of these symptoms are uncomfortable, even children do well with this method of testing. It is, however, a time-consuming process, and only a few substances can be tested during each session.

in 10 minutes, when symptoms are again noted. An allergic reaction is recognized where there is wheal growth and/or symptom change. Progressively weaker dilutions are then injected to discover a dose that relieves the symptoms and produces a negative wheal. The relieving dose is called a neutralizing dose, and treatment extracts are based on this amount. Taking the extracts on a regular basis prevents, blocks, or neutralizes reactions to the problem substance.

For sublingual provocative tests, the pulse is taken and baseline symptoms are noted. The test antigen is then placed behind the teeth, under the tongue, where it is rapidly absorbed by the sublingual blood vessels. In 10 minutes the pulse is measured again and symptoms are recorded. A positive reaction is noted if there are symptom changes and/or a change in the pulse. Progressively weaker dilutions are given until the pulse returns to its original level, or sta-

bilizes, and the provoked symptoms clear. Again, the relieving dose is called a neutralizing dose, and extracts can be made and used to control problem reactions.

When this test is used (intradermally or sublingually) to determine sensitivity to foods, the food should be eaten within 48 hours before the testing session. Intradermal and sublingual provocative neutralization can also be used to test sensitivity to chemicals, and is very effective for testing inhalants on people with pollen reactivity symptoms and low IgE levels.

The challenge dose for provocative testing may also be given nasally. A minute amount of powdered antigen is inhaled from the end of a toothpick in order to provoke symptoms. The neutralizing dose is then found by completing the test with intradermal injections, and extracts are made and used in the same way as for the intradermal provocative neutralization test.

■■ SERIAL DILUTION ENDPOINT TITRATION

This test is similar to traditional skin testing but goes a step further. Antigens diluted serially (1:5, 1:25, 1:125, and so on) are used for this test. First, a weak antigen dose is injected under the skin. If a wheal grows to two millimeters or more, it is considered a positive reaction. More injections are given (of either weaker or stronger dilutions, depending on the size of the first wheal) until a whealing pattern is obtained. This pattern is called progressive whealing.

The lowest concentration that produces a two-millimeter wheal growth is considered the treatment dose (endpoint) and this concentration is used in preparing the immunotherapy dose. The wheal produced by the next stronger dilution must be two millimeters or more larger than the first positive wheal. The wheal produced by the next weaker dilution should not grow.

▐▐ EAV TESTING

While EAV testing (electroacupuncture according to Voll) is being used extensively and successfully in Europe, it is conducted on only a limited basis in North America. Testing is done on an instrument that measures galvanic skin response. A vial containing a suspected allergen is placed in a receptacle in the instrument. The person being tested then holds a probe from the instrument in one hand while the tester uses a second probe to touch acupuncture points on the fingers of the person's other hand. An electrical circuit is thus completed between the person being tested and the measuring device. Any change from the calibration number on the meter indicates a problem reaction.

Foods, chemicals, inhalants, neurotransmitters, metals, nutrients, and many other substances can be tested in this way, and it is a rapid, painless, noninvasive method of screening for allergens. The accuracy of the results from this method compares favorably with, and can even exceed other methods of testing, although the skill of the tester is important.

In recent years computerized EAV instruments have been developed. The energy frequencies of the test substances are built into the computer and allow for extremely rapid screening and testing for numerous

antigens, including those that would be too toxic to test intradermally or subligually.

Several types of immunotherapy based on the results of EAV testing are possible. Homeopathic-type dilutions are usually used, and a treatment extract can be prepared for any substance tested. These extracts can be administered sublingually or intradermally and are usually taken once or twice a day.

▐▐ ENZYME POTENTIATED DESENSITIZATION

Enzyme potentiated desensitization (EPD) is a technique using small doses of allergens and the enzyme beta glucuronidase to desensitize people to allergies. The enzyme increases and alters the effects of the antigen. It is present in all parts of the body, and the dose given in the EPD injection is within the range of the enzyme concentrations normally present in the body. It apparently functions as a natural "messenger" in the immune system.

After testing, usually performed intradermally, and during which the allergens are identified, beta glucuronidase is mixed with antigens for foods, inhalants, or chemicals and given as an injection. Strict dietary and environmental control must be exerted two weeks before and after the injection, which may last for two to three months. Booster injections are given as required. The treatment length varies with the severity of the problems, taking as long as one or two years for some people.

People receiving benefit from the treatment may see results as early as a day or two after the injection. For others, benefits may

Holistic Approach

The best treatment for any disease process—whether it be an allergy to foods, chemicals, or inhalants, or an allergic response or illness caused by a bacteria, virus, parasite, fungus, yeast, or mold—considers the whole person, including mental, emotional, and spiritual aspects, as well as physical ones. In addition to testing and treating all aspects of an allergy, holistic medicine pays attention to improving immune function; achieving a healthy diet and adding nutrient supplementation as needed; making required changes in lifestyle, environment, and occupation; getting adequate exercise; and investigating past and present emotional or spiritual issues followed by appropriate therapy. (See chapter 24, Body, Mind, and Spirit.)

but rather as additional aids in the treatment and control of symptoms.

Symptom control is desirable, not only for the allergic person's comfort, but also to protect the immune system. If the immune system is constantly stressed by adverse reactions to foods, chemicals, or inhalants, its efficiency decreases over a period of time, and target organ damage can occur. Also, if the immune cascade is allowed to proceed unchecked, tissue damage will follow. Protecting the immune system with the use of extracts allows it to repair and heal.

Immunotherapy offers protection and relief from unwanted symptoms. The extracts are not physiologically addictive, as are some medications. Over a period of time, the frequency of use can gradually be reduced if symptoms do not occur. Many people can eventually remain symptom-free on one or two doses per week. Others heal sufficiently to stop treatment altogether.

not be apparent until three or four injections have been received over a period of six to nine months. Many people feel that this treatment has improved their lives enormously. Others receive no benefit from this treatment, and find that it actually makes them feel worse.

Immunotherapy Treatment

Because it is so difficult for the sensitive person to avoid or control exposures to all allergens, we have found immunotherapy treatment using extracts to be very helpful. They are used not as a panacea, substituting for dietary and environmental cleanup measures,

■ INHALANT EXTRACTS

Inhalant allergies as discussed in this book include allergy to pollens, terpenes, dust, dust mite, mold, animal dander, fibers, and tobacco smoke. Inhalant extracts allow individuals to be comfortable during pollen season and to endure exposures to such substances as animal dander, dust, and mold without symptoms.

Inhalant extracts may be made for immunotherapy from test results obtained by the scratch or prick test. However, the doses are chosen arbitrarily by the physician. Immunotherapy begins with a small dose, building up over a period of time until a protective dose is reached. It often takes a year to reach protective doses, and many individuals become sensitive to the glycerine and phenol that may be used as a stabilizer and preservative in these extracts.

Inhalant allergies can also be treated with immunotherapy based on the results of the RAST test, ALCAT test, scratch test, EAV testing, serial dilution endpoint titration, or provocative neutralization.

The following description of immunotherapy assumes the use of extracts based on results from either serial dilution endpoint titration or provocative neutralization tests. We have found these to be the most effective and safest immunotherapy method. In immunotherapy for inhalant allergies, the extracts contain small amounts of antigen, which will cause the body to produce IgG or blocking antibodies. These antibodies block allergic reactions when the person is exposed to the offending substance.

If a person has been tested by serial dilution endpoint titration, treatment extracts can be made based on the accurately determined treatment dose (endpoint). Relief from symptoms is immediate when the extract is administered because of its precise dose. This method is very accurate for testing inhalants in those individuals with high IgE levels. However, results for food and chemical allergies tested by this method are not accurate, because food and chemical allergies are not normally IgE mediated.

Regardless of the testing method, inhalant extracts may be given either by injection or sublingually. Some people obtain greater relief when the extracts are administered by injection. However, most people get significant relief from and prefer sublingual use of extracts.

Adequate control of symptoms is usually achieved by taking the extracts made from serial dilution endpoint titration weekly. In the height of pollen season, however, those who are acutely sensitive to pollen may have to take extracts more often. While pollen extracts are generally necessary only during pollen season, some people have better symptom control if they take them year round.

These extracts may be taken at home, as needed. This is possible because the exact treatment dose has already been determined, and there is no danger of anaphylactic shock. Over a period of time desensitization to inhalants will take place regardless of whether the extracts are taken by injection or sublingually.

Those who have low IgE levels and who have been tested for inhalants by provocative neutralization may take their extracts either sublingually or by injection and they may be self-administered, as there is no danger of anaphylactic shock, because the precise treatment dose has been determined. These extracts are usually taken twice a day, but may be repeated as often as need for symptom control.

Because exposures to animals, dust and dust mites, and molds occur throughout the year, extracts for these substances should be taken continually. When the mold count is extremely high, or when molds are sporing, extracts may have to be used more frequently.

■ FOOD AND CHEMICAL EXTRACTS

The mechanism behind the neutralizing dose in food and chemical extracts has not yet been determined, but several theories currently exist.

- Blocking antibodies are produced to prevent the reaction.
- T-cells are stimulated to stop B-cells from producing antibodies to the offending substance.
- T-cell levels are increased, thus increasing resistance to various substances.
- Immune complexes are bound so a reaction cannot take place.
- Abnormal balance between two types of T-helper cells is corrected.

Food extracts allow those who would be severely nutritionally deprived because of numerous food sensitivities or allergies to have a more varied diet. Immunotherapy treatment for food sensitivities offers many advantages, but extracts can only be prepared from certain types of testing, including the RAST, scratch or prick test, EAV test, and provocative neutralization test.

Food extracts may be taken either by injection or sublingually. Injections are required every four days, while sublingual doses are usually given before exposure to the offending food. If foods are rotated in the diet, each sublingual food extract would be needed every four days. If foods are not rotated, food extracts may be required more frequently. Taking food extracts allows individuals to eat problem foods without having symptoms, as well as relieving acute food reactions.

People who would be confined to their homes in order to avoid chemical exposures can, with chemical extracts and a common-sense approach to exposures, lead normal lives. Chemical extracts also may be used either sublingually or by injection. Taking chemical extracts will prevent reactions to chemical exposures, as well as relieving acute reactions.

The number and levels of exposure to chemicals determines the frequency with which chemical extracts must be taken. Extracts may be repeated as needed for symptom control. Extracts for chemicals tested by provocative neutralization may be self-administered. There is no danger of anaphylactic shock with this type of extract because the precise dose has been determined.

■ HOMEOPATHIC REMEDIES

Homeopathic remedies can be used to treat allergies or sensitivities to many substances, regardless of the testing method used to determine the offending substances. Classical homeopathic remedies may be used, or special extracts of common food, chemical, and inhalant allergens can be prepared by diluting the substances homeopathically. These remedies and extracts are usually taken twice a day. Extracts may be repeated as often as needed for symptom control.

The following allergies and sensitivities may be treated by the indicated classical homeopathic remedies:

- Dust: *Bromium, Silicea, Sulphuricum acidum*
- Animal dander, especially cats: *Tuberculinum*
- Mold: *Blatta orientalis*
- Egg: *Ferrum metallicum, Natrum muriaticum, Sulphur, Tuberculinum*
- Milk: *Lac defloratum, Natrum carbonicum,*

Natrum muriaticum, Sulphur, Tuberculinum, Urtica urens
- Wheat: *Natrum sulphuricum, Psorinum*
- Chocolate: *Sulphur*
- Perfume: *Ignatia*
- Pollution in general: *Sulphuricum acidum*

Hands-on Testing and Treatment

Several hands-on methods developed by chiropractors are very effective for testing and treating allergies. Muscle or kinesiology testing can be used as a testing method with all of these techniques, and for some of them, bioenergetic (EAV) testing can be utilized. Treatment involves the application of acupressure to the back, as well as other procedures individual to each method.

All of the hands-on allergy treatments effectively treat many types of allergies as well as treating and helping with other problems, including emotional problems. For some people, the results are permanent. Other people report a recurrence of symptoms when their body changes dramatically, such as during pregnancy or a growth spurt in children. Acute emotional stress and intense emotions have adversely affected the permanency of treatment for some people.

▮▮ KINESIOLOGY TESTING

Kinesiology is a form of muscle testing and can be used to test for allergies to foods, chemicals, inhalants, and other substances. The person being tested holds the test substance in one hand (enclosed in a container so that the identity of the substance is not known during the testing), or it is placed on the abdomen. The tester pushes on the other outstretched arm. If the tester is able to push the arm down with less resistance while the test substance is held, the person being tested is considered to be allergic or sensitive to the substance. If the tester cannot push the arm down, or can do so only with great force, the person undergoing testing is considered to be nonreactive to the substance.

There are several different variations of kinesiology, including applied, clinical, biological, transformational, and others. While there are subtle difference in technique between these methods, all utilize changes in muscle resistance when the person being tested is exposed to the test substance. The accuracy of this testing depends on the skill of the tester. Some practitioners are extremely skilled and can obtain reproducible results, while others are unable to do so.

▮▮ BIOSET™

Dr. Ellen Cutler of Corte Madera, California, developed BioSET™, which consists of four branches of healing. These include specific organ detoxification, either muscle or bioenergetic testing for sensitivities and meridian evaluation, enzyme therapy, and an allergy elimination technique to remove allergies.

Allergies that can be treated include food, chemical, pollen, inhalant, microorganism, and many other allergies. This method involves treating points on the back while the patient holds a sample of the allergen. This reprograms the body to accept the allergic substance without triggering an allergic reaction. A period of avoidance after the treatment allows the treatment to be processed by the body and includes no contact of any kind with the allergic substance, including smelling, touching, or tasting.

After the avoidance time, the person is rechecked, and if the treatment was successful, as determined by retesting, the allergen will no longer provoke symptoms. Emotional blocks and other health problems can also be treated by this method.

▮ NAET

Nambudripad's Allergy Elimination Technique (NAET) developed by Dr. Devi Nambudripad of Buena Park, California, combines kinesiology, acupressure, and acupuncture to test and treat allergies. Foods, chemicals, inhalants, or any other substance that may be a problem can be tested and treated by this method, which reprograms the central nervous system to safely accept the substance.

Testing for the offending substance and the organs of the body it affects is done by kinesiology, while the person holds a sample of the allergen. Bioenergetic EAV testing may also be used to determine allergies. Treatment is done on the back by stimulating the acupuncture points of the affected organs with an activator (a chiropractic instrument used to stimulate specific points on the body) as the person continues to hold a sample of the allergen.

The allergen must be totally avoided for 25 hours after the treatment. It cannot be consumed, touched, or even smelled, or the person may lose the benefit of the treatment. If this happens, the treatment must be repeated.

After 25 hours the person is rechecked, and if the treatment held, the allergen will no longer provoke symptoms and the person can safely be exposed to the substance.

Foods are more easily treated by this method, but it is successful for other substances as well, including treatment for an allergy to another person. (Humans can be allergic to other humans because of a negative interaction of their energy fields, causing discomfort to one or both people. People who are allergic to each other frequently care deeply for one other, but will not feel well in the presence of the other person.) Emotional blocks may prevent this treatment from being successful, but these blocks can be removed, which then allows successful outcome of subsequent treatment.

▮ NET

Neuro Emotional Technique (NET) is another technique that involves basic muscle testing to determine and remove emotional blocks that prevent regaining of health. Developed by Dr. Scott Walker of Encinitas, California, it is a chiropractic technique that utilizes and treats the three sides of balance necessary for health—biochemical, structural, and emotional. It allows a person to experience a more permanent and rapid correction to health and emotional balance, as well as teaching new ways of dealing with emotional problems. Special modifications of this method also allow allergy testing for foods and other substances.

▮ TOTAL BODY MODIFICATION (TBM)

Dr. Victor Frank of Sandy, Utah, originated Total Body Modification (TBM), which combines kinesiology, chiropractic, and acupressure to treat and relieve physical and emotional problems. It is an adjunct to all existing chiropractic techniques used for the restoration and maintenance of the optimum health of patients. However, practitioners other than chiropractors are trained in this method and use alternative methods to the chiropractic adjustment portion of this treatment.

Dr. Frank believes that there are five basic causes of allergies in 80 percent of allergy patients, including a sugar metabolism disorder, amalgam fillings, mercury sensitivity, sensitivity to honey bees and all the foods they pollinate, and sensitivity to bee pollen.

An allergy protocol relieves allergy to foods, chemicals, inhalants, microorganisms and other substances. This protocol involves testing for the allergen with kinesiology, and treating the points for the affected organs or glands with acupressure. This allows the body's "computer" to reset and allows the body to accept the corrections made. Further treatment with histamine, antibodies, and other substances complete the protocol. No avoidance period for the substance treated is necessary.

CHAPTER 9

Food Allergies

What is Food Allergy?

Food allergy and intolerance to food are not new phenomena. Over 2,000 years ago, Hippocrates described food allergy: "To me it appears that nobody would have sought for medicine at all, provided the same kind of diet had suited men in sickness and in health." In describing different responses to eating cheese he further stated, "Let thy food be thy medicine and thy medicine be thy food." During the same time, Lucretius wrote: "What is food for one, is to others bitter poison." Moses Maimonides (1135-1204) said, "No illness which can be treated by diet should be treated by any other means."

■■ FOOD ALLERGY PIONEERS

In 1905 Francis Hare, an Australian physician, described many aspects of food allergy, including food addiction, obesity, and alcoholism, in his book *The Food Factor in Disease*. Hare's interest in the clinical effects of different food groups had begun earlier, in 1889. Although he did not recognize sensiti-

zation to specific foods, his description of allergic manifestations is an important contribution to the concept of food allergy or intolerance.

Dr. Arthur Coca of New York formulated the concept of hypersensitivity, in which an antigen-antibody response does not play a role. He also coined the word "atopy," used to describe reactions mediated by antigens and antibodies. Dr. Coca founded and was the first editor of *The Journal of Immunology*, and in 1942 he wrote the book *Familial Nonreaginic Food Allergy*. The layman's version of his concepts was published in *The Pulse Test* in 1956. In the 1930s, Dr. Coca discovered that a person's pulse will go up after exposure to an allergenic substance. While not perfect, the pulse test is still helpful in determining problem substances.

Dr. Albert Rowe, formerly of the University of California School of Medicine in San Francisco, California, is considered to be the father of the concept of food allergy. He realized that foods can cause a problem even

Maladapted	+ + + +	Manic, with or without convulsions
	+ + +	Hypomanic, toxic, anxious, and egocentric
Adapted	+ +	Hyperactive, irritable, hungry, and thirsty
	+	Stimulated but relatively symptom-free
	o	Behavior on an even keel, as in homeostasis
Maladapted localized response	–	Localized allergic responses
Maladapted systemic response	– –	Systemic allergic responses
Maladapted advanced stimulatory response	– – –	Brain fag, mild depression, and disturbed thinking
	– – – –	Severe depression with or without altered consciousness

(Adapted from *An Alternative Approach to Allergies* by Randolph and Moss)

though the reaction is not IgE mediated. He is best known for his elimination diets, which are still important in identifying and treating food allergy. He developed two standardized versions of the elimination diet: the cereal-free elimination diet and the fruit-free, cereal-free elimination diet. Dr. Rowe wrote six books. The most comprehensive, *Clinical Allergy Due to Foods, Inhalants, Contaminants, Fungi, Bacteria and Other Causes,* was published in 1937. His last publication, *Food Allergy: Its Manifestations and Control and the Elimination Diets—A Compendium,* which he co-authored with his son, appeared in 1972.

The phenomenon known as "dumb Monday" was described in the 1930s by Dr. Walter Alvarez of the Mayo Clinic, who was a victim of this problem. This phenomenon occurs when traditional, often repeated, Sunday menus cause symptoms on Monday. Allergic reactions to the foods consumed can cause cerebral edema (swelling), headache, mental confusion, and malaise, all of which cause one to feel "dumb" and to function poorly afterwards.

The concepts of masked and unmasked food allergy, cyclic versus fixed food allergy, the deliberate food test, and the rotation diet were all developed by Dr. Herbert Rinkel of Kansas City, Missouri. *Food Allergy*, by Drs. Rinkel, Randolph, and Zeller, describes these ideas in detail.

Dr. Theron Randolph of Chicago, Illinois was the first to begin taking a detailed, ecologically oriented history, and he initiated the practice of fasting followed by controlled feeding in a hospital setting. Dr. Randolph also developed the concept of allergy/addiction, which can apply to foods, chemicals, or drugs. He proposed the stages of addiction listed in the chart on this page.

Dr. Randolph believed that food allergy is one of the greatest health problems in North America, and that food/drug combinations are even more addictive than food alone. Alcoholic beverages are a prime example of the potential for allergy and addiction to a

Allergy vs Sensitivity

Food allergy has traditionally been defined as an antigen-antibody response, or a cell-mediated reaction to food. Food hypersensitivity, on the other hand, occurs when there is an adverse reaction to food but no antigen-antibody response.

In our clinical practice, we consider any adverse response to food to be an equal problem, regardless of whether it is "true allergy" (IgE-mediated) or a hypersensitivity reaction (see chapter 1, Our Immune System). A sensitive person cannot wait until all of the immunological mechanisms have been determined in laboratory analysis and double-blind studies before receiving treatment.

substance that has both food and chemical content. Dr. Randolph also maintained that two-thirds of symptoms diagnosed as psychosomatic are undiagnosed maladaptive reactions to foods, chemicals, and inhalants.

■ FACTORS IN FOOD ALLERGY

Over the last few decades, food allergy has become an increasing problem in North America. Not long ago, food variety was limited for most families, with the usual exposure being about 40 different items. Today, with refrigeration, quick freezing, and other food preserving techniques, our food choices are almost unlimited. Some people eat a wide variety of foods, while others limit themselves to 10 to 15 recipes that they use repeatedly. Some people, particularly children, may self-select and limit themselves to only three to five foods.

Discouraging breast-feeding and substituting cow's milk or commercial formulas has helped to foster several generations of food-allergic people. The belief that children outgrow their allergies is untrue—food sensitivity in adults occurs in direct proportion to age. There are more multiple food allergies found in boys than in girls. This pattern reverses in adulthood, when multiple food allergy becomes more common in women than in men. Dr. Coca believed that 90 percent of the population had food allergies, while today others estimate the number of food-intolerant people in North America at 60 percent of the population.

Other factors affecting both the incidence and severity of food allergies include hormonal imbalances, infections, metabolic diseases, emotional stress, seasons, altitude, and nutritional imbalances. Heredity and race also play a role in food allergy. Dr. John Gerrard, formerly of the University of Saskatchewan in Saskatoon, Canada has traced milk allergy through five generations. Blacks, American Indians, and Asians experience a higher incidence of milk intolerance.

■ TYPES OF FOOD ALLERGIES AND REACTIONS

Food allergy may be classified in several different ways. Rinkel used the terms cyclic and fixed in relation to food allergy. A cyclic food allergy is one that worsens with repeated exposure; total avoidance reinstates tolerance. For some, it will take only a few months to re-establish tolerance to a problem food; for others, it may take years. Most food allergies are cyclic—once the food can again be tolerated, resensitization can be prevented by avoiding overexposure to the food as it is added back into the diet. New sensitivities can be prevented by spacing exposures to all foods.

If re-exposure to a food still provokes symptoms after it has been totally avoided for two years, the food allergy is considered to be fixed or permanent. Eating the food will always cause a reaction unless food extracts are taken to prevent or block the symptoms. Meats, grains, vegetables, and fruits, in decreasing order, tend to be fixed allergies.

Food reactions are also classified as:

- *Occult (hidden):* Pathology (damage) is evident, but without obvious symptoms.
- *Immediate:* Symptoms are obvious within minutes.
- *Delayed:* Symptoms may not appear until the next day, or several days later.
- *Thermal:* Symptoms occur after ingestion of a specific food followed by exposure to cold, heat, or light.

Occult food allergy should be suspected when there is a history of chronic illness, vague complaints, and a family history of similar complaints. Lab work will be normal, but there will be a suspicious correlation between the consumption of certain foods, many times in a definite pattern each year. Symptoms will include those not usually associated with food allergy by most physicians. Sometimes called cyclic, systemic, or hidden foods allergies, this older term, occult food reaction, has now been replaced by the term delayed reaction.

Immediate reactions are generally medi-

ated by an antibody known as IgE. Food particles, either proteins or peptides (parts of protein), are absorbed through the wall of the gastrointestinal tract, unaffected by digestion. The body recognizes these undigested food particles as foreign molecules and so produces antibodies (immunoglobulin IgE). When these antibodies combine with the antigen, allergy mediators such as histamine are released from the mast cells, producing immediate symptoms.

Immediate symptoms include urticaria (hives), wheezing, eczema, rhinitis, swelling of the lips and face, or anaphylactic shock. These reactions are easily recognized as being precipitated by a specific food, since they are acute, obvious, and sometimes dramatic. Every year deaths are attributed to anaphylactic shock stemming from food reactions. However, these reactions are usually to specific foods such as peanuts or shellfish, and are the exception rather than the rule. Food reactions are generally uncomfortable but not fatal.

A delayed food reaction is usually mediated by IgG antibodies, and the majority of food allergies fall into this category. IgG antibodies against protein can usually be detected in the blood during a delayed food reaction. Symptoms include chronic headaches (frequently migraine); chronic indigestion or heartburn; fatigue; depression; failure to thrive; joint pain or arthritic-type symptoms; recurrent abdominal pain; canker sores; chronic respiratory symptoms such as wheezing or bronchitis; nocturnal enuresis (bedwetting); and bowel problems such as colitis, diarrhea, or constipation. This type of food reaction is frequently misdiagnosed and often untreated, because it is difficult to link the symptoms with any event or food. Food testing is imperative in order to diagnose this type of food allergy.

Thermal food reactions are those that occur only when a hot or cold temperature extreme is experienced after eating a food. Without the temperature stress, the person will have no reaction to the food. There are some people who react to the temperature alone, and will develop hives, particularly to a cold exposure of any type.

Adverse food reactions can also be caused by small molecules other than proteins or peptides that form free radicals or act directly on tissues as though they were drugs.

▌▌ ALLERGY/ADDICTION PHENOMENON

When a person experiences symptoms from an offending food, partial relief may be obtained by eating the same food again. Many are surprised to learn they are sensitive to such common foods as coffee, sugar, wheat, eggs, corn, or milk. They may insist that the physician or test results are wrong, because the substance in question is the one they use to ease their worst symptoms whenever they occur. Many report cravings for problem foods, and say they always feel better when they eat them. They experience withdrawal symptoms if they stop eating the food regularly.

This phenomenon is an allergy/addiction combined with a masked food allergy. People are unaware of the sensitivity because eating the problem food makes them feel better. When the food is eaten regularly,

Difficult Diagnosis

Delayed reactions make food allergies very difficult to identify. The person who begins to wheeze immediate after eating a given food, or who develops a headache within 15 minutes of a meal, has no trouble recognizing that a food is triggering the symptoms. However, a migraine headache the afternoon of the day after consuming chocolate is much harder to associate with eating the chocolate. A person who feels well when he or she goes to bed, but who wakes up with a migraine, is usually reacting to a food consumed at dinner.

masking occurs, with chronic, low-grade symptoms. Constant postnasal drip, afternoon headaches or sleepy spells, or "spaciness" may be the only evidence of the problem. Avoiding the food (or chemical) for 4 to 10 days will unmask the allergy, and subsequent re-exposure to the food will elicit acute symptoms.

Allergic responses can be unpredictable, however. A person sometimes tolerates a food that at other times provokes symptoms. The total toxic load of the body is the determining factor in this case. When allergens, stress factors, or infection have created an overload, the person is unable to tolerate the problem food. When the body's total toxic load is small, the food can be consumed with no reaction. Low-sensitivity foods can sometimes be tolerated separately, but not when eaten together.

ALLERGENICITY OF FOODS

All foods can cause reactions, but some are more potent allergens than others. Protein foods are more allergenic than nonprotein foods, as proteins are more difficult to digest than fats or carbohydrates. If digestion of proteins is not complete, the molecule absorbed into the bloodstream is too large. The immune system recognizes the large molecule as a foreign substance rather than as a nutrient and sets up a chain reaction to destroy the invader. An allergic person benefits from addressing the causes of incomplete or disrupted digestion and absorption of food. Common causes include:

- low stomach acid
- insufficient pancreatic enzyme production
- improper levels of bicarbonate in the small intestine
- infections of parasitic, bacterial, fungal, or viral organisms
- irritation of intestinal lining as a result of long-term untreated food sensitivities
- stomach or duodenal ulcerations
- nutritional imbalances
- disordered amino acid metabolism, as in the case of candidiasis
- leaky gut syndrome (see chapters 7 and 17 for more information)

Amino acids are produced in the body from the breakdown of proteins. With inadequate protein breakdown, an amino acid deficiency can result, despite adequate levels of high-quality protein in the diet. The consequences of an amino acid deficiency may be the difficulty or inability of our body to produce adequate levels of enzymes, hormones, antibodies, and immune factors. This becomes a vicious circle because adequate enzymes are not available to digest the next ingested protein.

The allergenicity of foods is also affected by the following:

- *Cooking:* Will reduce allergenicity by half. Raw foods are more difficult to digest, and poorly digested foods tend to be more allergenic.
- *Heating foods in oils (as in stir-frying):* Slows their absorption rate and reduces reactions.
- *Purity:* Foods contaminated by additives, pesticides, antibiotics, bacteria, and hormones can cause problems, when pure foods may not.
- *Prescription drugs:* Can provoke reactions to normally "safe" foods.

CROSS-REACTIVITY

Cross-reactivity between foods and pollens heightens symptoms for some people. Bananas, watermelon, zucchini, honeydew, cucumber, and other members of the gourd family cross-react with ragweed pollen, which means their allergy-producing proteins are identical. As a result, a person sensitive to ragweed could react with symptoms the first time he or she consumes watermelon, cucumber, or bananas. Birch pollen cross-reacts with potatoes, carrots, celery, hazelnuts and apples.

CONCOMITANT AND SYNERGISTIC FOODS

A concomitant food is one that causes reactions when another allergen, such as a chemical or a particulate inhalant (pollen, dust, or mold), is present. For example, if milk, milk products, or mint are consumed

SUBSTANCE OR CONDITION	PROVEN CONCOMITANT FOODS
Trees	
Cedar, juniper	Beef, yeasts (baker's, brewer's, malt)
Cottonwood	Lettuce
Elm	Milk, mint
Oak	Egg, apple
Pecan, hickory	Corn, banana
Mesquite	Cane sugar, orange
Grasses: All	Legumes: beans, peas, soybean, cottonseed oil
	Grains: wheat, corn, rye, barley, oats, rice, millet
Weeds	
Ragweed, short and western	Egg
Ragweed, giant	Milk, mint
Sage	Potato, tomato
Amaranth family (pigweed, carelessweed)	Pork, black pepper
Marshelder	Wheat
Dust	Oysters, clams, scallops
Candida	Cheeses, mushrooms, vinegars and other fermented or molded foods
Cystic breast disease	Coffee, chocolate, cola
Poison ivy	Pork, black pepper
Viral infection	Milk, mint, onion, chocolate, nuts

SUBSTANCE	POSSIBLE CONCOMITANT FOODS (IDENTIFIED BUT NOT VERIFIED)
Weeds	
Marshelder	Tea
Chenopods (goosefoot family, such as lamb's quarters, firebrush, Russian thistle, shadscale, and winterfat)	Egg, corn
Dust	Nuts
Influenza vaccine	Onion

(Adapted from a compilation by Dr. Dor W. Brown, Jr., Fredericksburg, Texas.)

while ragweed is pollinating, one may experience an allergic reaction. However, the person may not react to any of these foods when ragweed is not in season. Reactions to a concomitant food can occur up to six weeks after the pollen season is over.

A synergistic reaction is one that occurs to two foods eaten within the same meal. For example, a person may experience an allergic reaction when corn and banana are eaten together, but not when they are eaten separately. Often, when people who are careful with their diets still have reactions, it is because they are eating synergistic foods.

Proven Synergistic Foods
- corn and banana
- beef and yeast (baker's, brewer's, malt)
- cane sugar and orange
- milk and mint
- egg and apple
- pork and black pepper

Possible Synergistic Foods (identified but not verified)
- wheat and tea
- pork and chicken
- milk and chocolate
- cola and chocolate
- coffee and cola
- coffee and chocolate

▐▐ DISEASE SYMPTOMS ASSOCIATED WITH FOODS

There are many disease symptoms that are linked to specific food allergies.

- *Arthritis:* Arthritic pain and joint involvement are linked to sugar, wheat, pork, and the nightshade family, including tomatoes, potatoes, bell pepper, eggplant, chili pepper, tobacco, and pimentos. According to Dr. Jonathan Wright of Kent, Washington, the nightshade family must be avoided for six to nine months in order to determine the role of these foods in arthritis.
- *Asthma:* Can be triggered by almost any food allergen. Egg, milk, seafood, peanuts, chocolate, corn, and nuts are common offenders.
- *Bad breath:* Can be caused by an allergy to any food. Candidiasis is also suspect in cases of chronic bad breath.
- *Bulimia:* Certain foods have been found to cause cravings in bulimic individuals; wheat and sugar are two common ones.
- *Colitis:* Most frequently linked to milk, although it can be caused by wheat, corn, egg, chocolate, and nuts. Dr. Abram Ber of Phoenix, Arizona, believes that next to milk, tomatoes are the most important food to eliminate from the diets of those with colitis. Inability to digest starches and disaccharides (complex sugars) also contributes to colitis.
- *Duodenal ulcer:* Milk allergy is a major factor contributing to ulcer pain. Unfortunately, in the past, the most common for treatment for ulcers was to drink milk, which only exacerbates the problem.
- *Eczema:* Frequently due to a food allergy. In children, milk should be suspected first, although eczema can be triggered by many other foods, including fruits, chocolate, peas, beans, peaches, grains, and eggs.
- *Headaches and migraines:* May be triggered by foods or chemicals. Allergy to almost any food can cause a migraine. Eggs, wheat, milk, chocolate, corn, cinnamon, wine, pork, and nuts are common offenders.

- *Hives:* May be caused by reactions to chemicals or foods. Peanuts, eggs, shellfish, tomatoes, chocolate, nuts, spices, milk, and food additives are frequently to blame.
- *Hyperactivity:* Often due to food or food additive allergy. Sugars and corn are a major cause, but many other foods can be involved. Artificial colors and flavors as well as preservatives can also play a major role.
- *Nocturnal enuresis (bedwetting):* Again, milk is the most frequent offender, followed by wheat, corn, egg, orange, and chocolate. Constipation also plays a role in bedwetting.
- *Obesity:* Hypoglycemia often occurs after food allergens are consumed, triggering insulin release, uncontrollable hunger and eating to stop the hypoglycemia. Frequent overeating causes weight gain. Any food can trigger hypoglycemic symptoms, but carbohydrates are the most common offender. (See chapter 7 for more information on hypoglycemia.)
- *Recurrent ear infections:* Many children have recurrent ear infections, which begin with an allergic response very similar to that in upper respiratory infections. Almost any frequently eaten food, or a natural gas exposure, can trigger this reaction, but milk is the prime culprit. Wheat, egg, peanut, soy, and corn cause fluid behind the eardrum. Orange, tomato, and chicken cause fluid also, but to a lesser extent. Fluid behind the eardrum predisposes the child to ear infections.
- *Recurrent upper respiratory infections:* Linked to food allergy, recurrent infections cause the mucous membranes to become swollen. This makes it easy for microorganisms to begin colonizing the damaged mucus membranes. There are many possible offending foods, but milk, egg, corn, and wheat are common.
- Other symptoms of food allergy include acne, eye pain, conjunctivitis, restless legs, fatigue, excessive perspiration, abnormal body odor, learning disorders, and depression.

The disease symptoms caused by food reactions are many and varied. This list includes only a few of the possibilities. While any system in the body can be affected, most sensitive people have a target organ that is usually affected when an allergic reaction takes place. For some, there may be itching in the inside corner of the eyes. The stomach may be a target organ for others, with nausea, belching, heartburn, or vomiting accompanying their reactions. The intestinal tract may also be a target organ, with symptoms of abdominal pain, diarrhea, constipation, or mucus in the stool. Cerebral symptoms include confusion, stupor, anger, or depression.

Some experience the same symptoms each time they have a food reaction, regardless of which allergenic food is eaten. Others report different symptoms for each allergenic food.

▌▌ PHENOLIC FOOD COMPOUNDS

Phenolic food compounds (PFCs) are special aromatic compounds that occur naturally in all foods. They give characteristic colors, flavors, and odors to foods and help to preserve them. These compounds receive their name from the presence of a particular type of structure in their molecules called a phenolic ring, which is different from the phenol compound. Although these compounds are not considered to be antigens, some scientists believe they become antigenic after being consumed by susceptible people.

Dr. Joseph McGovern of Oakland, California has found evidence of immune suppression on exposure to phenolic compounds, as well as behavioral disturbances in children. Phenolic food compound exposure can also cause elevated prostaglandins and histamine, depressed serotonin levels, and abnormal immune complex formation.

Testing for phenolic food compounds is essential for food-sensitive people. Desensitization treatment with extracts of PFCs can dramatically and quickly lower the allergic load because they occur in so many foods. For example, gallic acid is the most important of all the PFCs, and it is found in 80 to 90 percent of all foods. Rutin and quercetin (both of which are also bioflavonoids) and coumarin are also in the majority of foods, but to a slightly lesser extent than gallic acid.

In our clinical experience, extracts of phenolic food compounds have been helpful for both food and inhalant allergies, because these compounds are also prevalent in plants and pollens. Most of our patients improve more if given both whole food extracts and phenolic food compound extracts.

In addition, treating for neurotransmitters often helps with food allergy, as several chemicals with a phenolic structure that function as neurotransmitters also occur naturally in some foods. For example, choline chloride occurs in chicken, and bananas and avocados are among the foods that contain dopamine. Norepinephrine is also found in bananas, as is serotonin. Serotonin is also found in avocados, tomatoes, and other foods. All fish contain histamine, and phenylalanine is in eggs, milk, and potatoes. Lobster, mutton, and pork are among the foods that contain octopamine. High-tryptophan foods include wheat germ, cottage cheese, duck, pork, and turkey. Many other foods contain smaller amounts of tryptophan. (See chapter 3, Our Nervous System, for more information on neurotransmitters.)

Many symptoms can be relieved with immunotherapy for phenolic food compounds. Relief from arthritis pains, abdominal bloating, headaches, insomnia, hyperactivity, asthma, respiratory allergies, depression, fatigue, and dermatological problems, as well as improvement in people with intellectual disabilities, autism, dyslexia, menstrual disorders, bowel dysfunction, chronic constipation, and arrhythmias have been reported as a result of treatment with phenolic food compounds.

The following are but a few of the phenolic food compounds that can be a problem. Treating for sensitivities to these compounds is helpful in lowering total allergic load and relieving allergic symptoms to the foods in which they are contained. Because many of them also occur in pollen, they will help with pollen allergies. The compounds discussed below are but a few of the phenolic food compounds.

- *Apiol:* Occurs in almonds, bay leaf, beef, carrots, cheeses, dill, fennel, horseradish, lemon, lettuce, milk, nutmeg, oranges, parsley, peas, peppers, soy beans, tomatoes, and walnuts.

Relative Degrees of Allergenicity of Foods

FOOD CAUSING REACTIONS:

MOST COMMONLY	OFTEN	SOMETIMES	SELDOM
Corn	Alcohol	Alfalfa	Apricot
Eggs	Apple	Amaranth	Beet
Milk	Bacon	Banana	Carrot
Soy	Beans, dried	Barley (malt)	Cranberry
Sugar	Beef	Celery	Grape
Wheat	Berries	Cherry	Honey
Yeast	Buckwheat	Chicken	Lamb
	Cheese	Chilies	Peach
	Chocolate	Cloves	Rabbit
	Cinnamon	Cottonseed	Salmon
	Coconut	Garlic	Salt
	Coffee	Lobster	Squash
	Fish	Melon	Sweet potato
	Lettuce	Mushroom	Tapioca
	Mustard	Oat	Taro root
	Nuts	Oysters	Tea
	Onion	Pear	Vanilla
	Orange (citrus)	Peppers	
	Peanut	Pineapple	
	Peas	Plums/prunes	
	Pork	Quinoa	
	Potato	Rice	
	Raisin	Sesame seed	
	Rye	Spices	
	Shrimp	Spinach	
	Tomato	Strawberry	
		Sunflower	
		Turkey	
		Vinegar	

Odors and handling of any food material can also cause symptoms.

(Adapted from Dr. Doris Rapp of Scottsdale, Arizona and Dr. Del Stigler of Denver, Colorado.)

- *Coumarin:* Found in 30 foods, among them barley, beef, cheese, corn, eggs, rice, soy, and wheat. Very important for grain and grass allergy.
- *Gallic acid:* Found in most foods and food coloring. Stomach ache or abdominal pain is a clue that gallic acid is a problem.
- *Malvin:* Any red, blue, or purple food contains malvin, which plays a role in rage attacks. Malvin is found in strawberries, blueberries, beets, eggplant, apples, raspberries, and other foods.
- *Phenylisothiocyanate:* Found in 20 foods, including beef, cheese, chicken, eggs, lamb, peanuts, soybeans, and others. Very helpful for people who react to beans.
- *Quercetin:* Occurs in nature with rutin and causes the yellow coloring in plants, but may also be red to rust in color.
- *Rutin:* Found in 50 foods, including apples, asparagus, barley, beans, cabbage, cheese, milk, peas, potatoes, spinach, squash, strawberries, turkey, wheat, yeast, and many other foods.

Testing for sensitivity to PFCs may be done by provocative neutralization, hands-on allergy testing, or EAV. (See chapter 8, Allergy Testing and Treatment.) Specially prepared charts called dot charts allow physicians and patients to look up the phenolic compound content of foods and pollens.

Common Allergenic Foods

Testing for problem foods is an important part of allergy diagnosis for all sensitive individuals. The foods listed below are so common that it is almost impossible to avoid them completely. We can control exposures to these foods when eating at home, but

---

Unexpected Food Allergens

Food allergens occur not only in the foods we eat but also in alcoholic beverages, nutritional supplements, medications, soaps, cosmetics, cookware, glues, toothpaste, paper, paints, printing inks, and many plastics. Therefore, simply limiting exposures to foods by "rotating" them (eating a food or any form of that food only once every four days) may not be enough protection for a hypersensitive person.

Treatment with food extracts or hands-on allergy treatment provides needed protection against unavoidable and accidental exposures to these foods.

---

when dining out it is very difficult to avoid them.

As a first priority, the seven basic foods for which all sensitive people should be tested are: wheat, yeast, corn, soy, eggs, milk, and sugar. Many people eat these foods three times or more a day unless they are controlling their dietary exposures.

The following foods should be tested as a secondary priority: beef, pork, chicken, tomato, and potato. Sensitivity to milk and egg are an indicator that beef and chicken must be tested.

Testing for foods other than those mentioned above is recommended if they cause symptoms, or if they are eaten more than twice per week. A food which is seldom or never eaten generally does not need to be tested.

Sources of Beef

FOODS:
Baby foods (some)
Gelatin products:
   Cakes
   Candies
   Ice cream
   Jell-O
   Pastries
   Puddings
   Pies
   Sherbets
Gravies and sauces
Meats:
   Brains
   Hamburger
   Heart
   Kidneys
   Liver
   Ribs
   Roast
   Steak
   Suet

Glandulars and enzymes
(read labels carefully or contact the manufacturer):
   Adrenal
   Heart
   Liver
   Pancreas
   Tallow
   Tongue
   Tripe
MSG (Monosodium glutamate)
Processed beef (products that contain beef or beef products, or those processed in the same machine as beef):
   Liverwurst
   Sandwich meats
   Sausages
   Wieners
Soups and bouillon

OTHER SOURCES:
Capsules (gelatin, all types; nutritional supplements in capsules)
Cattle dander
Drugs (injectable, processed from beef or containing beef fractions):
   Adrenal cortical extract
   Heparin
   Insulin
   Pancreatin
   Pituitary
   Spleen
   Thyroid
Glue
Vitamins containing liver as a base

∎ BEEF

Beef is the most common meat consumed in North America. There are more than 30 registered breeds of beef cattle. Beef is the muscle meat from steers (castrated males) 18 months old or older, and from heifers (young females that have not yet calved). Veal is meat from young calves between one week and 26 weeks old. People who are allergic to beef will also be allergic to veal.

Those who eat beef can suffer from allergy to the meat itself, to the grains fed to the animals, or to insecticides found in feed grains; antibiotics given to cattle to prevent infection; and steroids injected to increase fluid weight. Most organic beef comes from grain-fed cattle, and will have white fat rather than the yellow fat characteristic of grass-fed cattle. However, some drugs given to cattle to change metabolism and increase fat create hard, white fat that is totally saturated.

∎ CORN

Corn and maize (the corn species of maize, as distinct from the cattle feed crop called maize) are found in a large variety of foods. Because corn is used in many forms in the preparation of many types of foods, it is the most difficult of common allergenic foods to eliminate from the diet.

Corn may cause allergic symptoms as a contactant (talcs, bath oils and powders, starched clothing, and corn adhesives); as an inhalant (fumes from vegetable forms of corn as they cook); and as an ingestant (corn and corn products that are eaten). Some people can tolerate processed forms of corn such as corn flakes, cornmeal, and cornstarch without noticeable symptoms, even though they cannot tolerate fresh forms of corn (corn on the cob, canned, frozen). However, it is best for those sensitive to corn to completely avoid all of its forms.

Treating corn allergy by avoidance requires the complete elimination of corn, maize products, and all foods or products containing any form or amount of corn. Continuing to use forms of corn that produce only negligible or subclinical reactions tends to maintain a high degree of corn sensitivity. This reduces the possibility of a sensitive person ever being able to eat corn without experiencing symptoms.

Always read labels. When inquiring whether a product contains corn, ask about each item by name. For example, when checking a bakery product, ask if the product contains any corn flour, cornmeal, cornstarch, corn oil, corn sugar (dextrose), or corn syrup. Do not accept the word of untrained personnel until you have inquired using every specific name of the different forms of corn.

Vegetable oils need not be identified on commercial labels, so sensitive people must assume that commercial products contain-

ing vegetable oil may contain some amount of inexpensive corn oil. Sugars also do not have to be labelled as derived from corn, cane, or beet, which means avoiding all commercially sweetened products in order to totally eliminate corn from your diet.

The simplest way to avoid corn is to eat only fresh foods (other than corn) without any additives. Fresh meat, fruit, and vegetables are free of corn. Unsweetened, uncreamed, diet products packed in water are also usually free of corn.

■ COMMON FORMS AND USES OF CORN

• *Alcoholic Beverages:* All ale, beer, brandy, gin, whisky, and vodka manufactured in North America is usually fortified with corn. Most domestic wines contain corn except California wines with 13 percent alcohol content or less. California sparkling wines and California wines above 13 percent alcohol can be fortified with corn. Imported wines and brandies are usually corn-free.

• *Cornmeal:* Buckwheat, oatmeal, or cornmeal is commonly scattered on the hearth before panless loaves of bread are baked, or may be sprinkled on the baking pan. Remove this layer by cutting a quarter-inch off the bottom of the loaf (do not scrape it off). Cornmeal is also used in cereals, scrapple, mush, johnny cake, Indian pudding, and other recipes, as well as in batter for deep-frying.

• *Corn oil:* Corn oil, which is comparatively inexpensive, is used for deep-frying, in salad dressings, and in some margarines.

• *Cornstarch:* Cornstarch is used as a thickening agent in gravies, icings and frostings,

Sources of Corn

FOOD:
Ale
American brandies (both
  apple and grape)
Aspartame (NutraSweet)
Baby foods (most)
Baby formulas:
  Prosobee
  Similac
  Nutramigen
Bacon
Baking mixes:
  Biscuits
  Doughnuts
  Pancakes
  Pie crusts
Baking powders
Batters for frying
Beers
Beets (Harvard)
Beverages (carbonated)
Bleached wheat flours
Bourbon and other whiskies
Breads and pastries
Cakes
Candy:
  Box candies (all grades)
  Candy bars
  Commercial candies
Carbonated beverages
Catsups
Cereals
Confectioner's sugar
Cookies (some)
Corn chips and other appe-
  tizers

Corn syrup
Crackers (some)
Cream pies
Cream puffs
Dates (confection)
Deep-fat frying mixtures
Dextrin
Dextrose
Flour (bleached)
French dressing
Fresh corn (canned, frozen)
Fried foods
Fritters
Frostings
Fruit juices
Fruits and fruit pies (canned
  and frozen)
Fructose
Frying fats
Gelatin desserts
Gin
Glucose products
Graham crackers
Grape juice
Gravies
Grits
Gum (chewing)
Ham (cured, tenderized)
High-fructose corn syrup
Hominy
Hydrolyzed vegetable oil
Ice cream (some)
Ices
Inhalants (cooking fumes
  from fresh corn, popcorn)
Jams

Jellies
Jell-o
Juices (vitamin C
  "enriched")
Karo
Leavening agents (baking
  powders, yeasts)
Liquors (all American and
  imported):
  Ale
  Beer
  Brandy
  Gin
  Vodka
  Whiskey
Maize
Mannitol
Margarine
Meats:
  All meats cooked with
    gravies
  All processed luncheon
    meats
  Bacon
  Bologna
  Ham (cured or tenderized)
  Sausages (cooked)
  Wieners (frankfurters)
Milk (in paper cartons)
Monosodium glutamate
Mull-soy
Nescafé
NutraSweet
Pablum
Pancake syrup

Sources of Corn

Parched corn
Pastries (cakes, cupcakes)
Peanut butters
Peas (canned)
Pedialyte
Pickles
Pies (cream or fruit)
Popped corn
Posole
Powdered sugar
Preserves
Puddings:
  Blancmange
  Custards
  "Royal" pudding
Rice (coated)
Rice Krispies
Saccharin
Salad dressings
Salt:
  All iodized salt
  Salt cellars in restaurants
Sandwich spreads and
  meats
Sauces for:
  Fish
  Meats
  Sundaes
  Vegetables
Sauerkraut
Sausages (cooked or table-
  ready)
Seasonings (some)
Sherbets
Sorbitol
Soup:

Creamed
Thickened
Vegetable
Soybean milks
String beans (canned,
  frozen)
Succotash
Sugar (powdered)
Syrups (commercially
  prepared glucose and
  Karo)
Tacos
Teas (instant)
Tortillas
Vanillin
Vegetables:
  Canned
  Creamed
  Frozen
Vinegar (distilled)
Vitamin C "enriched" foods
and juices
Whiskies (Scotch, bourbon)
Wieners
Wines (American):
  Dessert
  Fortified
  Sparkling
Xanthan gum
Yogurt
Zein
OTHER SOURCES:
Adhesives on:
  Envelopes
  Labels
  Stamps

Stickers
Tape
Aspirin and other tablets
Cough drops
Cough syrups
Cups (paper)
Dentifrices
Envelopes (gum on)
Excipients or diluents in:
  Capsules
  Lozenges
  Ointments
  Suppositories
  Tablets
  Vitamins
Gelatin capsules
Gloves (powdered with talc)
Inhalants:
  Bath powders
  Body powders
  Starch (while spraying,
  ironing)
  Talcums
Linit (starch)
Medication (tablet form)
Paper containers:
  Boxes (containing moist
  products)
  Cups
  Plates
Plastic food wrappers
  (inside may be coated
  with cornstarch)
Talcums
Toothpaste
Vitamins

pies, sauces, and many other items. Many baking powders contain cornstarch as a filler. Starched clothing and bedding, and adhesives in shoes may contain cornstarch and cause contact allergic symptoms. Cornstarch is also dusted on many brands of paper cups and plates, waxed and plastic containers, and plastic bags to prevent foods from sticking to them. There are also aerosol starch preparations for home laundry use that contain cornstarch. When sprayed, these preparations may be inhaled as well as contacted by the skin. Sterile gloves are coated with talc, which contains cornstarch.

- *Corn sugar (dextrose) and corn syrup (glucose):* Corn sugar and syrup are derivatives of cornstarch. Corn sugar does not become sticky and imparts a smooth texture to candies. It is used in nearly all commercial chocolates and caramels, cough drops, hard candies, lozenges, and suckers. The malted preparations used in ice cream, candies, and cereals are also derived from corn and wheat. Most bacon, canned fruits, ham, ice cream, Jell-o, jams, preserves, processed cheese, and soft drinks contain corn sugar or corn syrup. Dextrose is the most common sugar used for intravenous fluids. Synthetic vitamin C, commercial citric acid, sorbitol, and mannitol are derived from corn sugar. Corn dextrins and adhesives are used on stamps and envelopes and many other products, and some cigarettes are blended with corn sugar.
- *Vinegar:* White or acetic acid vinegar, usually derived from corn, is used commercially in salad dressings, pickles, sauerkraut, and sauces.

▋▋ EGGS

Chicken eggs are the most commonly consumed eggs in North America. Raw eggs in the shell purchased at a store should always be displayed in a refrigerated case, as cold temperatures help maintain egg quality by slowing the loss of moisture and carbon dioxide. Upon arriving home, refrigerate eggs as soon as possible. Egg quality will decline more during one day at room temperature than during one week in the refrigerator. Raw eggs in the shell will keep in the refrigerator for at least three weeks after leaving the supermarket.

Refrigerator temperatures also inhibit further growth of bacteria. Dr. Robert V. Tauxe of the Centers for Disease Control in Atlanta, Georgia warns that the world supply of commercial chicken eggs is contaminated with salmonella. Each pore of an eggshell is 100 times larger than salmonella bacteria, allowing them to enter the egg easily. The rate of salmonella infection is escalating, causing an increase in cases of reactive arthritis (even mild cases of salmonella poisoning cause sore joints). Immunocompromised people and infants just starting on solid foods are especially high-risk groups.

Most of the contamination problems with eggs have been traced to powdered and frozen eggs, which are derived from cracked eggs of insufficient quality to be sold as raw shell eggs. If you are using powdered eggs, be certain that they have been pasteurized. Purchase only clean, raw eggs with un-

Sources of Egg

FOOD:	Egg whites	Omelets
Baby foods	Egg white solids	Ovaltine
Baked goods	Egg yolk solids	Ovomalt
Baking powder	Egg yolks	Pancake flour
Batters for fried foods	Escalloped eggs	Pancakes
Bavarian cream	French toast	Pastas
Boiled dressings	Fried eggs	Pastries
Bouillons	Fritters	Poached eggs
Bread	Frostings	Pretzels
Bread crumbs	Fruit pies	Puddings
Breaded foods	Glazed rolls	Quiche
Cake flours	Griddle cakes	Salad dressings
Cakes	Hamburger mix	Sauces
Candies	Hard-boiled eggs	Sausages
Coddled eggs	Hollandaise sauce	Sherbets
Consommés	Ice cream	Shirred eggs
Cookies	Ices	Soda (not root beer)
Creamed eggs	Icings	Soft-cooked eggs
Cream pies	Lecithin	Soufflés
Croquettes	Macaroni	Soups
Custards	Macaroons	Spaghetti noodles
Dessert powders and whips	Malted cocoa drinks	Spanish creams
Devilled eggs	Marshmallows	Syrups
Doughnuts	Mayonnaise	Tartar sauce
Dried eggs	Meat jellies	Waffles
Egg albumin (ovalbumin)	Meatloaf	Wines (may be cleared with
Eggnog	Meringues	egg white)
Egg substitutes (Egg	Muffins	OTHER SOURCES:
Beaters)	Noodles	Laxatives

cracked shells, and do not use an egg if it is stuck to the carton or if the shell is dirty, stained, or spotted with foreign material.

Because of the problem with salmonella contamination, raw eggs should not be eaten. You also risk becoming ill if you eat lightly cooked eggs, including soft cooked, soft poached, soft scrambled, sunny-side up, and French toast. To be safe, eggs and egg dishes must be heated through to 160°F.

It is also possible for eggs to contain other contaminants. Pesticide residues, an-

Yolk or White Allergy?

Although some people react to both the egg yolk and egg white, those sensitive to eggs are frequently allergic to the egg white. Symptoms in response to eating egg yolk may indicate a fat-intolerant disorder. The method of cooking sometimes determines whether eggs can be tolerated.

tibiotics from feed, and drugs given to chickens to boost laying can all be found in eggs. Eggs produced by free-range, organically raised chickens will not contain these contaminants, and are also less likely to be contaminated with salmonella because their living conditions are more hygienic.

Albumin, livetin, ovomucin, ovomucoid, and vitellin on labels indicate the presence of egg or egg components. When inquiring about egg content of food items, do not overlook the possibility of powdered eggs.

Eggs from other fowl (ducks, geese, and turkeys) and even turtle eggs may be substituted for chicken eggs in recipes, as people who are allergic to chicken may not be allergic to the eggs of other fowl. (Adjustments will have to be made to compensate for differences in the size of eggs.)

▌▌ MILK

The major components of milk are lactalbumin, casein, lactose (milk sugar), and cream. The lactalbumin component varies from species to species. For example, the lactalbumin of human milk is different from that of cow's milk, and both are different from the lactalbumin of goat's milk. For this reason, some people who react allergically to the lactalbumin component of cow's milk may be able to drink goat's milk without difficulty. People who are sensitive to all components of milk will be unable to tolerate milk from any animal source.

Any product containing milk, milk byproducts, or milk proteins and sugars will cause the same symptoms as milk, and should be avoided. Watch for these ingredients when reading product labels or checking contents of food served to you: butter, cream, butterfat, whipped cream, skim milk, powdered milk, condensed milk, evaporated milk, milk solids, whey, yogurt, casein, caseinate, sodium or calcium caseinate, lactose, sodium or calcium lactate, non-fat milk solids, or lactalbumin.

Most people believe they will not get enough calcium unless milk is part of their diet. However, humans are the only species of mammal that drinks milk after being weaned from the breast (except for some housecats, and they should not be given milk). The majority of the world's population receive less than half the calcium that North Americans are told they need and, on the whole, have strong bones and healthy teeth.

Dairy councils constantly extol the virtues of milk. These nonprofit, promotional, and educational organizations publicize the supposed nutritional benefits of milk and milk products. However, milk is not the "perfect food," as it is frequently advertised.

Sources of Milk

FOOD:
Au gratin dishes
Baby foods (some)
Baked goods
Batters
Butter
Buttermilk
Cakes
Calcium caseinate
Canned milk
Carob chips
Carob coatings
Casein
Cheeses (all)
Chocolate beverages
Chocolate creams
Cocomalt
Condensed milk
Cookies
Cottage cheese
Cream
Cream sauces
Creamed soups

Curds
Custard
Doughnuts
Dried milk
Evaporated milk
Filled candy bars
Flours (prepared, such as
   Bisquick)
Fritters
Gravies
Hot cereals (some)
Hot dogs
Ice cream
Ice milk
Kefir
Lactalbumin
Lactate
Lactoglobulin
Lactose
Malted milk
Margarines
Milk chocolate candy
Milk puddings

Non-dairy products (some)
Nougat candy
Omelets
Ovaltine
Pancakes
Powdered milk
Pudding mixes
Rarebits
Salad dressings
Sausages
Sherbet
Skim milk
Sodium caseinate
Soufflés
Sour cream
Stroganoff
Timbales
Waffles
Whey
Whipped cream
Wiener schnitzel
Yogurt

■ PROBLEMS WITH MILK

Many people have difficulty drinking milk because it contains lactose, known as milk sugar. An enzyme, lactase, is needed to digest the lactose. Many children gradually lose the lactase enzyme, usually between the ages of one and four, and so are no longer able to digest milk sugar. Eight percent of North American Caucasians lose the lactase enzyme, and between 50 to 70 percent of other specific racial groups lose their lactase enzyme. Symptoms of lactase deficiency, which may show up after milk is consumed,

include cramps and diarrhea. However, lactase-deficient people can usually eat yogurt and cheese, which contain enzymes that help digest the lactose. A commercial product called Lactaid is available to aid in the digestion of dairy products.

Milk can cause other problems. Some people become constipated when they consume milk. In one study of 100 children, half stopped bedwetting when milk was removed from their diets. Milk is a poor source of iron, and is a common cause of iron-deficiency anemia in children. In babies, milk can cause a microscopic loss of blood in the stools. In addition, children will often fill up with milk and then will not eat solid foods.

There is evidence to suggest a link between high milk intake and cardiovascular disease. Cow's milk is high in saturated fats and fatty acids. Ice cream and some cheeses are even higher in fat content. For example, whole milk contains about one gram of fat per ounce, while cheddar cheese contains about 10 grams of fat per ounce.

Cow's milk is a common food allergen; people may be sensitive to some or all of its components. Symptoms of milk allergy include vomiting, diarrhea, bloody diarrhea, asthma, runny or stuff nose, recurrent ear infections, rashes, hives, and hyperactive behavior. Studies have linked delinquency and behavior disorders to high milk intake. Infant colic is related to cow's milk formula or milk that a breast-feeding mother may be drinking. People with Crohn's disease improve after milk is eliminated from their diets.

■ CALCIUM REQUIREMENTS

The Recommended Daily Allowance for calcium for growing children is 500 mg for infants up to one year; 800 mg for children up to age 10; 1,200 mg for children up to 18; 1,000 mg for people 19 to 50; and 1,200 mg for people 51 and over. However, these figures were derived from experiments utilizing diets high in phosphorus. Processed foods and carbonated beverages are high in phosphorus. Phosphorus binds to calcium in the intestine, preventing its absorption. It also leaches calcium from the body. If your diet is low in phosphorus, you need take only about one-tenth the recommended amount of calcium, or 100 mg.

The ratio of calcium to phosphorus in cow's milk is 1.2:1.0. Breast milk contains 300 mg of calcium per quart and cow's milk has 1,200 mg of calcium per quart, yet infants absorb more calcium from breast milk. The calcium to phosphorus ratio in breast milk is 2:1, which emphasizes the importance of this ratio for proper calcium absorption. Milk and dairy products, poultry, meats, some fish, whole wheat, cereal products, peas, sunflower seeds, and dark green leafy vegetables have a low calcium to phosphorus ratio.

Increased phosphate (a form of phosphorus) intake has been noted to adversely affect the behavior of hyperactive and learning-disabled children. Children who drink more than 1.5 liters of soda pop per week are in danger of developing hypocalcemia (low calcium). This causes leaching of the bone that can lead to osteoporosis in later years. Peak bone mass occurs in teenagers. Bone mass decreases significantly in women after their twenties, particularly when they reach menopause.

Acid-forming diets increase calcium excretion. Meats, other high-protein foods, and most cereal grains, including wheat, are acid-forming; most vegetables and fruits do not have this effect. Nutrients necessary for the proper absorption and utilization of calcium include magnesium, manganese, potassium, zinc, and vitamin D.

■ SOURCES OF CALCIUM

There are many sources of calcium other than cow's milk. Good food sources of calcium are sardines, kidney beans, broccoli,

FOOD	CALCIUM (MG)
Swiss cheese	925
Cheddar cheese	750
Carob flour	352
Sardines	332
Turnip greens	246
Almonds	234
Corn tortillas (lime added)	200
Dandelion greens	187
Brazil nuts	186
White beans	144
Pinto beans	135
Cow's milk	131
Goat's milk	129
Tofu	128
Dried figs	126
Sunflower seeds	120
Salmon (canned in oil)	119
Sesame seeds (hulled)	110
Raw broccoli	103
Spinach	93
Cooked broccoli	88
Peanuts	69
Raisins	62

almonds, fish, seaweed, and soybeans. Other foods with high calcium content are listed below. The indicated calcium content is for 100-gram edible portions, or 3½ ounces.

Giving up milk defies our traditional training. We are conditioned to drink milk, but taste is acquired, and conditioning can be changed. Try using soy milk, goat's milk, nut milk, apple juice, or other juices on cereal. You will be pleasantly surprised. Soy milk, goat's milk, or water can be used as a substitute in cooking. (See "But the Recipe Says..." in chapter 10, Eating Safely, for milk substitutions.) Goat's milk should not normally be used for babies under four months old because of the immaturity of their kidneys. If goat's milk is used as the sole source of milk for an infant (and this is rarely recommended), it must be supplemented with folic acid and vitamin B_6 (pyridoxine).

Calcium may also be obtained by taking a calcium supplement. The best calcium supplement is one in which calcium is chelated (bound) to an amino acid to enhance absorption. The supplement should contain both calcium and magnesium in a ratio of 2 to 1, which is best for absorption and utilization. (Some magnesium-deficient people, however, require a supplement containing equal amounts of calcium and magnesium.) If you are allergic to milk, avoid calcium lactate, which is milk-based. Dolomite is poorly absorbed as a source of calcium and may contain a high lead content. Bonemeal sources of calcium are also not recommended because they are difficult to digest.

See additional information on calcium and magnesium in chapter 20, Treating Allergies with Nutrient Supplements.

▌▌ PORK

Pork, the muscle meat from mature hogs, is sold fresh, cured, or processed. It is the most frequently processed of all meats. Severely pork-sensitive people must avoid all forms of pork.

Although organic pork is safer and contains more nutrients, the animals are frequently grain-fed, which can cause reactions for those with grain allergies. Hogs fed on

Sources of Pork

FOOD:

Fresh pork:
  Brains
  Chops
  Cracklings or chitterlings
  Kidneys
  Liver
  Ribs
  Roast
  Sausage
  Souse (head cheese)
Cured pork:
  Bacon
  Ham
  Pickled pig's feet
  Pork rinds
  Salt pork
  Sausage
Processed pork:
  Canned meats ("potted" meats)
  Luncheon meats
  Mincemeat
  Spam
  Vienna sausage
Wieners
Baby foods (some)
Baked beans
Bakery products
Candy bars

Chinese and Polynesian foods
Cocktail dips
Fried foods in restaurants
Fritos
Frosting mixes
Gelatin
Ice cream
Instant foods (such as mashed potatoes)
Jell-o
Lard
Margarine
Mayonnaise
Mexican foods
Non-dairy creamer
Potato chips
Pre-breaded frozen foods
Prepared cake and pancake mixes
Processed cheeses (in jars and cartons)
Puddings
Salad dressings
Shortening
Soups with pork
Vegetables seasoned with salt pork
Vegetable stock

OTHER SOURCES:

Drugs:
  Calcium and magnesium stearates
  Capsules
  Heparin
  Tonics and pills for anemia (hog stomach contains an intrinsic factor)
Glandulars and enzymes (read labels carefully or contact the manufacturer):
  Adrenal
  Mixed enzyme products
  Pancreas
  Pancreatin
  Pituitary
  Thymus
  Thyroid
Glue
Glycerine (soaps, cosmetics)
Iron skillets and Dutch ovens that have not been thoroughly scoured after being used to cook pork

---

garbage (boiled for safety) are the least problematic source of pork for grain-sensitive individuals. However, the practice of garbage feeding is suspected of spreading trichinosis, cholera, and brucellosis. Pretreating garbage to destroy the organisms also destroys the necessary nutrient content. Pigs that are fed cooked garbage tend to be anemic and have stomach ulcers.

The quality of pork can be affected by antibiotics in feed, inferior feed quality, drugs, vaccines, overfattening, artificial environments, and poor management. The practice of administering drugs to pigs before slaughter slows muscle changes after death and keeps the flesh red.

Trichinosis, an infection of *Trichinella spiralis* worms, was once prevalent in the United States, and was spread through infected pork. However, with the advent of cooked garbage feed, better freezing procedures, improved hog-raising methods, and more stringent pork inspection, the incidence of trichinosis in the U.S. population is down to 4 percent. These infections result from consuming raw or undercooked pork or pork products, or improperly cooked ground beef that has been adulterated with pork. The advent of microwave cooking temporarily increased the number of trichinosis cases. People were unaware that pork cooked in the microwave could be undercooked.

Symptoms of trichinosis include submucosal inflammatory reactions, nausea, vomiting, diarrhea, fever, edema, hemorrhages under the fingernails, muscular pain, and congestive heart failure.

▮▮ SOY

Soybeans have been grown in Asia for centuries, especially in China, where they have provided the bread, protein, and oil. Since the beginning of the 19th century, American farmers have grown soybeans for livestock, feed, or for fertilizer.

Chemists have also found many uses for soybeans, which are proving to be a bonanza. Ford Motor Company uses byproducts of soybeans to make plastic window frames, steering wheels, gearshift knobs, distributors, upholstery fabric, and other

parts. Rubber substitutes and lecithin in leaded gasoline are also made from soybeans. (See next page for Sources of Soy.)

Expect many new food and industrial uses of soy. If you remember that soybeans are used as flour, oil, milk, nuts, and meat extenders, it will be possible to anticipate most new food contacts. Soy products have steadily grown more popular as part of the human diet, including tofu, miso, soy milk, and soybeans. When purchasing prepared foods, consider soy as a possible ingredient if the label says vegetable oil, vegetable broth, or textured vegetable protein.

Eating in restaurants almost always means a soy exposure, as most restaurants and fast-food chains cook with soy oil or flour. Soybean flour containing only 1 percent oil is now used by many bakers in dough mixtures for breads, cakes, rolls, and pastries, to keep them moist and fresh several days longer. The roasted beans are often used in place of peanuts on breakfast rolls. Some biscuits and several crisp crackers also contain soybean flour.

▮▮ SUGAR AND ALL THINGS SWEET

North America has turned into a land of "sugarholics." We eat huge quantities of sugar, in the form of refined sugars added to foods we choose to eat and naturally occurring sugars in fruits and vegetables. Much of the sugar we eat is "hidden" sugar—we are unaware that we are consuming it. Foods that were once unsweetened are now sweetened, and others that previously were sweet have been elevated to higher levels of sweetness.

Hidden sugars are primarily the result of

Sources of Soy

FOOD:
Artificial meats and nuts
Baby foods (some)
Bakery goods
Cake mixes (may contain
    artificial fruit made from
    soy)
Candies:
  Caramels
  Carob chips
  Chocolate chips
  Hard candies
  Nut candies
  (Lecithin, derived from
    soy, is used in candies to
    prevent drying and to
    emulsify fats.)
Cereals
Fried products:
  Corn chips
  Potato chips
  Tortilla chips
Ice cream (dairy and tofu)
Margarine and butter sub-
    stitutes
Meats:
  Canned meats and fish
  Hamburgers (fast food)
  Luncheon meats
  Pork-link sausages
Milk substitutes:
  Infant formulas
  Non-dairy creamers
  Soy milk
Nuts:
  Any roasted in soy oil

Soy (formed to look like
    other nuts)
Soybeans (toasted, salted,
    and used as nuts)
Oils (Crisco, Spry solid or
    liquid)
Pastas:
  Macaroni
  Noodles
  Spaghetti
Peanut butter (some)
Processed cheeses (some)
Salad dressings (may con-
    tain soy oil, but list only
    vegetable oil on the
    label)
Sauces:
  Lea & Perrins
  Soy sauce
  Steak sauce
  Tamari
  Teriyaki sauce
  Worcestershire sauce
Soups (may contain soy oil
    and/or lecithin)
Soy products:
  Miso
  Natto
  Tempeh
  Tofu
Tuna (packed in vegetable
    oil)
Vegetables:
  Margarine or oil on
    vegetables
  Soy sprouts

OTHER SOURCES:
Adhesives
Automobile parts
Blankets
Candles
Celluloid
Cloth
Clothing
Coffee substitute
Cosmetics
Custards
Diet aids
Dog food
Enamels
Fertilizer
Fish food
Fodder
Glycerine
Illuminating oil
Lecithin
Linoleum
Lubricating oil
Make-up
Massage creams
Nitroglycerine
Paints
Paper finishes
Paper sizing
Printing ink
Soap
Telephones
Textile finishings
Toys
Varnish
Vitamins

industrial practices that are largely unfamiliar to the public. For example, the sugar content of meat is increased by feeding sugar to animals before slaughter to improve the flavor and color of the meat, and by adding it to the meat itself as it is prepared in packing houses and restaurants. Any dish prepared with ground meat may contain added syrups to help minimize shrinkage and to improve flavor, juiciness, and texture.

The presence of hidden sugars should be suspected in the following items, either because their manufacturers are not required to list the sugar content, or because the sugars are listed in such a fashion that the consumer does not recognize them as sugars.

- bouillon cubes
- breadings for fried or baked poultry and meats
- canned and frozen vegetables
- catsup
- convenience foods
- cottage cheese
- dry roasted nuts
- frozen and canned entrées
- gravies
- instant coffee
- instant tea
- iodized salt
- luncheon meats
- mixes to stretch chopped beef
- peanut butter
- potato chips
- salad dressings
- soups
- weiners (frankfurters)
- cigarettes

When sugar is listed in the ingredients, the exact percentage is difficult to determine.

Sugar appears on labels under many names; the "ose" ending of words indicates a sugar. All of the following items are sugars:

- brown sugar
- corn syrup
- corn syrup solids
- dextrose
- fructose
- glucose
- grain syrups (wheat, rye, rice)
- high-fructose corn syrup
- honey
- malt syrup
- maltodextrin
- mannitol
- maple syrup
- molasses
- raw sugar
- sorbitol
- sorghum
- sucrose
- turbinado
- xylitol

Sugar, like alcohol, is rapidly absorbed and floods the system, predisposing the sensitive person to severe reactions and addictions. In a study done by Dr. Timothy Jones of Yale University, adults and children were given proportionately equal doses of glucose, the form of sugar to which all carbohydrates in blood are metabolized. The children received 20 teaspoons of glucose, the sugar equivalent of two 12-ounce colas. The blood glucose levels in both the adults and children recorded similar highs and lows, but the adrenalin levels of the children were twice as high as those of the adults. More of the children felt weak and shaky. As a result of this study, Dr. Jones advises that children

Sugarholics—and the Consequences

The average North American consumes approximately his or her own weight in sugar each year, the national average being over 130 pounds of sugar per person. High sugar intake has been linked to dental caries, obesity, diabetes, coronary heart disease, hypoglycemia, and behavioral problems. Sugar depletes the body of specific nutrients, including the B vitamins, magnesium, chromium, manganese, and other minerals. Ingesting sugar also destroys the germ-killing ability of the white blood cells for four hours.

Our body machinery is designed to cope with about 2 teaspoons of sugar per day. If we eat additional amounts of sugar—such as a piece of apple pie, with 19 teaspoons of sugar—it disrupts our body's "sugar equilibrium." These disruptions stress our body and overload the adrenal gland and pancreas, which are critical to allergy control.

not be given sweets on an empty stomach. He also suggests that the increase in adrenalin could be linked to the hyperactivity some children display after eating sweets.

Young children eat small amounts of food and are dependent on this food to obtain the nutrients they need. Eating sugar, which has little nutritional value, adversely affects their appetites, thus decreasing their intake of nutrients. Sweets should also never be used as a reward food.

There is no completely safe sweetener—all have drawbacks or side effects. While honey or maple syrup used in small amounts are better than refined sugars, fruit juices are probably the best choice for sweeteners. Although allergy extracts are available for sugar, it is healthier to avoid it.

The following sweeteners are in common use in North America.

▌SUCROSE

Sucrose is the most commonly used sugar in our food supply. It can be refined from both sugar cane and sugar beets, and the resulting sugars have identical structures. However, many hypersensitive people can distinguish one from the other by their reaction to the small residues of the source plants. Sucrose stimulates the production of fat in the body, particularly in women using contraceptive drugs. It also increases tooth decay, and there is always an increase in diabetes mellitus in populations when their sugar consumption goes up.

Beet and cane sugars are used as:
- fermentation mediums in baked goods, contributing to the color, flavor, and quality of the crust; retention of moisture; and extension of shelf life
- curing agents for processed meats
- preservatives in fruits, jellies, jams, and preserves
- sweeteners in canned goods
- bulking agents in ice cream, baked goods, and confections
- "bodying" agents in soft drinks
- preservatives in medications
- ointments

▌CORN SWEETENERS

Over half of the cornstarch milled in North America is used to produce corn sweeteners. They are used extensively by the food industry because of their low cost and because a sweeter mix is obtained when they are combined with sucrose.

Corn sugar carries all of the allergenicity of corn, and many corn-sensitive people react to it more quickly than to other components of corn. As the food industry has stepped up its use of corn sweeteners and cornstarch, sensitivities to corn have risen. Corn-sensitive people must avoid products containing dextrose, glucose, sorbitol, and mannitol (generally made from dextrose).

Corn sugar found in infant formulas can produce eczema and gastrointestinal upsets in corn-sensitive babies, and diarrhea in all infants.

Corn sweeteners:
- add body and texture to soft drinks
- add chewiness to confections and chewing gums
- are used in maple, nut, and root beer flavoring for beverages, ice creams, candy, and baked goods
- are used in processed meats, hams, bacon, fish products, and sausages
- help retain bright colors in preserves, cured meats and catsup
- absorb moisture to keep hard candy from becoming sticky
- inhibit crystallization of other sugars
- ferment easily, which aids brewers and distillers

▌DEXTROSE

Dextrose, maltose, corn syrup, and corn sugar are derivatives of cornstarch. Dextrose, in addition to the uses listed above, is an ingredient in intravenous solutions commonly used in hospitals. Many corn-sensitive patients react to these IVs, experiencing problems that are commonly attributed to "surgical complications." For example, Dr. Kendall Gerdes, of Denver, Colorado, reported a case of a woman who developed bronchospasm after receiving IV dextrose.

▌GLUCOSE

Glucose is a commercially processed sugar derived from cornstarch, occurring naturally in grape and corn sugar. Its name can be misleading, since blood sugar is also referred to as glucose. It is frequently labeled as corn syrup because the public at one time thought it was a sugar derived from glue.

Glucose is a dangerous sweetener because of its low sweetness level. It is only one-fifth as sweet as sucrose, and so large quantities can be absorbed without a person being aware of its presence in food.

Glucose is frequently used to flavor ground meat dishes, luncheon meats, and hams, as well as to extend maple syrup.

▌HIGH-FRUCTOSE CORN SYRUP

High-fructose corn syrup is commercially produced from dextrose. A 42 percent solution of this syrup is as sweet as sucrose. Because it is considerably cheaper than sucrose—and because supply is not subject to the fluctuations of the sugar market—the use of high-fructose corn syrup has increased drastically since the 1970s. Since two major cola companies switched to high-fructose corn syrup in 1980, it has become an ingredient in all soda pops.

High-fructose corn syrup is not safe for corn-sensitive individuals or for diabetics.

High-fructose corn syrup contains some glucose, with the amount varying from product to product, and glucose is the sugar that diabetics are least able to utilize.

It is sometimes very difficult to identify the source of the fructose in a given food item because of the confusion between crystalline fructose and high-fructose corn syrups.

Processors use high-fructose corn syrup in:
• baked goods and icings
• carbonated and non-carbonated beverages
• cereals
• chocolate milk, eggnog, yogurt, ice cream, and sherbet
• diabetic and reduced-calorie foods
• jams, jellies, and preserves
• salad dressings, pickles, and catsups
• table syrups and liquid table sweeteners
• wines

■ FRUCTOSE

Fructose or levulose is the natural sugar found in fruits, vegetables, berries, and honey. The fructose commonly sold in stores is usually processed from cane or beet sugar, not from fruits. Fructose is twice as sweet as sucrose and it dissolves readily in water. It also absorbs water, which helps to keep baked goods and confections from drying out. It does not crystallize during storage and shipment, and is an excellent masking agent for the bitterness of saccharin. (See artificial sweeteners, below.)

Fructose is slowly metabolized in the liver into glucose, which then requires insulin for use in the body. Although the glucose is released slowly, it does not represent any particular advantage for diabetics, as has been claimed. Metabolic disturbances occur in both normal and diabetic individuals when fructose is used in intravenous solutions. It also matches sucrose in contributing to tooth decay.

Fructose is used in many processed foods, including:
• breakfast cereals
• cake and cookie mixes
• candies and chewing gums
• gelatin and frozen desserts
• jams and preserves
• jellies
• lemonade and tea mixes
• peanut butter
• protein supplements and other beverage powders
• puddings
• salad dressings and mayonnaise

■ RAW SUGAR, BROWN SUGAR, TURBINADO SUGAR, AND MOLASSES

To make sugar, juice is squeezed from sugar cane with rollers and then boiled in a vacuum pan until the sugar crystallizes. The liquid that does not crystallize becomes molasses, and the newly formed crystals (still coated with molasses) are raw sugar. When the molasses is removed from these crystals, they are referred to as refined, and become white table sugar.

Raw sugar may be contaminated with insecticides, smoke residue, bacteria, dirt, fibers, lints, mold, sand, lice, waxes, and yeast. If the raw sugar is washed and centrifuged, some but not all dirt will be removed, along with some solid materials and bacteria. The resulting product is marketed as turbinado sugar if it meets the minimum sanitary level set by the government.

Raw sugar produced in North America is usually white sugar with traces of cane or beet pulp replaced. "Unrefined" or "natural" on labels is meaningless, as the raw sugar has gone through several refining processes.

When molasses is further processed, more crystals form, which are yellow to brown in color. This is "brown sugar," which tends to clump because it still has a molasses covering. However, brown sugar is often more refined than white sugar. Its deep color frequently has been added, rather than being from molasses residue.

The molasses is processed numerous times to extract all possible sugar. The remaining syrup is blackstrap molasses, the waste product of sugar manufacturing. It carries most of the mineral matter and all of the gum, ash, dirt, and indigestible matter present in the unprocessed sugar. Molasses, which is 30 percent sucrose, is not a source of natural sugar, nor is it a good source of iron. True blackstrap molasses is not sold for human consumption, but to produce industrial alcohol for rum and yeast, and for animal feed. There are products called blackstrap molasses that are sold for human consumption, but because of their high iron content they tend to be bitter in spite of the 30 percent sucrose.

The quality of molasses depends on the maturity of the sugar cane, and on whether the processor intends that molasses or sugar should be the primary product. Many food processors use molasses blends that may also contain corn, wheat, or soy constituents. Read labels carefully when purchasing molasses.

Unsulfured molasses is made from the juice of sun-ripened West Indian cane. Blending of products from various places produces a uniform molasses, which is aged for a year or two. Sulfured molasses is a byproduct of sugar refining made from immature cane. The cane is treated with sulfur during the sugar extraction process, and a sulfur residue remains in the molasses.

▌ HONEY

Bees gather nectar, which is 80 percent sucrose. By using a digestive enzyme, invertase, they convert the nectar to two simple sugars: glucose and fructose. This mixture is called invert sugar and requires no digestion by humans. The ratio of fructose to glucose varies for different honeys.

Dissolved aromatics give each honey its own distinctive flavor and appearance. The remaining components in honey are water, a small amount of bee pollen, sucrose, dextrin, gums, and a few minerals, vitamins, and enzymes.

Honey ripened in the hive will have a smooth mellow flavor and a moisture content of less than 17 percent. Green honey, which has been removed from the hives too early, has a moisture content of over 20 percent, a bitter flavor, and will ferment easily. If honey is extracted from the hive with mild heat, it will retain some of its nutrients. Prolonged heat exposure breaks down enzymes and proteins and impairs color and flavor.

Honey is graded by clarity; the greater the clarity, the higher the grade. This grading has no significance other than measuring the size of particles filtered out. It bears no relation to quality.

Honey labeling is a neglected problem. Terms such as natural, old-fashioned, country style, organic, or undiluted are meaningless. Labels citing the source of honey are not accurate because honey is frequently blended, and bees do not visit just one type of plant. The problem that blended honey poses for the allergic person is the possibility of hidden, unlabelled allergens, not its quality or taste. Honey may also be adulterated with corn syrup or cheap sugars.

Honey may also contain some contaminants, such as traces of sulfa drugs and antibiotics used to control bee diseases. Empty combs may be fumigated with mothballs. Honey from certain plants can also be poisonous. However, these problems are not widespread—generally, honey is a safe food. As a nutrient source, however, it is highly overrated. Raw honey may be hazardous to infants under one year of age because it may contain botulism spores, which have caused the death of some babies.

▌ MAPLE SYRUP

Maple syrup is processed from maple tree sap. Maple trees are tapped by scoring the bark, and the sap is collected in buckets that hang beneath the scar. The syrup must be collected when the tree chemistry is in the "sweet water" stage. If it is collected when the tree is producing substances used for tree growth, the sap becomes "buddy" and is useless for table-grade syrup. After collection, the liquid is filtered and concentrated for marketing.

Paraformaldehyde pellets are used to kill bacteria to help keep the tap holes open. The pellets increase both production and profits by allowing the trees to be tapped earlier and permitting the sap to run for longer periods of time. The formaldehyde from the pellets supposedly evaporates during processing, and maple syrup producers are not required to state on their labels whether their syrup is from the sap of a pellet-treated tree.

Maple syrup grading is based on appearance rather than taste, with color the prime factor. Many households use pure maple products. However, many products that people think are pure are actually blends. Generally, however, most people prefer the taste of the blends. Beware of maple syrup blends that may contain corn, cane, or beet components, which may be allergenic for you. Many products contain only imitation maple flavor and none of the real thing. Read the label!

The predominant sugar in maple syrup is sucrose. While maple syrup does contain some nutrients, they are not present in sufficient amounts to be nutritionally advantageous. As with molasses and honey, maple syrup should be considered to be a flavoring agent rather than a food.

▌ SORGHUM

Sorghum is a grain that is cultivated for human food and animal feed. It can be processed into sugar, syrup, and starch. In North America only 23 percent of the sorghum crop is used for human consumption, whereas in Asia and Africa the majority of the crop is consumed by humans. It is now possible to separate the sugar from the sorghum starch so that it can be crystallized.

While this crystalline sugar could help reduce our dependency on foreign sweetener sources, it is a moral question as to whether a crop traditionally earmarked for human nourishment and animal feed should be used to satisfy our cravings for sweets.

▌ MALT

Malt is a sprouted grain, usually barley, although malts can be made from other grains. The grain is roasted under low heat, then ground and made into either syrup or powder. The malt contains the sugars, salt, and protein from the grain. Bakers use malt extract to impart flavor and color to baked goods, as well as barley malt syrup, which has a dark color and a strong flavor. Some malt is used in dough; its enzymes break down the flour starches to become sugars, which serve as yeast food. These same enzymes play comparable roles in fermenting beer and other malt beverages. Some bakers also use malt extract, which has a good flavor, but is not very sweet. Malt is considered a food additive, and while it is on the GRAS list (generally recognized as safe) some people are allergic to malt.

▌ MALTODEXTRINS

Maltodextrins are hydrolyzed (degraded) carbohydrates. They are less sweet than dextrose, and are processed either from corn or maize. They are relatively bland and very soluble, and they inhibit crystallization. Maltodextrins are used to convert liquid flavors into dry powders. They are found in many dehydrated products, such as:

- doughnut, cake, cookie, and icing mixes
- instant coffee, tea, and cocktail mixes
- powdered citrus drinks
- soup and gravy mixes
- spice blends, seasonings, and salad dressing mixes

Maltodextrins are also used in:

- frozen desserts
- frozen eggs
- infant foods
- jelly beans
- marshmallows
- peanut butter
- sausages
- whipped toppings

▌ GRAIN SYRUPS

Wheat, rye, and rice syrups are used to reduce the necessity for other sugars and colors. Alternatives to malted barley syrups and blends, they add sweetness, enhance flavor and color, and add body and sheen to such cereal-based products as baked goods, snacks, breakfast cereals, and pet foods. Each syrup has its own distinctive flavor, color, and sweetness level, and they all withstand baking at high temperatures.

▌ RARE SUGARS: SORBITOL, MANNITOL, AND XYLITOL

Rare sugars are non-glucose carbohydrates called sugar alcohols. While they are initially metabolized in the liver, independent of insulin, they are eventually converted to glucose, which does require insulin. In limited amounts, rare sugars are safe for diabetics. They are absorbed poorly because we do not have the proper enzymes to process them.

Sorbitol is found naturally in berries, apples, pears, cherries, plums, seaweed, and algae. It can be used to mask the bitter aftertaste of saccharin (see Artificial Sweeteners below) and to provide the illusion of body in low-calorie drinks. Sorbitol itself, however, is not low calorie as frequently advertised, and it can affect our body's ability to absorb and utilize certain drugs and nutrients, particularly B vitamins. Sorbitol can also cause diarrhea if consumed in large amounts, either in one large dose or slowly over the course of a day. Commercial sorbitol is made from dextrose (corn). It is used in:

• alcoholic and nonalcoholic beverages
• baked goods, frostings, and gelatin puddings
• fats and oils
• frozen dairy products
• poultry, fish, meat, and nut products
• processed fruits
• snack foods
• sweet sauces, seasonings, and flavorings

Mannitol is found in many plants and plant extracts, but is usually derived from seaweed. Mannitol is poorly digested by our body, and in relatively small amounts can cause diarrhea. In intravenous feedings, it has been associated with a wide range of problems. Mannitol can also induce or worsen kidney diseases. It leaves a cool sweet taste in the mouth and is used in:

• antacid tablets
• breath fresheners
• chewing gum
• children's aspirin tablets
• cough and cold tablets
• sugarless candies

Xylitol is made from xylose, a wood sugar. It can also be obtained from corn cobs, peanut shells, wheat straw, cotton seed hulls, and coconut shells. Xylitol has the same sweetness level as sucrose and leaves a pleasant, cool taste in the mouth, but can cause diarrhea if consumed at high levels.

Intravenous xylitol infusions have been prohibited in Europe and North America, and in tests they produced liver injury and calcium oxalate crystals in the artery walls of the midbrain. It is still used in North America in chewing gum. Xylitol is also marketed as a crystalline sugar, but its cost—around $17 per pound—should keep its usage low.

■ ARTIFICIAL SWEETENERS

Artificial sweeteners are non-nutritive, non-caloric sweeteners that have been synthesized in a lab. They are intended to help decrease sugar and calorie intake, and to be safe for diabetics. However, artificial sweeteners increase appetite in general and interfere with the taste, enjoyment, and satisfaction obtained from eating foods high in complex carbohydrates. They also increase our preference for fat intake and interfere with our body's ability to select foods containing the nutrients it needs.

■ POLYDEXTROSE

Artificial sweeteners add sweetness to products, but not bulk. This is a problem in the manufacture of frozen desserts, instant puddings, cakes, and hard candies. Polydextrose is a bulking agent consisting of dextrose, sorbitol, and citric acid. It is a suitable replacement for sucrose, carbohydrates, and fats in many food products. However, the sorbitol content of polydextrose can cause a laxative effect if more than 50 grams a day are consumed.

■ ASPARTAME

Aspartame is about 200 times sweeter than sucrose and can intensify the taste of other flavors and sweeteners. It cannot be used in heated products, however, since high temperatures cause aspartame to break down. It also loses its sweetness after long storage.

Aspartame is composed of two amino acids, phenylalanine and aspartic acid, which are linked together with a molecule of methanol. When aspartame is broken down in our bodies, this molecule of methanol is released by the small intestine into the bloodstream. The methanol is converted to formaldehyde and is further degraded. In sufficient amounts, methanol and formaldehyde can cause neurological damage, eye damage, or blindness. The phenylalanine in aspartame is not safe for those with phenylketonuria (inability to oxidize a metabolic product of phenylalanine).

Taking large amounts of aspartame over time can upset the amino acid and neurotransmitter balance in our bodies. Thousands of side effects have been documented after aspartame use. Among the reported symptoms are headaches, dizziness, confusion, depression, blindness, tinnitus (ringing in the ears), nausea, diarrhea, urticaria, frequent urination, tremors, abdominal pain, shortness of breath, chest pain, convulsions, slurring of speech, and many others.

There is concern about the amount of aspartame being consumed by children. Research has shown that aspartame can slow neurological response to the point where a child will begin to miss a baseball that he or she previously would have hit.

The Food and Drug Administration (FDA) and G.D. Searle (its chief manufacturer) still maintain that aspartame is safe. However, the circumstances under which aspartame was approved by the FDA are at best open to question because of conflict of interest. Aspartame is marketed as Nutra-Sweet and Equal.

▮ SACCHARIN

Saccharin is a non-nutritive, synthesized sweetener that is 300 to 500 times sweeter than sucrose. Its commercial fate is uncertain, however, because of cancer found in animals that were fed high amounts of saccharin. It is a weak carcinogen, but more importantly, saccharin is a co-carcinogen (a substance which assists the progress of cancer). Because of conflicting studies, a ban on saccharin has been delayed to provide additional time to gather data and study new evidence.

Saccharin frequently contains other sweeteners to mask its bitter aftertaste. These masking sweeteners are important to allergic people because they are frequently derived from corn. Saccharin is also an appetite stimulant because of its capacity to lower blood sugar.

▮ WHEAT

Wheat is the staple grain in North America. While there are over 30,000 varieties of wheat, only one (Triticum aestivium) is grown for consumption here. It is referred to as common wheat, and further classified as spring wheat or winter wheat, depending on when the seed is planted. Wheat is also classified as hard or soft, depending on the amount of gluten in the grain. Hard common wheat is 10 to 13 percent gluten and is difficult to mill. Soft common wheat is 6 to 10 percent gluten, contains more starch, and is more easily milled. Hard durum wheat, also called semolina, is the hardest wheat of all. It represents only 5 percent of the total wheat crop of North America.

Wheat contains more gluten than any

Sources of Wheat

FOOD:

Alcoholic beverages (including beer, gin, whiskey)
Baby foods (some)
Barley malt
Batter-fried foods
Biscuits
Bisquick
Bologna
Bouillon
Bran
Bread, unless labelled wheat-free
Bread crumbs
"Breaded" products
Bread stuffings
Bulgur
Buns (hot dog and hamburger)
Cakes
Candy
Cereals
Chocolate
Cocoa
Cold cuts
Cookies
Cornbread
Cracker crumbs
Crackers
Cream of wheat
Croutons
Doughnuts

Dumplings
Farina
Flours (wheat flour can be bleached, unbleached, enriched, or unenriched)
Fried food coating
Gluten
Graham crackers and flour
Granola (many contain wheat bran)
Gravies
Hamburger mix
Hamburgers (fast food restaurants may add wheat)
Hot dogs with wheat filler
Ice cream (thickening agents)
Ice cream cones
Liverwurst
Macaroni
Malt products
Malted milk
Matzos
Mayonnaise
Monosodium glutamate (MSG)
Muffins
Noodles
Ovaltine, Postum
Pancake mixes
Pasta

Pastries
Pepper, synthetic
Pies
Pita pockets
Pizza
Popovers
Pretzels
Puddings
Pumpernickel bread
Rolls
Rye bread
Sauces
Sausages
Soups
Soy sauce, tamari
Spaghetti noodles
Tortillas
Vermicelli
Waffles
Wheat germ
Yeasts (some)

OTHER SOURCES:
Garlic capsules
Hand creams and lotions
Lip gloss
Make-up (many contain wheat germ oil)
Shampoos
Vitamins

other grain. Gluten is a water-soluble mixture of sticky proteins. When wheat is made into a dough, the sticky property of gluten traps gas bubbles from the leavening agents and causes the dough to rise. Rye, barley, spelt, kamut, and oats contain some gluten, while corn, rice, teff and millet contain none.

Gluten intolerance is known as celiac disease or non-tropical sprue. Various theories exist to explain its cause, including missing enzymes to process gluten, a metabolic error, or an immunological disorder. Gluten intolerance can appear at any age and is a lifetime disorder. Symptoms of gluten intolerance are malabsorption, irritable bowel syndrome, diarrhea, pale malodorous stool, nausea, vomiting, poor appetite, headache, pallor, anemia, weight loss, skin rash or scaling, muscle spasms, and joint pain.

Some celiacs do not tolerate millet, and many of them are also intolerant of other foods, such as milk. Although buckwheat is not a true grain, some sources state that it contains gluten and some celiacs cannot eat it. Other sources state that it is the high rutin content of buckwheat that causes the problem.

Total avoidance of gluten is necessary for the control of gluten intolerance. Unfortunately, gluten is difficult to avoid in processed foods. It is used as a starch, binder, formulation aid, emulsific filler, bulking agent, stabilizer, shaper, thickener, and glaze, and as an aid for forming tablets. Because of these uses, even foods labeled "wheat-free" may contain gluten.

On page 130 is a partial list of sources of wheat/gluten. It is best to read labels carefully before purchasing an item and to inquire about food content in restaurants when you are in doubt.

▮▮ YEAST

Yeast (a one-celled fungus) is a widely used ingredient in many foods, medications, and vitamins. It converts sugars to alcohol and carbon dioxide in a fermentation process. This property of yeast is essential to both bakers and brewers in manufacturing their products. The carbon dioxide causes dough containing gluten to rise; the alcoholic content of beers and liquors results from the fermentation of grains and other substances.

Yeasts and molds have common carbohydrates in their cells that may cause cross-reactivity in hypersensitive people.

New Problems with Foods

In recent years, modified foods that have been developed by humans are causing problems for the food-sensitive person. These include genetically modified foods, irradiated foods, and designer foods. In spite of all efforts to halt the continued development of these products, their use appears to be increasing. People with food sensitivities must carefully investigate the sources and handling of all their foods.

▮▮ GENETICALLY MODIFIED (GM) FOODS

Genetically modified (also called genetically engineered) foods are a result of genetic engineering in which the genetic material (DNA) inside the cells of the food has been manipulated to block or add desired traits. Supposedly beneficial genes from another species, including other plants, animals, bacteria, and viruses, are implanted into the plant to provide benefits or improvement. Among the desired benefits are increased shelf life, less need for pesticides, and enhanced nutritional value.

Proponents of genetically manipulated food claim that it is "substantially equiva-

Sources of Yeast

The following products contain naturally occurring yeast or yeastlike substances. Yeast may also be added in the manufacturing or preparing process—always be sure to read labels!

FOOD:

Barbecue sauce
Black tea
Bread crumbs
Breads
Bread stuffings
Buns (hot dog and hamburger)
Buttermillk
Cakes and cake mixes
Canned refrigerated biscuits and rolls
Catsup
Cheese (all types, including cottage cheese)
Citric acid (almost always a yeast derivative)
Coffee (regular and instant)
Cookies
Crackers
Doughnuts
Dried fruits of all kinds (dates, figs, prunes, raisins)
Dried roasted nuts
Enriched farina, cornmeal, and corn grits
Fermented beverages of all types:
  Beer
  Brandy
  Gin
  Ginger ale
  Root beer

Rum
Whiskey
Wine
Vodka
Flour ("enriched" with vitamins made from yeast)
Fruit juices of all types, whether frozen or canned (only homemade are yeast-free)
Grapes (The mold on grapes and thus in grape products may sometimes bother a person allergic to yeast)
Herb teas
Malted products of all types (candy, cereals, malted milk drinks)
Meat, fish, or fowl fried in cracker crumbs or breading
Melons (watermelon, honeydew melon, and especially cantaloupe have mold on the skin surface)
Milk fortified with vitamins
Monosodium glutamate (may be a yeast derivative)
Morels
Mushrooms

Pastries
Peanuts, peanut products
Pistachios
Pizza
Prepared foods containing cheese (such as macaroni and cheese)
Pretzels
Rolls (homemade or canned)
Salt-rising bread
Sour cream
Soy sauce
Sprouts
Tamari
Torula (a type of yeast used in health foods)
Truffles
Vinegars of all types (apple, distilled, grape, pear)
Vinegar may also be used in the preparation of the following foods and may not be included on the label:
Baby cereals
Barbecue sauce
Barley cereal
Catsup
Chili and peppers
Horseradish
Mayonnaise
Mincemeat
Mustard

Sources of Yeast

Olives	OTHER SOURCES:	Tetracyclines
Pickles	The following items contain	Any others derived from
Salad dressings	substances that are derived	mold cultures
Sauerkraut	from yeast or have yeast as	Vitamins (unless otherwise
Spices (cinnamon, pep-	their source.	stated on label):
per)	Antibiotics:	All multiple vitamin cap-
Tomato sauce	Chloromycetin	sules, powders
	Lincocin	All vitamin B capsules
	Mycin drugs	Tablets containing vitamin
	Penicillin	B made from yeast

---

lent" to conventionally produced food. However, Marc Lappé of the Center for Ethics and Toxics in Gualala, California, compared genetically modified and unaltered soybeans that had been cultivated under similar conditions, and sprayed according to their usual schedule. The modified beans contained an average of 12 to 14 percent less isoflavones, the chemicals that give soybeans some of their therapeutic value. While isoflavone content can vary with weather, location, and seed variety, this study does indicate that genetic variation can also affect it. In addition, the Food and Drug Administration (FDA) approved modified soybeans based on nutritional analysis performed before the crops had been sprayed, and no studies have compared the beans after they have been sprayed. Genetically modified soybeans now make up half of the American soybean crop.

Scientists usually insert a "marker gene" into the plant along with the desired gene, so they can test whether the gene splice was successful. The most commonly used marker is a bacterial gene for antibiotic resistance, and most GM food contains such a gene. This raises the possibility of contributing to antibiotic resistance, since bacteria readily exchange antibiotic-resistant genes. These genes could transfer into pathogenic bacteria, making them resistant. It is also possible that antibiotic-resistant genes could be transferred in the digestive tract to bacteria. This phenomenon would increase the already serious problem of antibiotic-resistant organisms in disease.

Many plants are modified for insect resistance, virus resistance, and herbicide tolerance, each of which poses an environmental risk. Insect-resistant crops all contain a gene from the bacteria *Bacillus thuringiensis,* which causes the plant to produce an endotoxin in its leaves and fruit. Corn, cotton, potatoes, tomatoes, and rice are frequently modified with this gene. However, these plants can be toxic to beneficial as well as harmful insects. The ultimate result could upset established ecological balances.

Genes from virus-resistant crops can mix with natural plant viruses to create new viruses that can be even more serious. If the gene for herbicide tolerance escapes into

Allergenic Genes

One of the most serious dangers of GM foods for people with food allergies is that the transferred portion can cause a food that was formerly safe to become allergenic for a sensitive person. For example, in March of 1996 researchers and the University of Nebraska in the United States confirmed that an allergen from Brazil nuts had been transferred to soybeans. The genes from the Brazil nuts were implanted into the soy in an attempt to make them taste nuttier and to improve their protein content. People who were not allergic to soy, but who were allergic to Brazil nuts, reacted to the genetically modified soy. Fortunately, the product was withdrawn from the market by its developer.

weeds, it could result in herbicide-tolerant weeds that would be difficult to control.

It is essential for people with allergies to know what their food contains. In North America at this time, genetically modified foods do not have to be labeled, nor do they have to be tested for safety. These foods can be in many different products, including powdered infant formula, pasta, muffin mixes, soft drinks, cooking oil, taco shells, and veggie burgers. Supermarkets and natural foods retailers do not know what percentage of their goods contains GM material. In Europe, genetically modified foods are being withdrawn from the market. Because of public outcry, some natural foods markets in North America are taking steps to assure that none of the foods they sell contain GM products. However, these markets represent a very small proportion of food suppliers.

▮▮ IRRADIATED FOODS

Fighting food spoilage is an ongoing problem for food suppliers. Chemical techniques and temperature control are frequently utilized to combat this problem. However, food irradiation is being increasingly used to prolong shelf life. Irradiation kills insects, bacteria, fungi, and viruses, making fumigants and chemical preservatives no longer necessary.

Irradiation is done by three methods: gamma rays, X-rays, and electron beam radiation. According to the FDA, when food is irradiated, there is a slight loss of nutrients but the food is basically unchanged. It does not become radioactive, and the FDA does not consider irradiation a food additive. However, irradiation can bleach and change the color of the food, as well as destroying vitamins and other nutrients. It also destroys natural antioxidants and causes an off flavor in fatty foods.

Unique radiolytic products (URPs), chemical molecules that have never before been analyzed, are produced when food is irradiated. The health risk from some of the URPs is unknown, as is their potential for contributing to food allergy. However, some known radiolytic products are carcinogenic. In addition, some microorganisms found in food are relatively resistant to radiation.

Present laws do not require labeling of irradiated foods if they are used in a mixture; only whole food that is radiated and then sold unchanged must be labeled. The FDA has approved irradiation of wheat, wheat flour, pork, potatoes, spices, and whole fruits and vegetables. Until recently, only spices were irradiated in significant amounts in the United States. However, new rules that took effect in February of 2000 allow the irradiation of raw beef, pork, and lamb. Most meatpackers have plans to begin testing the market for irradiated ground beef.

▌▌ DESIGNER FOODS

Designer foods are intended to reduce the risk of disease in people who eat particular foods, such as margarine. Most of the current products are formulated to reduce heart disease and its currently recognized marker, blood cholesterol levels. These products include designer margarines that aid in the reduction of cholesterol.

The designer margarines contain phytosterols, a form of cholesterol that occurs in plants. Phytosterols compete with dietary cholesterol to be absorbed in the intestine, and are reported not to create the same sort of blockages in blood vessels as does cholesterol.

These margarines and other designer foods can be used in lines of food products, such as cookies, crackers, and other snack foods. For people with food allergies, these designer foods create a new exposure and new risks.

There is also concern that designer foods can interact dangerously with prescription drugs, or cause overdoses with additive effects. For example, some foods have added herbs, such as St. John's wort and echinacea. People eating the food and supplementing with the herb may find it difficult to keep track of the dose they are receiving. Some of the herbs added to drinks would also interact with prescription medications.

CHAPTER 10

Eating Safely

How Can We Eat Safely?

After food testing is completed, you may feel like saying: I cannot be allergic to that many foods. What am I going to eat? There is nothing left for me to eat. What am I going to do? I'm going to starve! You've taken away all of my favorite foods. I don't have time to shop for exotic foods and prepare complicated meals.

Except in extreme cases, most people will find there are more foods that they can eat than those they cannot eat. While people may have to limit the number of times they can eat a given food to which they are allergic, unless they have life-threatening symptoms when exposed to the food, they will not have to avoid it entirely.

In this chapter you will find out how to safely eat foods, both from an allergy perspective, as well as from a healthy, nutritional perspective. You will develop a creativity about eating that you never thought possible, and you will lose none of the enjoyment. You will be eating differently, but very well.

Eat clean food that has been purchased wisely and cooked properly. Quality food, preferably fresh organic food, will not have the contaminants found in food raised with herbicides, pesticides, and chemical fertilizers. Organic meats will be from free-range animals and will not contain residues of hormones and drugs.

Fresh food is preferable to frozen and canned foods, although frozen food contains more nutrients than canned food. Fresh organic fruits and vegetables, in addition to the nutrients needed for optimum health, also contain the food enzymes needed to help digest them. Whole grains still contain their nutrients and fiber.

Proper food preparation is essential for a healthy meal. Oven broiling or baking produces a healthier dish than frying, which adds saturated fats to the food. Charcoal broiling and smoking foods over an open fire deposit a coat of chemicals on the surface of the food, as well as exposing the food to carcinogenic chemicals in the smoke. Steaming vegetables retains more of their nutrients than does boiling. The high heat of stir-frying locks in nutrients. When oil is used, it coats the food, making it less allergenic for some people. Remember that heat destroys enzymes, and eating raw fruits and vegetables allows the benefits of food enzymes.

Avoid sugar, salt, white flour, saturated fats, alcohol, caffeine, and artificial sweeteners. Also avoid processed foods to which flavors, colors, and preservatives have been added. Most processed foods are low in fiber and high in salt, sugar, and fat. Food processors and manufacturers add many things to food, and it is essential that you have the knowledge to read any food label accurately.

▮▮ READING LABELS

The safest foods for allergic people to eat are fresh, organically grown fruits, vegetables, and meats. However, because many of us are unable to grow our own food, and because top-quality food is not always available, we are forced to buy commercial and some processed foods. It is important to learn to read food labels intelligently, to recognize food additives, and to use this information to make wise food purchases.

▮ RECOGNIZING ALLERGENS AND ADDITIVES

The first aim in reading labels is to identify any food that is an allergen. Foods may be listed by their common, usual names, or they may be described by their "food component" names. For example, zein, which is corn protein, appears on labels, as does whey, which is a milk component. Familiarize yourself with the food lists to learn the various ways common food allergens are listed on labels.

Reading labels can also help to determine the presence of food additives that may cause reactions. A food additive is a substance or mixture that has been added to aid in production, processing, packaging, or storing the food. Chance contaminants are not considered food additives. Contrary to popular belief, food additives are not a modern invention. Adding chemicals to food began thousands of years ago when it was first discovered that salting meat would make it last longer.

Over 10,000 intentional additives are currently used in foods. Many people are allergic to even the smallest amounts of these compounds. Inconsistent labeling makes it difficult to determine whether the offending substances have been added to food. If in doubt, always write to the packer or manufacturer. Explain that you have allergies and must know more about the product in order to be able to use it.

The laws governing packaging and food processing state that labels must:
- identify the product in a language the consumer can understand
- identify the manufacturer, packer, or distributor
- declare the quantity of contents, either in net weight or volume
- list the ingredients in order of the amount used by weight. An item that lists sugar first or second will have a very high sugar content.
- accurately represent the contents of the container, if a picture of the product is used on the label

In some cases, relatively few food additives need to be listed on labels. For over 300 "standard" foods (those for which the government has written chemical recipes), no ingredients need to be listed. Manufacturers can choose among many alternative standard chemicals without having to indicate on the label which is used. Only if the processor substitutes or adds a nonstandard chemical must they indicate that fact on the label. For example, ice cream, considered a standard food, can have up to 30 additives that do not have to be indicated on the label. Similarly, if monosodium glutamate is used in canned vegetables, it must appear on the label, but it may be added to mayonnaise and salad dressings without being listed if a standard recipe is followed. It is impossible for consumers to know whether the absence of additives on a label means that none are present, or whether it means the food is covered by a standard recipe and contains numerous additives.

Consumer demand for uniform appearance and flavor in food products has played a large role in the increased use of food additives in recent years. To meet this demand, food processors and manufacturers are using increasingly more additives. Most are unfamiliar chemicals with no nutritional value. Some additives are quite harmless, but the safety of others is in question, despite testing that has been done on them. Frequently, additives are used to conceal the inferior quality of food, to heighten the appearance of damaged food, and to make the food more attractive to the consumer.

Chemical additives used in food processing must make the food more easily available, improve shelf life, enhance nutritional value, increase quality or customer acceptability, or facilitate the food's manufacture or preparation.

While not all artificial additives are harmful for everyone, many of them do cause problems. For example, the common additives tartrazine and benzoic acid can increase hyperactivity levels in children. Natural additives are generally safer, but are not universally tolerated. The additives discussed in the summary below are but a few of the many types used in the food industry in packaging and processing, and in restaurants. (For more information on specific compounds, see Recommended Books.) It should be obvious that eating fresh fruits, vegetables, and meats, together with cooking "from scratch," are vital for people with allergies!

▌ PRESERVATIVES

About 100 chemicals called "antispoilants" are used to help prevent microbiological growth and chemical deterioration. They include antioxidants, "mold" inhibitors, fungicides, sequestering agents, and general-purpose preservatives such as sulfur dioxide and propylgallate. Preservatives prevent changes affecting color, flavor, texture, or appearance. Traditional preservatives include salt, sugar, vinegar, spices, and wood smoke; however, wood smoke is no longer considered to be safe.

Common antioxidants used today include butylated hydroxyanisole (BHA), used in lard, shortenings, crackers, soup bases, and potato chips; butylated hydroxytoluene (BHT) used in potato chips, dry breakfast cereals, fresh-frozen pork sausage, and freeze-dried meats; and benzoic acid, used in margarine. BHA can cause allergic reactions, and affects the liver and kidney function. BHT may be more toxic to the kidney than BHA, and it is prohibited as a food additive in England. Benzoic acid is a mild irritant to the skin and can cause allergic reactions including asthma, red eyes, and skin rashes.

❙ ACIDS, ALKALIS, BUFFERS, AND NEUTRALIZERS

To ensure product appearance and quality, the acidity or alkalinity of processed foods must be maintained. Acids and alkalis are added to foods for this reason. Acids provide tartness in candies, jams, gelatin desserts, sherbets, carbonated soft drinks, and fruit juices. Alkalis are used in confections, cookies and crackers, baking powder, creamed cottage cheese, ice cream, prepared pancake mixes, biscuit and muffin mixes, and bleached flours.

Buffers and neutralizing agents help to control acidity or alkalinity by absorbing or "neutralizing" excess acid or alkaline substances. Buffers are added to many processed foods, including breakfast cereals, baked goods, jellies and jams, and canned vegetables.

❙ MOISTURE CONTENT CONTROLS

Substances that prevent loss of moisture are called humectants. Glycerine, propylene glycol, and sorbitol absorb moisture from the air and are frequently used as humectants. As glycerine is used, it is nontoxic and nonirritating, but some people are sensitive to it. Propylene glycol is classified as GRAS, but people may be sensitive to it. Sorbitol consumed in excess can cause diarrhea and gastrointestinal symptoms. Calcium silicate

and dextrose are added to prevent table salt from caking due to moisture absorption from the air.

❙ COLORING AGENTS

Both natural and synthetic food colorings are used in processed foods to heighten acceptability and attractiveness. However, color can also be used to conceal damage or inferior quality.

Synthetic food colorings are preferred in the food industry over natural ones because of their better coloring power, uniformity and stability, and lower cost. Synthetic coloring agents, however, can cause serious problems for an allergic person. Those sensitive to petrochemical hydrocarbons will usually react to one or more of the certified food colorings.

Food colorings are added to thousands of foods, including baked goods, soft drinks, fruit juices, ice cream, gelatin desserts, maraschino cherries, oranges, sweet potatoes, sausages, prepared mixes, processed meats, cheeses, butter, cream, margarine, breakfast cereals, candies, jellies, and pet food.

❙ FLAVORINGS

A wide variety of flavorings is used in processed foods, including spices, natural extracts, oleo resins, essential oils, and the numerous synthetic flavors produced by chemists. Flavoring agents are the most common food additives. There are over 2,000 flavoring agents in use, of which only 500 are natural.

Flavoring agents produce or modify the flavors of foods. Foods that lose their original flavor as a result of processing generally require flavoring agents to make them palatable. Flavorings are added to baked goods, beverages, candy, cottage cheese, fruit-flavored toppings, gelatin, ice cream, liquor, pickles, processed meats, puddings, shortening, and many other food items.

Flavorings—whether natural or synthetic—can pose a problem for the allergic person. Imitation (synthetic) flavorings contain very little, if any, natural materials. Unless a flavoring agent is made entirely from natural materials, it is considered to be an imitation.

Flavor enhancers are also added to foods, the most common being monosodium glutamate (MSG) and maltol. Flavor enhancers usually add no flavor of their own to foods, but heighten or modify existing flavor. Some researchers believe as many as 80 percent of our population will react to monosodium glutamate, with symptoms ranging from migraine headaches to a feeling of fatigue.

▮ PHYSIOLOGICAL ACTIVITY CONTROLS

Physiological activity control chemicals serve as ripeners or antimetabolic agents for fresh foods. Ethylene gas is used to speed the ripening of bananas; this gas is highly flammable and can asphyxiate at high levels. However, the average consumer is not exposed to large quantities. Maleic hydrazide prevents potatoes from sprouting and is highly toxic to humans. It has caused genetic damage in plant and animal systems, and the FDA residue tolerance for potato chips is 160 ppm.

Some physiological activity controllers are nontoxic enzymes of natural origin. Enzymes are used in fermentation and in the manufacture of bread, artificial honey, and frozen milk concentrates. Allergic people do not usually react to these enzymes.

▮ BLEACHING AND MATURING AGENTS

Bleaching agents are used to improve the appearance of food products, while maturing agents hasten their maturation. Both bleaching and maturing agents are added to flour. Fresh ground flour is pale yellow, and slowly becomes white with storage. Processors add agents to the flour to accelerate its aging process, which improves its baking qualities and reduces storage costs, spoilage, and the possibility of insect infection. These agents can reduce the nutrients in the food.

▮ PROCESSING AIDS

Processing aids include sanitizing agents that remove bacteria and debris from products; clarifying agents that remove extraneous materials; emulsifiers and emulsion stabilizers that help to maintain a mixture and assure consistency; texturizers, stabilizers, or thickeners that are added to products to provide "body" and maintain a desired texture; and whipping agents or propellants in cans.

Sorbitan derivatives are a processing aid used to retard "bloom" on the surface of chocolate candy. Calcium chloride is added to canned tomatoes to prevent them from falling apart, and sodium nitrate and nitrite are used to develop and stabilize the pink color of meats. Many people are allergic to these-meat processing aids, and some are known carcinogens.

Since artificially sweetened beverages lack the "thickness" normally contributed by sugar, bodying agents or thickeners may be added to correct this problem. Some processors simply increase carbonation to make up for the lack of body.

■ A NEW FOOD ADDITIVE

The "fake fat" olestra, an indigestible fat substitute, is a new type of food additive. Olestra contains no fat or calories and is made from sugar and vegetable oil, usually soybean or cottonseed. Its structure prevents digestive enzymes from breaking it down, and the body absorbs neither the fat nor the sugar. However, olestra causes unpleasant side effects in many people, including bowel urgency, diarrhea, cramps, and involuntary soiling of clothes. The FDA has downplayed the label notice that states, "Olestra may cause abdominal cramping and loose stools."

Food Management

Food management is necessary to help you find your way to better health. Many people with diagnosed food allergies refuse to change their eating habits, with the following results.

If you maintain your regular diet, there is no chance for body repair, leading to increased debilitation and the gradual decline of health. When you continue to eat foods to which you are allergic, without using allergy extracts or following a rotation diet, you will experience reactions with every meal and snack. Continued masked reactions over a long period of time will weaken your immune system, which can ultimately lead to degenerative diseases and increased infections.

Children with untreated food allergies may suffer frequent earaches, eczema, bed-

---

Enriched?

If natural nutrients have been removed and then replaced during processing, the food is labelled as enriched. Enrichment can also mean that yeast has been added. However, added nutrients always fall short of the number of nutrients removed in processing.

A fortified food is one with nutrients added to make it more nutritious than it was before processing.

---

wetting, asthma, hyperactivity, learning or discipline problems, and many other symptoms. Adults whose allergies are left untreated may have frequent headaches, "spaciness," spells of sleepiness, arthritis, depression, postnasal drip, sinus symptoms, hypoglycemia, frequent infections, and many other maladies. Both children and adults may experience outbursts of temper as a result of untreated food allergies.

Because your enzyme functions are unable to repair, your digestive processes will suffer, and will gradually degenerate. Improperly digested food is antigenic to your body and will cause an increase, over time, in the number of foods to which you are allergic. The situation becomes a vicious circle.

There are four basic approaches to controlling food allergies, which will be discussed in detail in the following section.
• Avoidance and retesting
• Allergy extracts
• Rotation diet
• Hands-on allergy treatments

Temporary Discomfort for Long-term Gain

Avoiding a food allergen allows our body to revert to a more normal state, which may initially be uncomfortable. Think of these feelings of discomfort as withdrawal symptoms. You may experience strong cravings for various foods. Whatever your withdrawal symptoms may be, they will last only a few days, and then you will begin to feel better.

■ AVOIDANCE AND RETESTING

This approach allows the best immune system repair, but nutrition may suffer if too many foods must be avoided.

Foods that cause violent symptoms must be eliminated from the diet completely for a minimum of 30 days, perhaps longer depending on your health and the foods involved. Study the food lists in the previous chapter to learn unsuspected sources of food ingredients. Avoid all forms of the food, for even the smallest amount can cause reactions as severe as those caused by a regular serving.

At the end of the avoidance period, you are ready to test your tolerance of the food. Re-introduce only one food at a time every four days, by eating a regular serving *once* for either lunch or dinner. If you experience no symptoms within 48 hours, then it is safe to try the food again in four days. If you still have no difficulty, you may add the food to your diet on a four-day rotation.

However, if you experience symptoms every time you eat the food, avoid it again for six months, and then try it with a 10-day interval between exposures. If you experience symptoms with each exposure to the food, it is possible that: 1) you have had inadvertent exposures when you thought you were avoiding the food; or 2) you have a fixed or permanent food sensitivity. With a fixed food sensitivity, you will react every time you eat the food, regardless of how long you have avoided it or how little of it you eat.

■ ALLERGY EXTRACTS

Taking allergy extracts for foods to which you are allergic will lead to some immune system repair, but it will be slow since the body continues to be exposed to the same food. No enzyme repair will occur unless extracts are combined with another approach, such as the rotation diet.

■ ROTATION DIET

This approach allows moderate immune system repair and better nutritional support. Rotation also prevents food reactions and allows enzyme function to repair. The rotary diversified diet, now more commonly referred to as the rotation diet, was developed by Dr. Herbert Rinkel of Kansas City, Missouri. It is based on the fact that it usually takes four days for food components to "clear" our bodies. For some it may take seven to ten days for the food to clear, but for most of us four days is sufficient. On the rotation diet, a food is eaten, and is then not repeated until it has cleared the body, preventing a cumulative effect from consuming offending foods.

Foods, both animal and vegetable, are divided into families according to their common biological and botanical properties. On a rotation diet, these families are assigned and spread out over four days so that each day offers a selection of meats, vegetables, and fruits. Each day's selections are treated like a menu in a restaurant. You may choose only from what is on the menu for that day, omitting foods that are listed for another day.

For the more sensitive person, and for those who have a slower clearing time, the food families may have to be spread out over a seven-day or even ten-day rotation. While this means fewer foods to choose from each day, it prevents overlapping and allows these people to rotate foods safely.

The strictness with which you follow a rotation diet depends on the severity of your food allergies and symptoms. Some people can eat only one food per meal, and cannot repeat the same food during a 24-hour period. Others are able to eat several foods in a meal and repeat foods if the meals are separated by a number of hours. The easiest way to begin is to start your rotation day with supper and end it with lunch the following day. If you cook extra portions for supper, you will have "leftovers" for breakfast, lunch, or the freezer.

▎ "BORROWING" FOODS

There are many different versions of the rotation diet. If you have chosen a diet in which there are too many foods permitted on one day and not enough on another day, you can change the order of rotation. You may switch foods from one day to another, but you must move an entire food family at once and leave it on the day to which it was

> ### Rotation Bonuses
>
> *A rotation diet prevents new food allergies from developing due to overexposure to a particular food; it preserves tolerance for foods to which a person is not sensitive; and it aids in identifying food sensitivities. Each time the cycle repeats, symptoms on a given rotation day signal an unidentified problem food. With only a few specific foods being consumed on a particular day, it is easier to identify the food allergen.*

moved. Otherwise, you will find you are no longer rotating.

For special occasions, you may temporarily "borrow" a food by using the following method: skip the food on the cycle just before the special occasion. Then eat the food for the special occasion. Skip the food on the next cycle, and add it back on the subsequent cycle. This method will allow you to cope with the diet on special occasions. However, beware of accommodating too many such occasions, or you will no longer be truly rotating.

▎ ROTATION BASICS

Keep rotation meals very simple, and use only good-quality, additive- and preservative-free foods. Even though you may not have to eat single-food meals, try to limit the number of foods you consume at one sitting. Choose simple recipes and make any necessary substitutions. Remember, unless a food is permitted on a given rotation day, you should not eat it on that day.

• *Grains:* If you are strictly rotating, grains

may be consumed only on the day you eat foods from the grass family. For some whose sensitivities will permit, a grain may be eaten every other day, or gluten and non-gluten grains may be alternated. Corn, rice, teff and millet are the non-gluten grains; wheat, rye, barley, spelt, kamut, and oats all contain gluten in varying amounts. Buckwheat is not a grain, but it does contain some gluten. (For more information about gluten content in foods, see Wheat in chapter 9, Food Allergies.) Now that amaranth, quinoa, spelt, kamut, and teff flour are available for baking, finding a bread substitute is not as difficult as it was several years ago. Bean flours are available and they make good pancakes and waffles. Potato flour can also be used to make bread substitutes.

- *Butter, Margarine, and Oils:* In addition to wanting a bread for each rotation day, some people long for butter or margarine each day. Butter is allowable only on beef/milk days. Since most margarines contain whey combined with vegetable oil, they do not really fit in on any rotation day. An interesting margarine/butter substitute for vegetables is the "oil of the day" in which spices for the day have been marinated.

- *Cheese:* Many people are "cheese-aholics" and eat cheese every day. However, cheese made from cow's or goat's milk is allowed only on beef/goat/milk day. Soy cheese, which is made from soy milk, may be used on legume day. It is not a yeast/mold exposure as are cheeses cultured from milk because rennet is used to convert the soy into cheese.

- *Seafood and Poultry:* Because of the number

of seafood/fish families, some type of seafood is a possibility for each rotation day. Duck, chicken, and turkey are in separate families but are so closely related that it is best to separate them by a day.

- *Spices, herbs, and teas:* These must be rotated in the same way as other foods. However, you may "float" spices or seasonings if you wish. For example, some people like onion and garlic, which are in the same family, for special dishes. They "save" the onion and garlic and use them only for these dishes, which they eat only once or twice a month. However, asparagus, chives, and leeks are also in this family. If you "float" onions and garlic, be careful that you have not eaten asparagus, chives, or leeks on another day of the same rotation cycle.

- *Alcohol:* Alcoholic beverages do not fit well into rotation diets. The fermented bases for these beverages include grains, fruits, coconut, potatoes, cactus, and juniper. All alcoholic beverages contain ethanol, yeast, and some type of sweetener. Beet and cane sugar, honey, or corn syrup are used for the sweeteners. Beer and wine may contain sulfites.

Keeping a notebook helps to make following a rotation diet easier. Keep your menu for one to two weeks (or for a length of time convenient for you) in the notebook. Your menu should include both meals and snacks, written out in detail. Also, you should note cooking plans—what to thaw, what to cook in advance—which will help when you are making your shopping list. You should also note any symptoms that occur on specific days either on your menu or on a record sheet in your notebook. This will enable you to identify additional problems.

Another helpful technique, particularly if you have children, is to "color-code" the rotation days. Snacks, freezer meals, shelves, or kitchen cabinets can be color-coded to correspond to rotation days. Children and family members can then easily find the food and snacks allowed on any given rotation day.

Even though all family members may not have allergies, it is easier on the person preparing the meals if the whole family rotates foods, so that only one menu need be cooked. A rotation diet is a healthy, balanced way to eat and includes meats, vegetables, and fruits from which to choose each day. The whole family can benefit from following a rotation diet; it will help identify allergies, prevent new allergies from forming, "protect" currently tolerated foods, and prevent any cumulative effects from eating a food or food group too often.

Easing into rotation gradually will probably make your family more cooperative—and perhaps even unaware that changes are being made. Start by rotating the protein portion of the meal (chicken, beef, fish, pork). After this has become commonplace in your menus, work on rotating vegetables, and then fruits. Leave grain rotation until last, because it is a bit more difficult. Alternative grains do not provide the same texture to baked goods as our old standby, wheat.

The benefits afforded by a rotation diet can make eating an exciting experience. You will be eating high-quality whole foods, which will help to improve your health. You will be avoiding prepared mixes containing additives and harmful chemicals that can cause reactions and fatigue. Your palate will be able to appreciate the wonderful subtle tastes of foods you have never noticed before. As your health improves from your dietary changes, your quality of life will improve. Exciting times are ahead! For more information on rotation diets, see Recommended Books).

▮ SAMPLE ROTATION DIET
The following chart provides an example of a rotation diet used by one family. Listed below are the foods that were used in the rotation menus that follow. There are other foods listed in the original diet, but these are the foods that this family chose.

Day 1

ANIMAL PROTEIN		VEGETABLES	
Milk products,	Suet	Mushrooms	Cucumber
cheeses	Crab	Eggplant	Squashes
Goat's milk, goat	Lobster	Pepper	Pumpkin
cheese	Prawn	Bell, sweet	Potato
Beef	Shrimp	Chili	
Veal	Ocean catfish	Avocado	HERBS & SPICES
Lamb	Sardines	Tomato	Basil
	Catfish species		Bay leaf

HERBS & SPICES
(cont.)
Cayenne pepper
Chili powder
Cinnamon
Marjoram
Mint, peppermint
Oregano
Paprika
Poppyseed
Rosemary
Sage
Spearmint
Summer & winter
savory
Thyme

SEEDS & NUTS
Hickory nuts
Pecans
Walnuts
Brazil nuts
Pumpkin seeds

FAT & OILS
Butter
Suet
Avocado
Walnut

FRUITS
Watermelon
Cantaloupe
Honeydew
Apple
Pear
Pomegranates
Dried currants
Grapes
Raisins

BEVERAGES
Grape
Apple
Pear
Milk

SWEETENER
Raisin
Sage Honey

OTHER
Yeast
Cream of tartar
Potato meal
Potato starch
Wine vinegar
Cider vinegar

Day 2

ANIMAL PROTEIN
Clams
Scallops
All bass
All perch
Walleye
All trout
Salmon
Chicken
Chicken eggs

VEGETABLES
Water chestnuts
Carrots
Celery
Sweet potato
Artichoke
Endive
Lettuce

HERBS & SPICES
Anise
Caraway
Celery Seed
Chervil
Coriander
Cumin
Dill
Fennel
Nutmeg
Parsley
Tarragon

SEEDS & NUTS
Coconut
Filberts
Sunflower seeds

FATS & OILS
Safflower oil
Sunflower oil

FRUITS
Dates
Coconut
Pineapple
Banana
Rhubarb
Blackberries
Boysenberries
Raspberries
Strawberries
Persimmons

BEVERAGES
Coconut milk
Pineapple juice
Strawberry juice
Chamomile tea
Chicory

SWEETENER
Date sugar

OTHER
Buckwheat
Artichoke heart
meal
Sunflower seed
meal
Coconut meal

Day 3

ANIMAL PROTEIN
Flounder
Halibut
Sole
Turbot
Duck (meat and
eggs)
Goose (meat and
eggs)
Pork

VEGETABLES
Asparagus
Alfalfa sprouts
Onion
All beans
All peas

Soybeans
Jicama
Okra

HERBS & SPICES
Garlic
Chives
Vanilla beans

SEEDS & NUTS
Peanuts
Cashews
Pistachios
Sesame seeds

FATS & OILS
Peanut oil

Soy oil
Sesame oil
Cottonseed oil

FRUITS
Figs
Grapefruit
Lemon
Lime
Orange
Tangerine
Kiwi
Papaya

BEVERAGES
Soy milk
Grapefruit

Orange
Lemon
Lime
Tangerine
Papaya
Hibiscus

SWEETENER
Clover honey

OTHER
Carob
Soy flour
Peanut flour
Sesame seed (meal)

Day 4

ANIMAL PROTEIN
Whitefish
Pike
Turkey
Turkey eggs

VEGETABLES
Yam (true)*
Turnips
Beets
Spinach
Olives
Broccoli
Brussels sprouts
Cabbage
Cauliflower
Chinese cabbage
Radish
Watercress

HERBS & SPICES
Allspice
Cloves
Ginger
Horseradish
Mustard seeds
Turmeric

SEEDS & NUTS
Chestnuts
Macadamia nuts
Almonds

FATS & OILS
Apricot oil
Almond oil
Canola oil
Olive oil

FRUITS
Apricot
Peach
Plum
Cherries
Blueberries
Cranberries
Guava

BEVERAGES
Apricot
Cherry
Peach
Plum
Cranberry
Guava

SWEETENER
Maple syrup or
sugar

Beet
Sugar

OTHER
Arrowroot starch
Tapioca starch/flour
Grains**
Barley
Corn
Kamut
Millet
Oat
Rice
Rye
Spelt
Teff
Triticale
Wheat
Quinoa (See note)

---

*True yams are a tropical vegetable. Most yams in our grocery stores are a variety of sweet potato and not true yams.
**Although grains are listed only on this day, they may be used on other days in several different ways.

Note: Quinoa is not a grain, but a seed that can be used as a grain substitute. It is on this day's rotation because it is in the same family as spinach. Amaranth is also a seed that can be used as a grain substitute. It is in a family by itself and not related to any other food. It can be assigned to any day where it is needed.

▌SAMPLE MENUS

This version of a sample diet begins the rotation day with the evening meal and goes through lunch the next day. Dinner leftovers can be used for lunch or breakfast. Grains are rotated every other day.

This is a very simple menu designed to give you an idea of some possibilities. See Recommended Books for sources of more information.

Day 1

DINNER	BREAKFAST	LUNCH
Sliced roast	Wheat cereal	Hamburger patty
Sautéed squash in oil with	Milk	Sliced cucumbers
green chile (grated cheese optional)	Raisins	and tomatoes
Roasted cubed potatoes		Apple, yogurt, and
		walnut salad

JUICE: Apple, grape, pear
SNACKS: Watermelon
Dried fruits
Trail mix (raisins, nuts, dried apples or pears)
Frozen melon balls or grapes

Day 2

DINNER	BREAKFAST	LUNCH
Roasted chicken	Scrambled eggs	Salmon on lettuce
Salad with lettuce, celery,	Carrot and celery sticks	
carrots, chestnuts, and	Pineapple and banana slices	
sunflower seeds		
Baked sweet potato		

JUICE: Pineapple
SNACKS: Fruit juice "Popsicles"
Fresh coconut
Strawberry banana smoothie

Day 3

DINNER	BREAKFAST	LUNCH
Baked flounder	Nut butter on rice cakes	Lentil soup
Orange kiwi salad		
Steamed asparagus		
JUICE: Orange, grapefruit		
SNACKS: Ice cream (soy-based)		
Roasted soybeans		
Fruit juice "Popsicles"		
Pistachios		

Day 4

DINNER	BREAKFAST	LUNCH
Sliced turkey with gravy	Fruit tapioca	Tuna on spinach salad
Stir-fried broccoli and cauliflower		Apricots
Peaches		
JUICE: Black cherry, peach, or plum		
SNACKS: Toasted almonds, macadamia nuts		
Trail mix (dried fruit and nuts)		

(Based on and adapted from If It's Tuesday It Must Be Chicken by Golos and Goldbitz.)

▌▌ HANDS-ON ALLERGY TREATMENTS

Hands-on allergy treatments discussed in chapter 9 allow some people to eat without restrictions. However, this does not mean that they should not eat a healthy diet. For example, "junk food" is not healthy for anyone, with or without food allergies.

Even for people treated with a hands-on allergy treatment technique, we recommend the principles of a rotation diet. Eating the same foods over and over can wear out enzyme systems in the body. This causes improperly processed foods, which can lead to more allergies that will have to be addressed and treated. Eating a variety of foods following the principles of a rotation diet avoids both exhausting enzymes and the development of new allergies. However, the diet may be able to be more modified and lenient than the diet of an untreated person or a person taking allergy extracts.

▌▌ "BUT THE RECIPE SAYS…": LEARNING HOW TO SUBSTITUTE FOODS

Following a rotation diet means that you will have the opportunity to create new recipes, something that many of us have never tried.

Once you have learned about your family's food sensitivities, cooking will take on a new dimension. Rotating foods means that traditional recipes can seldom be used just as they are. Substitutions for many ingredients may be necessary. This can seem to be an overwhelming problem at first, but there are resources available, and adapting recipes does become easier with time. The challenge and reward of creating satisfying, delicious meals for yourself or your family—plus the pleasure that comes from seeing them regain their health and positive outlook—make the time invested in the kitchen very worthwhile.

Fortunately, you are not the first person to attempt food rotation. Many good books with helpful hints and recipes are available. (See Recommended Books.) At first, the foods, recipes, and menus may seem strange to you, but in time you will find that the unadulterated taste of high-quality food is wonderful. Your tastes, and those of your family, will become accustomed to new delights that you might not have otherwise tried.

The following are substitutions that you may use in recipes. You will find that substituting ingredients will cause variations in the texture and consistency of your recipes, but this is a part of the pleasure of expanding your cooking horizons.

▌ BEVERAGES

▌ *Coffee*

• Use 1 or 2 Tbsp. fig syrup to 1 cup hot water. Commercial coffee substitutes are also available at health food stores. They are made from several different substances, including roasted grain, which grain-allergic people will not tolerate. Read labels to be certain you tolerate these substitutes.

▌ *Soda Pop*

• Make your own: mix carbonated spring water with fresh or concentrated fruit juices, or herbal teas.

• Commercial "sodas" made from pure fruit juices and carbonated water are available.

▌ *Smoothies*

• Blend ice cubes and fruit juice until smooth. Add fresh fruit for extra flavor and thickness.

• If you tolerate them and they are on your rotation day, try adding soy milk or rice milk.

▌ CONDIMENTS

▌ *Catsup*

• Catsups sweetened with honey or rice syrup are available.

▌ *Mayonnaise*

• Several egg-free, cholesterol-free, honey-sweetened mayonnaise products made with cold-pressed oils are available.

• For a tasty, no-fail, egg-free mayonnaise that may be substituted for oil, sweeteners, and spices, follow this recipe: In a blender, place 3 Tbsp. soy milk powder and 1/2 cup water. Blend well. Add 1 Tbsp. maple syrup or honey, 1 tsp. sea salt, and one green onion bulb, finely chopped. Mix. Slowly add 1 cup oil and continue blending on low until mixture is thick. Add 1/4 cup lemon juice, blend, and refrigerate. This mayonnaise is not as thick as commercial products. Yields 1 1/2 cups.

▌ *Salt*

• Most brands contain dextrose (corn) and chemicals. Try using spices, sea kelp, or soy sauce (read labels). Non-iodized salt does not contain corn.

❙ *Vinegar*

- Vinegar contains yeast and should be avoided by those who have candidiasis or a yeast allergy. Substitute lemon or lime juice in an equal amount for vinegar.

❙ EGGS

❙ *As Binders*

In most recipes, substitutes can replace eggs without many changes. However, this depends on the recipe.

- Eggs can easily be replaced with 3 Tbsp. puréed fruit or vegetable for each egg required in the recipe.
- 1 Tbsp. flaxseed mix may be substituted for each egg. Flaxseed mix can be made by blending until smooth 1 cup ground flaxseeds to 3 cups water. This mixture keeps well in a covered container in the refrigerator.
- Two parts arrowroot powder, one part tapioca flour, and one part slippery elm powder makes an effective binding mixture. Use 1 Tbsp. of this mixture with 2 Tbsp. water to replace each egg.
- Many recipes work well when 2 Tbsp. oil beaten with 1 Tbsp. water is used to replace each egg.
- When needed for binding, one egg equals 2 Tbsp. of this blend: one part bean flour and two parts water, heated in a double boiler for an hour. Refrigerate in a covered container.
- For binding, one egg = 1/2 tsp. baking powder and 2 Tbsp. bean flour.

As Leavening Agents

- For each egg to be substituted (not more than two), beat together 2 Tbsp. carbonated water with 2 tsp. baking powder.

- Try substituting 1 Tbsp. bean flour and 1 Tbsp. oil for each egg.
- Another substitution is 1/4 cup tapioca starch for each egg.

Certain brands of commercial egg replacer available at health food stores may also be substituted for eggs.

❙ GRAINS

❙ *Biscuit Mix*

- For each cup of biscuit mix, use 1 cup flour, 1 1/2 tsp. baking powder, 1/2 tsp. sea salt, and 1 Tbsp. oil or shortening. Mix these ingredients well.

❙ *Bread Crumbs*

- Crushed whole-grain cereals or whole-grain crackers work well.
- Crushed chips—rice, corn, potato, sweet potato, or taro—make a good substitute.
- Any dried 100 percent grain bread, or any ground nuts or seeds, may be used.

❙ *Flour*

- Any type of flour may be substituted for wheat flour. When baking with alternative flours, the texture of the product will differ with each flour. Alternative flours should almost always be sifted before measuring, as this helps improve texture. Use the same amount the recipe indicates for wheat flour, but vary the amount of liquid to achieve the desired consistency. You may also have to adjust the temperature to prevent burning, particularly when baking cookies.

❙ *Flour in Gravy*

Follow your usual recipe for gravy and substitute one of the following for each tablespoon of wheat flour:

- 1/2 Tbsp. arrowroot powder

- ½ Tbsp. rice starch or flour
- 1 Tbsp. buckwheat flakes or flour
- cooked, puréed, starch vegetable
- powdered brewer's yeast (very strong taste)
- 2 Tbsp. tapioca flour
- ½ Tbsp. potato starch or flour
- ½ Tbsp. cornstarch
- 1 Tbsp. barley or rye flour

▮ *Non-Wheat Based Crackers*
- Norwegian flatbread
- Rice cakes, or rice crackers
- Some brands of Rye Krisp (read labels)
- Oat cakes

▮ MILK AND DAIRY PRODUCTS

All recipes work well with milk substitutes. In fact, interesting textures and tastes can be discovered with each substitute that is used.

Each item in the following list of milk substitutes is equal to 1 cup of milk:
- ½ cup plain yogurt plus ½ cup water
- 1 cup goat's milk
- 1 cup fruit juice
- 1 cup rice milk
- 1 cup soy milk
- ½ cup nuts blended with water to make 1 cup
- 1 cup water
- water with ½ tsp baking soda and lemon or lime juice or vinegar
- 1 cup vegetable liquid
- 1 cup tomato juice for casserole-type dishes

▮ *Soy Milk*
- Mix 1 cup soy flour, or any bean flour, with 4 cups water. Place the ingredients in the top of a double boiler and let them sit for two hours. Bring the mixture to a boil and simmer for 20 minutes. Cool and strain. Sweeten if desired, and keep the mixture in the refrigerator. Soy milk mixes are available at most health food stores, but be sure to read the label.

▮ *Artichoke Milk*
- In a saucepan, combine 2 cups water and ½ cup artichoke flour. Mix together with an electric mixer. Bring the mixture to a boil and simmer for 20 minutes. Cool and sweeten if desired.

▮ *Coconut Milk*
- In 2 cups water, soak 1 cup unsweetened shredded coconut. Mix in a blender until very smooth and strain if desired. Milk drained from fresh coconut may also be used.

▮ *Nut Milk*
- Use one part water to ½ part nuts. Grind nuts or seeds in a blender. Add water and blend the mixture until smooth. If desired, add sweetener and vanilla. Commercial nut milk mixes are available at health food stores.

▮ *Potato Water*
- Use water from cooked potatoes in place of milk. This is useful in baking and making sauces.

▮ *Zucchini or Other Vegetable Milk*
- Blend one medium, peeled zucchini in a blender until smooth. Pour the liquid into a pan and heat on low. Add 2 Tbsp. sweetener and one beaten egg (the egg can be omitted) to the mixture, stirring constantly for about 10 minutes. If the mixture is overcooked, it will separate. Should this happen, pour the mixture into a blender and blend until smooth. Use as a milk substitute in recipes, or just chill and drink.
- Alternatively, peel and cut a zucchini into chunks, and then liquify in a blender. The

pulp and seeds will constitute a thick liquid that can be frozen.

▮ *Powdered Milk*

• Try equal amounts of soy milk powder or powdered goat's milk, both available at health food stores.

• In some recipes, commercial nut milk powder can be substituted. It works well in icings.

▮ *Evaporated Milk*

• If tolerated, try evaporated goat's milk.

▮ *Buttermilk*

• Substitute 1 cup plain yogurt, soy milk, rice milk, or milk. To curdle, add 1 Tbsp. lemon or lime juice.

▮ *Chocolate Milk*

• To your choice of milk or milk substitute, add carob syrup to taste, or try the following non-dairy carob milk recipe: In a blender, blend 1^1/$_2$ cups nut milk, 3 Tbsp. roasted carob powder, 5 chopped dates or figs (or use raisins), 1 Tbsp. nut butter, and a dash of pure vanilla (optional). Chill and serve. Makes 2 cups.

▮ *Whipped Cream*

• A whipped cream substitute can be made by adding a sliced banana to one egg white. Beat until stiff, and the banana will dissolve. (*Caution:* Uncooked egg can be a source of *Salmonella* contamination. If you use this recipe, use only clean eggs with uncracked shells.)

▮ *Cottage Cheese*

• Tofu pressed between paper towels and crumbled is a good substitute.

▮ *Cream Sauce*

• Steam cauliflower until tender. Place it in a blender, and blend until smooth. Gradually add vegetable, meat, fish, or poultry broth until thick and creamy. Add ^{1}/$_2$ Tbsp. oil and spices if desired. Makes about 1 cup.

• A beautiful green sauce can be made using broccoli, peas, or spinach in the above recipe.

• Melt meat, fish, or poultry fat in a pan and add flour until the mixture becomes pasty. Slowly add broth and stir until desired consistency is obtained. Add spices if desired.

▮ SWEETENERS

▮ *Confectioner's Sugar*

This contains 3 percent cornstarch. Substitute:

• non-instant dry milk powder

• goat's milk powder

• maple syrup granules, ground to powder in a blender

▮ *Molasses*

• Use equal portions of fig syrup or rice syrup.

• Try equal portions of all-fruit syrups.

▮ *Sugar*

• Honey, sorghum, maple syrup, and fruit syrups may be substituted for sugar, but use only half the amount called for in the recipe. Be sure other liquids are decreased (^{1}/$_4$ cup for each cup of liquid sweetener).

• Date sugar and maple syrup granules are also good substitutes. Use ^{1}/$_2$ to ^{3}/$_4$ cup date and maple sugars to 1 cup sugar.

▮ DESSERTS AND CHOCOLATE

▮ *Chocolate Syrup*

• Blend ^{1}/$_2$ cup roasted carob powder, ^{1}/$_2$ cup honey or maple syrup, 1/3 cup water in a blender. Bring to a boil in a saucepan, stirring constantly. Boil for one minute. Remove from heat and beat in 1/3 cup tolerated margarine. Refrigerate syrup when cooled.

- Carob chips can also be used. Melt in a double boiler until smooth, and pour over ice cream or desserts.

❚ *Cocoa (unsweetened)*

- Use equal amounts of carob powder in place of cocoa.

❚ *Gelatin*

- Soften 2 Tbsp. agar-agar in 1 cup juice. Add the mixture to 2 cups hot liquid and boil for two minutes. Add sweetener if desired. When set, add fruit and nuts (if tolerated).

❚ *Ice Cream*

- If milk is a problem, soy-based and rice-based products are available.
- To avoid refined sugar exposures, look for products sweetened with maple syrup, rice syrup, or fruit syrups.
- If chemicals and preservatives are a problem, try homemade ice cream. Combine one quart half-and-half cream with 1/2 jar of Knudsen flavored syrup and mix in an ice cream maker. "Clean" store brands of ice creams are also available.

❚ *Icings*

- Blend mashed bananas with yogurt.
- Try unsweetened whipped cream with pure concentrated juice or a touch of carob powder if milk products are not a problem.
- Try cream cheese blended with maple syrup if milk products are not a problem.
- Use a regular icing recipe and substitute, as in the following adapted recipe:

The recipe calls for	Substitute
3 Tbsp. butter	3 Tbsp. oil
2 Tbsp. unsweetened cocoa powder	2 Tbsp. carob
1 1/4 cups instant powdered milk	1/2 cup puréed almonds
1/4 cup water	same
1/3 cup mashed banana	same
1/4 tsp. lemon juice	same
1/4 tsp. vanilla	same

❚ *Popsicles*

- Freeze unsweetened fruit juice in paper cups or molds, or purée and freeze fresh or frozen fruits.
- To make creamsicles, add yogurt or milk to puréed fruits and freeze.
- Blend one cup plain yogurt, 1/4 cup carob powder, and 1/4 cup sweetener. Freeze and enjoy!

❚ MISCELLANEOUS

❚ *Baking Powder*

Most brands contain cornstarch. Corn-free powders are available at health food stores, or you can try making your own with the following recipes.

- Mix well 1 cup baking soda, 1 cup cream of tartar, and 1 cup arrowroot powder. Store in a covered container.
- Mix well 3/4 cup cream of tartar, 9 Tbsp. baking soda, and 6 Tbsp. potato, rice, or tapioca starch. Store in a covered container.
- Mix well 1/2 lb. rice or potato starch, 1/2 lb. cream of tartar, 5 oz. baking soda, and 1 oz. potash or tartaric acid (found at pharmacies). Sift these ingredients several times and store in a covered container.

❚ *Bouillon Cubes*

- Undiluted meat, fish, poultry, or vegetable drippings may be frozen in ice cube trays and used in place of bouillon cubes.
- Another substitute is 1 Tbsp. soy sauce or 1 Tbsp. yeast in powder or flake form (*Caution:* Soy sauce frequently contains wheat).

❚ *Cornstarch*

- Arrowroot may be substituted for cornstarch in recipes that will not be heated.

- Use 2½ Tbsp. potato starch or tapioca starch for 1 Tbsp. cornstarch.
- Flour works well in place of cornstarch for thickening sauces and gravies.

I *Flavored Extracts*

These usually contain sugar and alcohol, but extracts without sugar and alcohol are available.

- Vanilla flavor can be obtained by leaving a vanilla bean in honey. Use small amounts of the honey in a recipe that calls for both sweet and vanilla tastes.

I *Shortening*

- All soy margarines or oils used in equal measurement work well as butter or shortening substitutes.
- Melted animal fat of any kind may be used. Poultry fat adds flavor, but goose and duck fat are softer and more moist than butter. Pork and beef fat have about the same texture as butter; lamb fat stays very firm at room temperature and has a stronger flavor.

■■ EATING OUT

More North Americans are eating out than at any other time in history. Many people eat 35 percent of their meals in a restaurant, and in cities some of the population eats out 75 percent of the time. For people with food allergies, eating out can be a challenge because they lose the measure of control they have over their diet when they eat at home. However, with care and planning, you can eat out safely, at parties, banquets, fine restaurants, and even at fast-food restaurants.

I PARTIES AND BANQUETS

Many people turn down dinner party invitations and do not attend banquets because of their food allergies. This is unfortunate because several types of precautions will allow participation in these events, and enable you to eat without triggering an allergic reaction. For scheduled events, manipulate your rotation so that you can eat part, if not all, of the planned menu. (See Borrowing Foods, discussed earlier in this chapter.) Manipulating your rotation and avoiding your more severe allergens will allow you to eat safely on these special occasions.

For parties and banquets, call the host or caterer ahead of time and inquire about the planned menu. Briefly explain your problem and why you are inquiring. Many hosts and caterers are willing and even eager to try to help you and welcome suggestions and hints about what you can safely eat. Any time you are asked to make suggestions about what you can tolerate, remember the wonderful adage KISS—Keep it simple, stupid! Do not give anyone a long list of your food allergies. Tell them *only* the main foods that you really need to avoid, the ones that give you the most severe symptoms. Also tell them some simple things to cook that you can tolerate. Many people are totally unfamiliar with food allergies and are unable to think of and plan for alternatives. Volunteer to bring your own food if necessary, but keep in mind that you may want to take enough to share!

If the host or caterer does not volunteer to help you, or cannot or will not help you, you still have several options. If there will be nothing you can eat, and if you cannot manipulate your rotation, have your meal before you go and take a small bag of tolerated

Fast Food Disaster

Fast foods are a nutritional and allergic disaster. Saturated fat, cholesterol, and sugar provide most of the excess calories. Fast-food meals always contain one or more major food allergens, as well as additives and preservatives. Despite this, the average North American seems willing to pay for convenience, spending more than $400 a year for fast foods. Every second, 200 customers order one or more hamburgers at a fast-food restaurant.

More formal restaurants usually present less of a problem for people with food allergies than fast-food restaurants. They serve a larger variety of better-quality foods with fewer additives, salt, and sugar. The menus are more flexible, and changes can be made at your request. However, it is possible to eat at fast-food restaurants. Keep in mind that the food available may not be as healthy for you as you would like, and you will be unable to request variations or changes in your food.

▌ FAST FOODS

Fast foods are the major contributors to America's overconsumption/undernutrition eating pattern. The smell of grease in most fast-food restaurants tells us that fat is probably the biggest offender. The deep-fat fryer may contain highly saturated beef fat or hydrogenated vegetable oils. The continual heating and reheating of the vegetable frying oils converts the oil molecules to trans fatty acids, a form that is injurious to our body metabolism. Chicken and fish, which are coated with batter that absorbs large amounts of these frying fats and oils, may contain more fat than a hamburger. Still more fat is added by the use of condiments such as mayonnaise, sauces, and salad dressings.

Nearly all the items on fast-food menus contain large amounts of salt (sodium chloride). All foods contain some natural sodium, but 90 percent of our sodium comes from salt added to foods at the time of manufacture or consumption. Some fast-food sandwiches contain $1/2$ to $3/4$ tsp. of salt, more than half the daily recommended

nuts or fruit to discreetly munch on. Never stay home because of your allergies! Go and enjoy socializing even if you cannot eat.

▌ EATING AT RESTAURANTS

Asking the right questions may be the most important aspect of eating out safely. Calling ahead and talking to the chef or manager can prevent many problems. This allows you to find out the ingredients in any dish you might wish to order. Keep in mind that simple dishes with fewer ingredients will be more easily tolerated. Many times a chef will volunteer to prepare something special to meet your needs.

You can also question the person who serves you regarding the contents of the dishes when you order, and a competent server will endeavor to find out the answers to your questions. However, many servers have no understanding of food allergy and are unaware of the importance of the accuracy and completeness of their answers.

sodium intake. Milkshakes may contain as much as 300 mg of sodium, 100 mg more than is in 10 potato chips. It is extremely difficult to determine by taste how much sodium foods contain. French fries, though they taste quite salty, frequently contain less sodium than do the burgers (salt is added to the outside of the French fries just before they are served, increasing their salty taste).

Sugar is also added to many poor-quality fast foods to improve appearance and taste. For example, molasses and corn syrup mixes are added to hamburger meat to reduce shrinkage and improve color, flavor, and juiciness. French fries may have a sugar coating that turns brown when it is immersed in hot grease. The batters on fried foods always contain some sugar, often sucrose, but more frequently they are corn sweeteners. Soft drinks, the most common beverage at fast-food restaurants, are the greatest single contributor of sugar to our diets. Excess sugar will disrupt blood sugar levels, cause pancreatic overload, disrupt the function of neurotransmitters in the brain, and contribute to the likelihood of dental cavities.

The combination of salt and sugar in fast foods can cause problems for patients with high blood pressure. Hidden sugars are a hazard for diabetics. Perhaps what is most dangerous, however, is that fast-food fans develop larger appetites for salt and sugar, then crave and eat more salt and sugar on all foods.

Soft drinks sold at fast-food restaurants often contain the stimulant caffeine. Colas usually contain caffeine, and clear or light-colored drinks do not, with the exception of Mountain Dew and Surge. Root beer usually does not contain caffeine. Too much caffeine can cause anxiety, irritability, muscle twitches, upset stomach, insomnia, rapid heart rate, and nervousness, as well as depleting B vitamins. Prolonged use or overuse of caffeine overstimulates adrenal function, which can lead to adrenal exhaustion. Although a can of soda has only one-third of the caffeine found in one cup of coffee, its effect on a child's body is the same as the coffee would have on an adult. A child who drinks several sodas in a day may have trouble sleeping, as well as exhibiting symptoms of hyperactivity, because of the caffeine.

Fruits, vegetables, and whole grains are necessary sources of fiber in our diets, and are rarely included on fast-food menus. Salad bars are the exception and do provide small amounts of fiber, particularly if beans, one of the best sources of soluble dietary fiber, are offered. A few fast-food restaurants offer whole-grain or multigrain buns. However, the percentage of whole grain in the buns is low and some contain brown food coloring rather than whole grains. A diet consisting largely of fast foods provides very little of the fiber needed for good digestion.

Fast foods are also low in nutrients, particularly vitamin A, biotin, folic acid, B_5, calcium, iron, copper, magnesium, B_6, and vitamin E. Salad bars can offer some foods with vitamin A, such as broccoli, carrots, red peppers, and yellow squash, and orange juice and potatoes contain vitamin C. The calcium-containing foods, such as cheese and milkshakes, are also high in fat. There is some iron in hamburger patties and in some foods at the salad bar, such as green leafy vegetables and sesame seeds. However, a steady diet of fast foods and junk snack foods can lead to serious nutritional deficiencies.

I *Fast Food Allergens*

The many common allergens found in fast foods create problems for the allergic person.

- *Beef:* In hamburgers and most Mexican food; the major meat served at all restaurants. May also be in frying oil.
- *Corn:* May be hidden in meats as a flavor additive; flour or starch may be added to the batter of deep-fat fried foods. Corn provides the chief sweetener in soft drinks, and may also be added to dressings and sauces as grain vinegar.
- *Egg:* May be in the batter of deep-fat fried foods, or in salad dressings and sauces, breads, doughnuts, pasta, or ice cream.
- *Milk:* Used in cheese on sandwiches, in garnishes, in milkshakes, ice cream, soups, doughnuts, and hot dogs. Milk solids, lactose, and whey are added to breads, desserts, salad dressings, and sauces.
- *Potatoes:* May be in salads, or served as baked potatoes or French fries.
- *Soy:* May be in hamburger patties. If the hamburger has a special name that does not include the word hamburger, soy and other extenders may be added. The most common oil used in all restaurants, soy is also used in cheeses.
- *Sugar:* Occurs in desserts, soft drinks, and batters on fried foods.
- *Tomatoes:* Used frequently in sandwiches,

pizza, and spaghetti sauce, or served at salad bars.

- *Wheat:* Makes up the batter of deep-fat fried foods; used in sandwich bread and buns, pizza crust, and pasta.
- *Yeast:* Occurs in sandwich bread and buns, cheese, doughnuts, hot dogs, pizza crust, barbecue sauce, catsup, mayonnaise, and mustard.

In addition to common food allergens, fast foods also contain chemical additives. Artificial colorings are used to increase visual appeal. MSG (monosodium glutamate), a flavor enhancer, is frequently added to batters for breaded foods, salad dressings, gravy, soups, and croutons.

At one time, sulfites were used extensively to preserve the color and freshness of fruits and vegetables. Because of several fatal allergic reactions to sulfites, restaurants may no longer add sulfites to their menu items. However, some foods may have sulfites added at the manufacturing level, particularly potatoes, stuffing, beer, wine, breaded shrimp, lime juice, and maraschino cherries.

BHA and BHT are antioxidant chemicals that may be used in beverages, ice cream, baked goods, soup bases, lard, shortening, and dry breakfast cereals. Aspartame, an artificial sweetener, is also found in some fast foods.

Recently, many fast-food chains have made an effort to reduce the fats in their foods. They have switched from saturated beef fat to vegetable oils for all products except French fries. Unfortunately, this causes a trans fatty acid exposure, which is harmful to health. Some companies are also seeking to eliminate dyes, particularly yellow dye #5, which is highly allergenic.

Because ingredients may change daily in traditional restaurants, they are not required to label their food. However, fast-food restaurants produce standard products that could easily have ingredient labels on their wrappers or boxes. Because of allergy problems and nutritional concerns, such labels would be advantageous for the consumer. However, there are no government requirements for this, although government agencies do acknowledge that the restaurant industry has changed since 1938, when labeling rules were formulated. The restaurant industry is generally opposed to labeling, although some fast-food restaurants have voluntarily disclosed the ingredients in their food.

For an allergic person, it would be best to avoid eating at fast-food restaurants. If you are sensitive to the basic foods (corn, wheat, eggs, soy, yeast, milk, and sugar), it will be almost impossible for you to avoid these ingredients. One possibility, of course, is for you to take food extracts. If you can do so without symptoms, you might occasionally visit a fast-food restaurant on only a very limited basis. Even with the use of extracts, it is easy to overload. Fast-food menus are definitely not part of rotation diets!

❙ *Surviving Fast Foods*
If you do eat at a fast-food restaurant, use the following guidelines to help make your meal as healthy as possible.

- Eat at restaurants where there is a salad bar. Eat only the fresh vegetables and the beans; use the dressings sparingly and avoid the pickled condiments.
- Order less than you want in order to conserve on calories. Avoid anything labeled big, deluxe, or whopper.
- Try to avoid fat by seeking out foods that are baked or broiled. Ask for the sauces, mayonnaise, cheese, and bacon to be omitted. If you order something deep-fried, peel off the batter or breading. Do not order "extra crispy."
- Ask that salt not be added to your meal. Avoid salted condiments, processed meats, and cheese.
- Reduce calories and sugar by avoiding soft drinks and desserts.
- If you suspect you will react to the restaurant water, bring your own from home.
- If the restaurant does not serve fruit that you can eat for dessert, bring fresh fruit from home.
- Ask if the restaurant has an ingredients list for their foods. Read it carefully to avoid surprises.
- Instead of eating at the restaurant, take food home from the drive-in window or take-out counter and serve it with healthy beverages, fruit, and vegetables.

CHAPTER II

Common Chemical Sensitivities

What is Chemical Sensitivity?

Since the mid-19th century, the development of modern chemistry and the refinement of laboratory techniques and equipment have radically changed our lives.

Chemical warfare agents were used toward the end of World War I, and after World War II the chemical revolution began in earnest with the formulation of thousands of new chemicals and compounds. While modern chemistry has given us wonderful products, it is not entirely a blessing. Over 500 billion chemicals are manufactured in North America each year, of which 500,000 are in common use. These chemicals have found their way into our homes, our food, our water, and our air, and, ultimately, into our bodies. Chemicals and their cumulative effects have a serious impact on our health.

The understanding of chemical sensitivity has developed slowly, as an adjuvant to studying food allergy. Dr. Albert Rowe of Oakland, California, discovered in the 1930s that many of his patients had multiple fruit sensitivities. Rather than displaying an allergy to fruits in a particular family, these patients were allergic to all fruits. In the early 1950s, Dr. Theron Randolph of Chicago, Illinois found that the problem was caused by chemical contamination of the fruit rather than a true fruit allergy, because unsprayed fruits were tolerated by these patients.

Dr. Randolph is the father of the concept of chemical allergy. He first described chemical susceptibility in 1951, and in 1953 he outlined the effects of natural gas on sensitive people. In 1962 Dr. Randolph published *Human Ecology and Susceptibility to the Chemical Environment*, which identified the environmental chemicals—including indoor and outdoor air pollution, food additives and contaminants, cosmetics, toiletries, and drugs—responsible for a wide range of physical and mental illnesses. The concept of chemical allergy or susceptibility was born. Dr. Randolph used the term susceptibility to avoid debate over whether reactions to chemicals were allergies in the classical sense or hypersensitivity. Regardless of the mechanism, reactions to small doses of chemicals can cause severe symptoms.

Chemicals enter our body through the

mouth and nose, and through direct skin contact. Chemically sensitive people acquire their susceptibility because of hereditary and genetic factors, lowered immunity, and inadequate or damaged body detoxification mechanisms. Chemical susceptibility usually develops as a result of repeated, low-level exposure to a number of chemicals over a period of time. Such susceptibility might also be initiated by a massive, overwhelming exposure to a chemical spill or fire, pesticide spray, or general anesthesia.

Dr. Bill Rea of the Environmental Health Center in Dallas, Texas has noted that patients develop chemical sensitivity after:

- repeated low doses of a chemical over a long period of time. Cumulative effects of these doses will eventually result in small doses triggering symptoms.
- a massive, overwhelming exposure to a chemical that can cause acute symptoms and later may cause chronic symptoms. Subsequent exposures to the same or different chemicals will trigger more severe or additional symptoms.
- exposure to small amounts of a chemical after a trauma such as an automobile accident, surgery, immunizations, severe injury, or childbirth.
- an acute infection, which may be bacterial, viral, fungal, or parasitic.

TYPES OF CHEMICAL EXPOSURES

There are many types of chemical exposures. Air pollution is one type, and indoor air exposures differ from outdoor exposures. In recent years, indoor air pollution has become increasingly more important as a health hazard. We are also exposed to chemicals in the food and water we consume, and any medications we take are chemicals. Clothing and personal care products are additional chemical exposures.

INDOOR CHEMICAL AIR CONTAMINANTS

Any chemical that pollutes the indoor environment is dangerous for the chemically susceptible person. Unfortunately, buildings themselves are frequently the largest contributors. Building materials, unless carefully selected, can be very toxic. For example, a significant amount of formaldehyde is found in building materials and is dangerous to humans, even in low concentrations. Carpets may contain large amounts of formaldehyde, and also trap dirt, dust, and mold.

Furnishings such as drapes and upholstered furniture emit chemicals from dyes, stain protectors, and surface treatments. Foam padding in upholstered furniture decomposes when it becomes old and emits toxic chemicals. Wood furniture can outgas chemicals from stains, varnishes, and waxes, as well as formaldehyde from particleboard construction.

Combustion products from natural gas, fuel oil, coal, and heating systems fill the air. Gas stoves, hot water heaters, and dryers, as well as oil fumes (generated by running motors), contribute further to the problem. Fresh paint, cleaning supplies, deodorants, disinfectants, detergents, plastics, and insecticides all add to the toxic chemical pool.

With the advent of more energy-efficient buildings, these indoor contaminants are trapped in our homes and workplaces. The workplace is becoming increasingly con-

Illness and Pollution Correlation

After the reunification of Germany in 1990, there was a tremendous decline of air pollution levels in East Germany in a short period due to the closure or conversion of manufacturing plants and the conversion of heating fuel from coal to central gas heat. Two surveys conducted by the GSF Institute of Epidemiology in Germany in the middle 1990s showed a decrease in respiratory illnesses that corresponded with a decrease in air pollution. When the total suspended particulates and sulfur dioxide in the air decreased, so did the rates of bronchitis, ear infection, colds, and illnesses accompanied by fever.

taminated by the use of photocopiers, computers and printers, correction fluid, and carbonless paper.

■ OUTDOOR CHEMICAL AIR CONTAMINANTS

Outdoor air often is not safe to breathe. Traffic exhaust and smog raise outdoor pollution to dangerous levels in our cities. Despite government regulations and monitoring, some industries contribute to outdoor pollution. Oil refineries, wells, and storage tanks pollute the air for miles around them. Indiscriminate spraying of crops, forests, orchards, gardens, and lawns adds still more chemicals to the air. Paving and resurfacing roads and tarring roofs contaminate outdoor air. Woodstoves and fireplaces emit smoke

from chimneys, fouling outdoor and indoor air.

Natural events also contribute to outdoor air pollution. Forest fires, dust storms, volcanic eruptions, natural gas, marsh gas, meteorological phenomena, terpenes from plants, ammonia from biological decomposition, and floods add many chemicals to the outdoor air. Control measures are more limited, if not impossible, for these natural events.

■ CHEMICAL CONTAMINANTS OF FOOD AND WATER

Our most intimate connection with the toxic environment is through the food we eat. Intended to nourish our bodies, our food frequently is a source of chemical exposures. Residues of pesticides, fertilizers, and chemicals used to hasten ripening may be on our produce. Processed foods contain preservatives, additives, artificial flavorings and colors, which are all chemicals. Animals raised for slaughter in feedlots may have been given antibiotics or hormones to keep them disease free and make them mature for market faster. Other chemicals find their way into our food from the containers in which they are packaged.

In some areas, chlorine and fluoride are added to drinking water that may already be contaminated by fertilizers and pesticides or high mineral content leached from the soil. Inadequate or nonexistent sewage treatment may also contribute to water pollution. Some water is contaminated by disease-causing microorganisms, as well as algae.

■ DRUGS AND MEDICATIONS

As pharmacology flourishes, reactions to drugs and medications become more fre-

Common Chemical Allergens

Sources of Problem Chemicals	Chemical to Test for
Perfumes, solvents, artificial flavorings, tea, raspberries	Benzyl alcohol
Tap water for drinking, showers or baths, or dishwashing; water in swimming pools or hot tubs; laundry bleach; disinfectants	Chlorine
Water for drinking, showers or baths, or dishwashing; hot water in tubs, swimming pools; toothpaste; dental fluoride treatment	Fluoride
Clothing or fabric stores, carpets, mobile homes, new homes or additions, paneling or particleboard, fresh paint, fresh concrete, glues and adhesives, air deodorizers, insecticides, hairsetting lotions, facial tissues, wood smoke	Formaldehyde
Cosmetics, liquid and bar soaps, furniture polish, cough drops, toothpaste, hand lotion, vitamins (soft gelatin capsules)	Glycerine
Car exhaust; gas heat, stoves, or furnaces; oil heat or furnaces; airport fumes	Petrochemicals (gas or diesel)
Car exhaust; gasoline; perfumes; liquors; gas heat, stoves, or furnaces; oil heat or furnaces; wood smoke; cleaning agents; airport fumes	Ethanol
Perfumes, aftershaves, cosmetics, newspapers, canned foods, computers, aspirin or sulfa drugs, wood smoke, waterbeds, glues and adhesives	Phenol

quent. Adverse reactions to all classes of medications have been reported, which may be due to the substance itself, to the vehicle of the drug, or to the preservative. Many sensitive people are losing their "drug umbrellas"—drugs that are still safe for them to take, which they keep in reserve. As their immune system dysfunction increases, they react to more and more drugs. Many are unable to tolerate any antibiotics or local anesthetics, and there are no reserve medications under their "umbrellas."

In addition, many people have a high toxic body burden. Their detoxification systems are so overloaded that their body, particularly their liver, cannot process any medication. To the overworked detoxification mechanisms, the medication is just another chemical that must be metabolized. These people can tolerate few, if any, medications.

■ CLOTHING AND PERSONAL CARE PRODUCTS

With the advent of synthetic fabrics, reactions to clothing, bedding, and upholstery have become common. Natural fabrics can also cause reactions because of detergents,

Society's Canaries?

Chemically sensitive people in our society can be compared to the canaries used in coal mines during the last century. Miners would take caged canaries into the mine shafts with them to act as sensors. If the canaries became sick or died, the shafts would immediately be evacuated. Death of the birds indicated the presence of methane gas.

The chemically sensitive are those whose detoxification pathways and immune systems have been damaged by overexposure or subtle, cumulative exposure to harmful chemicals. These people are the sensors of our polluted air, water, and food. They are the early warning signs that we must clean up our home and work environments.

dry-cleaning fumes, plasticizing starches or sizing, fabric dyes, or gas dryer residues. The rubber in elastic can also be a problem for some people.

Most personal care products are no longer natural or biological in origin. They are now entirely formulated in laboratories, and most contain harsh chemicals that may sensitize a susceptible person.

■ TYPES OF CHEMICAL REACTIONS

According to Dr. Randolph, reactions to chemical allergens may be seen as part of a maladaptive process. When susceptible people are exposed to chemicals, their bodies adapt after the first exposures and no symptoms are obvious. As exposures to chemicals continue, however, adaptation to our total load slows down. The maladaption then spreads to related chemicals and even to foods. Chronic symptoms begin to develop, and the cumulative damage causes a gradual decline in health.

Some chemical reactions are IgE mediated, which means that they involve an antigen-antibody response. Rashes, hives, and skin eruptions are symptoms common to this type of reaction. More research is needed to uncover the exact mechanism of most reactions. As with food reactions, some chemical reactions are immediate and the offending substance can be identified.

Some chemically sensitive people experience reactions that differ from an acute, immediate response. These chemical reactions are delayed, making the connection to a particular chemical exposure unclear. These reactions are occult or hidden, where damage is caused but no symptoms are obvious. Thermal reactions are those triggered by cold, heat, or light following a chemical exposure.

The toxicity of most chemicals is determined by animal studies. While these studies are helpful, they are not absolute. Animal physiology differs from human physiology, making the effects of a chemical different. Human drug doses that are simply extrapolated, based on weight, from animal doses, may not be accurate.

■ SYMPTOMS OF CHEMICAL SENSITIVITY

The brain is the primary target organ in chemical reactions. Chemicals are deposited in fat cells, and the brain has a very high fat content. Smooth muscle is also a major responder in both food and chemical sensitivities. However, chronic symptoms and illness resulting from maladaption to various environmental elements can affect any system or organ of the body.

- *Cerebral:* Confusion, depression, anger, "brain fag," inability to concentrate, apathy, emotional instability, mental fatigue, light-headedness, and lethargy. Extreme reactions can result in psychosis, disorientation, regression, and sometimes hallucinations, delusions, and amnesia.
- *Respiratory:* Coughing, bronchitis, asthma, chest pain, and "air hunger."
- *Gastrointestinal and urinary:* Excessive thirst, eating or drinking binges, diarrhea, constipation, urgency and frequency of urination, nausea and vomiting, gas, dry mouth, bad or metallic taste in the mouth, abdominal pain, difficulty swallowing, heartburn, and gallbladder symptoms.
- *Neurological:* Headaches, neck aches, nerve pain, fainting, restless legs, and numbness.
- *Ear, nose, and throat:* Ringing in ears, dizziness, cough, itching inside ears, hypersensitivity to noise, rhinitis, nasal obstruction, and stuffy nose.
- *Skin:* Hives, acne, blisters, eczema, itching, and burning.
- *Eye:* Vision disturbances, watery eyes, light sensitivity, eye pain, swelling around eyes, and drooping, itching, swollen, or red eyelids.
- *Musculoskeletal:* Fatigue, muscle pain, cramps, weakness, joint pain, stiffness, lack of coordination, arthritis, and neck aches.

Chemical reactions can also have cardiovascular effects. Dr. William Rea has shown that angina symptoms can be triggered in nonatherosclerotic patients by exposures to various chemicals. Other cardiovascular symptoms include heart pounding, racing, palpitations and irregular beats; edema; fainting; flushing; pallor; phlebitis (vein inflammation); and purpura (hemorrhaging under the skin).

Chemically susceptible people can be "masked" to chemicals, just as people can be masked to food allergies. For example, sensitive people can always identify a fresh paint smell as a problem, because it is not often encountered, but they may not recognize that the odor from a gas range is problematic because they are exposed to it daily and have become masked. If they avoid all natural gas exposures for four to seven days, symptoms will appear upon their return to the natural gas sources.

People may be addicted to chemicals just as they may be addicted to allergenic foods. Those who are chemically addicted may say they love the smell of gasoline, nail polish, or fabric softener. As a child, one of our patients used to eat her father's lunch leftovers, which reeked of the oil refinery in which he worked. She eagerly awaited his return so she could eat this contaminated food and she confessed it was the high point of her day. It is significant that her father felt so sick from his work exposures that he was unable to eat all of his lunch.

Chemically sensitive people have an extremely acute sense of smell and are more aware of odors and chemicals than those who are unaffected. However, they may not

Anxiety Response to Chemical Exposure

Often, there is an emotional component to a chemical reaction. For many people, the reaction to the chemical triggers an anxiety response, in addition to the physical symptoms. They may become fearful and anxious, dreading their symptoms, and worrying that they may pass out, stop breathing, or have a seizure. Because of this anxiety response, they may become hypervigilant in trying to avoid exposures and in protecting themselves.

detect the very chemical or odor that is triggering a reaction. When exposed to chemicals, sensitive people should always breathe through their mouth since chemical fumes entering the nose can directly affect the brain through interconnecting nerve pathways. Chemicals entering the body through the mouth must circulate through the bloodstream and pass through the blood-brain barrier before affecting the brain.

Those with chemical sensitivities are often misunderstood by friends, relatives, coworkers, and physicians, who tend to label them as lazy, troublemakers, or, worst of all, crazy. Many physicians immediately recommend psychiatric help or counseling after listening to their patients' symptoms, and employers suspect psychological problems rather than symptoms from chronic chemical exposure. Chemically sensitive people

can suffer a lifetime of impaired health unless they find proper diagnosis and treatment. They can become unable to work, and even existing comfortably can be difficult for them. However, there is hope. The following information includes ways that chemically susceptible people can help themselves.

Common Sources of Chemical Exposure

All of us face unavoidable chemical exposures at home, school, and work. You should be tested for the chemicals listed below if you experience any of the problems associated with them. Chemical neutralizing extracts or hands-on allergy treatment for specific chemicals can help control your symptoms.

▮▮ BENZYL ALCOHOL

Benzyl alcohol has a faint, sweet odor and a burning taste. It occurs naturally in tea, raspberries, jasmine, hyacinth, ylang-ylang oils, Peru and Tolu balsams, and storax (a gum used in perfumes).

Benzyl alcohol is used as a topical antiseptic, a local anesthetic, and a preservative in injectable medications. It is used frequently as the scent extractor in perfumes, as the flavor extractor in synthetic flavorings, and in many manufacturing processes.

Vomiting, diarrhea, and central nervous system depression are caused by ingesting large doses of benzyl alcohol. Stronger solutions are corrosive to the skin and mucous membranes. If you are sensitive, it is possible to avoid products that contain benzyl alcohol.

Sources of Benzyl Alcohol

Acne medications	Ice cream	Grape
Anesthetic (local)	Ices	Honey
Antiseptic (topical)	Nylon dyes	Liquor
Artificial flavorings	Ointments	Loganberry
Baked goods	Perfume	Muscatel
Ballpoint pen inks	Photographic chemicals	Nut
Beverages	Preservative in medications	Orange
Candy	Raspberries	Raspberry
Chewing gum	Solvents	Root beer
Cosmetics	Synthetic flavorings and	Rose
Cough drops	scents:	Vanilla
Ear drops	Blueberry	Violet
Gelatin desserts	Cherry	Walnut
Heat-sealing polyethylene	Floral	Tea
films	Fruit	

■ CHLORINE

In its elemental state, chlorine is a yellow-green gas with a suffocating odor. Because it is a very reactive element, it does not occur in a free state. It is found abundantly in compounds with other elements, in the form of chlorides. Chlorides have properties and actions that are totally different from those of chlorine. Some chlorides, such as salt (sodium chloride), are not harmful and may even be beneficial.

Other compounds of chlorine release small amounts of chlorine gas when put in water, resulting in chlorine exposure. Reactions can occur to chlorine fumes rising from hot or cold running tap water. Symptoms include red eyes, sneezing, skin rashes, fatigue, abdominal pain, fainting, or dizziness. Taking a shower, washing dishes, or even washing your hands exposes you to chlorine.

Higher concentrations of chlorine can cause skin eruptions; heart swelling; severe respiratory tract irritation; swelling of the throat; delirium; coma; circulatory collapse; vomiting; erosion of the mucous membranes; and pain and inflammation in the mouth, throat, and stomach.

If you are chlorine-sensitive, set your drinking water out in an open glass bottle for 24 hours to let the chlorine dissipate. This should be done in a well-ventilated room or outside so that you are not exposed to the chlorine as it disperses. *Do not* store water in plastic containers, as it will absorb chemicals from the plastic. A water purifier may be used to remove the chlorine from your tap water, but it may be wise to supplement your diet with minerals since some filters also remove trace minerals.

Swim team members have a higher incidence of asthma than the general popula-

Sources of Chlorine Gas and/or Compounds

Aging and oxidizing agents	Processing of meat, fish, vegetables, and
Anesthetics	fruit
Antiseptics	Production of organic and inorganic
Bleaching of flour	chemicals
Bleaching of textiles and wood pulp	Refining of oil and sugar
Bleaching powder (Ajax, Comet)	Shrinkproofing of wool
Cleaning agents	Water sources:
De-tinning and de-zincing iron	Bathtubs
Disinfectants	Hot tubs
Fire extinguishers	Municipal water systems
Industrial preparations of various com-	Sewage systems
pounds (dyes, plastics, and synthetic	Showers
rubber)	Spas
Laundry bleach	Swimming pools
Metallurgy	

tion. Chlorine neutralizing extracts taken before a bath or shower—and before *and* after a swim or hot tub session—help to prevent chlorine reactions.

▌▌ FLUORIDE

Fluoride is the name given to a class of fluorine compounds. In its elemental state, fluorine is a pale yellow gas. It is the most active of all elements, and so is found only in combination with other elements.

Dietary sources of fluorides include a wide range of foods, depending on regional fluoride-content variations in the soil and water supplies.

Fluorides are plant-toxic pollutants because they accumulate in the leaves. These plants are then toxic to the animals and humans that eat their leaves. This type of plant contamination commonly occurs near ore smelters, refineries, and industrial plants that manufacture fertilizers, ceramics, aluminum, glass, and bricks.

Water is the greatest source of fluoride exposure for most people in North America. In many communities, one part of fluoride per every million parts of water is added to aid in reducing dental caries, which has provoked an ongoing argument. Studies done in New Zealand, Japan, Canada, and Michigan have shown that fluoridated communities do not have lower levels of dental caries than the general population. The studies were done over a 10- to 15-year period, and results were compared to those from areas with unfluoridated water supplies. Some research demonstrates that fluoride actually damages teeth by interfering with the proper formation of proteins that make up the structural framework of growing teeth.

Excessive amount of fluorides can be toxic to us, causing fatigue, weakness, mot-

Sources of Fluorides or Fluorocarbon Derivatives

Aluminum refining	Propellant in aerosol sprays
Cutting steel	Refrigerants
Fire extinguishers	Rocket fuel
Insecticides	Rodenticides
Isotope separation	Soil-release agents
Lubricants	Solvents
Plastics	Textile treatments

tling of the teeth, wrinkling of the skin, a prickly sensation in the muscles, kidney and bladder disorders, constipation, vomiting, itching after bathing, excessive thirst, headaches, arthritis, gum disease, nervousness, diarrhea, hair loss, skin and stomach disorders, numbness, brittle nails, sinus problems, mouth ulcers, vision problems, eczema, bronchitis, and asthma. Too much fluoride can also reduce vitamin C levels, weaken the immune system, cause birth defects, and damage enzyme systems.

The following sources of exposures are, or contain, fluorides:

- *Ammonium fluoride:* Used as wood preservative
- *Antimony fluoride:* Catalyst for organic reactions
- *Boron fluoride:* Catalyst for organic reactions
- *Calcium fluoride, hydroflurosilicic acid, potassium fluoride, sodium fluoride, sodium silicofluoride:* Used to fluoridate water
- *Chlorine trifluoride:* Fluorinating agent
- *Cobaltic fluoride:* Fluorinating agent
- *Cryolite:* Solvent for aluminum oxide
- *Fluoride lasers:* Some, such as the Krypton fluoride (KrF) laser, contain fluoride as part of the medium

- *Fluorite:* Used as metallurgic flux
- *Fluorspar:* Used to prepare fluoride
- *Freon:* Refrigerant and propellant in spray cans
- *Hydrofluoric acid:* Used for etching glass, as a solvent, and as a catalyst in gasoline production
- *Magnesium fluoride:* Used in the optic industry to improve light transmission in glass
- *Sodium fluoride:* Insecticide and disinfectant
- *Sodium silicofluoride:* Used in water and toothpaste to prevent tooth decay (two parts/million)
- *Stannous fluoride, tin difluoride, fluoristan:* Used in toothpaste and as a fluoride treatment to prevent tooth decay
- *Sulfur hexafluoride:* Gaseous electrical insulator
- *Teflon:* Non-stick compound

▌▌ FORMALDEHYDE

Formaldehyde is a potent chemical manufactured from methanol, natural gas, or lower-petroleum hydrocarbons. At normal temperatures, it is a colorless, pungent gas, which irritates the eyes, nose, and respiratory tract. Other types of formaldehyde are trioxane, a crystalline solid form of formaldehyde; paraformaldehyde, a colorless, granular form of formaldehyde with the same irritating qualities; and formalin, an aqueous solution of formaldehyde. Formalin is the major form in which formaldehyde is marketed, containing 37 to 50 percent formaldehyde, stabilized by a water solution of methanol.

Annual formaldehyde production is measured in billions of pounds. The resinous compounds formed when formaldehyde is combined with other chemicals make it particularly important commercially. It has many industrial uses:

- to set dyes
- to waterproof fabrics
- as a germicide, disinfectant, and fungicide
- in tanning and preserving hides
- in printing and photography
- in manufacturing building materials
- in manufacturing artificial silks, cellulose esters, dyes, organic chemicals, glass mirrors, explosives, and resins

Formaldehyde is a major, continuous indoor pollutant. Its odor can be sensed at levels as low as 0.05 parts per million (ppm). How much constitutes a safe level of formaldehyde exposure is the subject of debate. Most people are unaware of formaldehyde if levels are maintained at 0.1 ppm, which is the safety standard. Health hazards are associated with this level and many people are calling for the standard to be reduced, since chemically sensitive people are affected by this and lower levels.

Indoor levels of formaldehyde can vary from day to day, and from hour to hour, according to fluctuations in temperature and

Average Concentrations of Formaldehyde

SOURCE	PPM
Outside air	0.003
Textile manufacture	0.1–1.4
Clothing stores	0.13
Stores unpacking new clothing	0.14–0.25
Treated paper	0.14–0.99
Fertilizer production	0.2–1.9
Fabric stores	0.60
Mobile homes	0.80
Plywood industry	1.0–2.5
Wet biology laboratories	1.70
Hospital autopsy rooms	2.2–7.9
Cigarette smoke	50.00

humidity. When relative humidity is between 50 and 60 percent, indoor formaldehyde levels peak, while on cold days they are usually lowest. Adequate ventilation in any building is important to reduce the indoor formaldehyde level.

Concentrations of formaldehyde also depend upon the type of building construction. Mobile homes have the highest concentrations—regardless of age, a mobile home contains formaldehyde. By the time a mobile home is two years old, its formaldehyde level will have dropped 20 to 30 percent; that level will be maintained for 10 or more years. Again, indoor ventilation is extremely important to lower formaldehyde levels.

There are many sources of formaldehyde exposure in our homes. To reduce overall exposures, do not use items containing formaldehyde, such as:

- air fresheners
- cosmetics and deodorants (some)
- glues
- insecticides
- leather
- mothballs
- paints
- soaps and shampoos (some)
- spray starch
- vinyl

Because new clothes, drapery and upholstery fabrics, and electronic equipment (televisions, computers, stereos) outgas, or dissipate, a significant amount of formaldehyde, these items should be aired completely before use. Thoroughly wash new clothing before wearing it.

Carpeting is a significant, constant source of formaldehyde exposure that increases when carpets are wet. Formaldehyde is used to set the dye and added to the backing to stiffen the jute. It takes at least three years for carpet to outgas the majority of its formaldehyde. Despite the age of the carpet, however, some formaldehyde will always outgas. In recent years, manufacturers have attempted to reduce formaldehyde levels in carpet, and some have successfully done so.

Wood and composite paneling are another formaldehyde source. It takes about 18 months for paneling to outgas the major portion of formaldehyde. Like carpeting, paneling will continue to emit this chemical.

Particleboard (used in furniture, bookshelves, subflooring, home construction, and cabinet shelves) and plywood used in homes are significant formaldehyde sources. Particleboard outgases more form-aldehyde than plywood, and its release from these materials increases with moisture and heat.

Combustion produces formaldehyde. Gas stoves and heating systems, fireplaces, kerosene space heaters, and wood-burning stoves will cause problems for chemically sensitive people.

Because cigarette smoke contains extremely high concentrations of formaldehyde, chemically sensitive people should not smoke or allow smoking in their homes or cars.

Formaldehyde is also found in our food supply. Freshly caught fish may be washed with formaldehyde solution to prevent bacterial growth. Chicken may be dipped in a formaldehyde wash to whiten the skin. Formaldehyde may be used as a preservative in flour, and some maple syrup contains form-aldehyde from the pellets used on maple trees to keep taps open. Meat from animals given feed containing formaldehyde will be contaminated. At one time, formaldehyde was added to milk and eggs to increase shelf life, but this practice was discontinued due to health problems caused by this chemical exposure.

■ SYMPTOMS OF FORMALDEHYDE EXPOSURE

Formaldehyde is extremely toxic. Exposures at concentrations from 0.1 to 5 ppm can cause asthma, contact dermatitis, nausea, chronic headache, diarrhea, memory lapse, fatigue, drowsiness, eye and respiratory tract irritation, nosebleeds, dry and sore throats, insomnia, and disorientation.

Higher exposures (10 to 20 ppm) may produce coughing, tightening in the chest, a

Sources of Formaldehyde

Acrylic, wool, and nylon fibers
Adhesives
Aerated waste
Aerosol insecticides
Agricultural seeds
Air and furnace filters
Air fresheners
Animal feed
Antihistamines
Antiperspirants
Antiseptics
Anti-slip agents
Anti-static agents
Automotive exhaust
Bactericides
Barber and beauty shop disinfectants
Binders and mineral wool insulation
Binders for sand foundry cases
Binding agents for machinery casting
Binding on paper bag seams
Biology laboratories
Brake drums
Butcher paper
Buttons
Car exhaust
Carpeting
Catalytic heaters
Chalk
Chemistry laboratories
Chewing gum
Chickens (may be washed with formaldehyde to whiten the skin)
Chipboard
Cigarettes and cigarette smoke
Clothing
Clothing stores
Coated papers used for cartons and labels
Coatings for appliances
Concrete or plaster
Cosmetics
Cotton fabric (some)
Cut flower arrangements (some)
Dental fillings
Deodorants
Detergents (some)
Dialysis units
Disinfectants
Disposable sanitary products
Drapery fabrics
Dry cleaning (disinfectant in cleaning solutions)
Dyes
Electric shavers and mixers (in housing)
Electrical insulation parts
Electronic equipment
Embalming fluid
Enamels
Explosives
Fabric stores
Fabrics (used to improve color stability, wrinkle and shrink resistance, water repellency, moth proofing, and flame retardation in both synthetic and natural fabrics)
Facial tissues
Fertilizers (nitrogen)
Fiberboard
Fish (used as a preservative rinse on fresh or frozen)
Flame retardants
Flock adhesives
Floor coverings
Flour (preservative)
Foam insulation
Formica
Foundries
Fuels
Fungicides
Fur
Furniture adhesives
Gas stoves
Glass manufacturing
Glues
Gum (chewing)
Hair setting lotions
Hair permanent preparations
Hardeners
Hardware or hardware stores
Hospital bed sheets
Incinerators
Insecticides
Instant coffee
Insulation (urea-formaldehyde foam: fiberglass, and wool)

Sources of Formaldehyde

Kerosene stoves	Newsprint	Resins
Lacquers	Non-woven binders	Rubber hose production
Laminates	Nylon fabric	Sanforized cottons
Latex paint	Oil-based paints	Shampoo (some)
Lawn and garden equipment	Orthopedic casts and bandages	Soap
Leathers	Paneling	Soap dispensers
Lubricants (synthetic)	Paper products	Softeners
Maple syrup (some)	Particleboard	Solvents
Mascara	Pesticides	Sporting goods
Meat smokehouses	Phenolic thermosetting resins	Spray starch
Melamine tableware		Sterilizing solutions in barber and beauty shops
Mildew prevention	Photochemical smog	Tires
Mimeographed paper	Photographic developing solutions	Toilet seats
Mineral wool production		Toothpaste
Mobile homes	Plaster	Utensil handles
Molding compounds	Plastics	Vaccine preparation
Mothballs	Plumbing fixtures	Vinyl resins
Mouthwash	Plywood	Water filters
Mushroom farms	Polishes	Water softening chemicals
Nail hardener	Preservatives	Waxed paper
Nail polish and undercoatings	Razor blades	Waxes
	Reclaimed paper products	Wood-burning stoves
Napkins	Refrigerator hardware	Wood finishes

sense of pressure in the head, and heart palpitations. Exposures at 50 to 100 ppm and above can cause serious injury or death.

Chronic or long-term health problems remain after formaldehyde exposure stops. It is a suspected carcinogen and it may be implicated in SIDS (sudden infant death syndrome) since most infant furniture is made of particleboard. We need more research to determine the role of low-dose formaldehyde exposure in chronic health problems and cancer.

Many people are sensitive to formaldehyde. There is strong evidence that it interferes with the functioning of the immune and detoxification systems, which causes sensitivities to an increasing number of substances. This is called the spreading phenomenon. An untreated formaldehyde sensitivity becomes worse with time so that one reacts to lower formaldehyde concentrations.

Formaldehyde exposures are a greater problem for those with candidiasis (yeast in-

Sources of Glycerine

Adhesives	Freckle removal lotions	Plastics
Animal fat:	Furniture	Polishes:
Beef	Glues, cements	Floor
Chicken	Hand lotion	Furniture
Lamb	Inks:	Nail
Pork	Ballpoint pen	Shoe
Antifreezes	Copy machine	Polyurethane foam (auto
Astringents	Felt-tipped pen	dashboards, carpets, floor-
Capsules (soft gelatin)	Permanent marking	ing, furniture, mattresses,
Coconut	Printers' ink	pads, seat cushions)
Cosmetics (especially cake	Rubber stamp	Regenerated cellulose
or compact form)	Stamp pad	Shaving creams and lotions
Cough drops	Water-soluble	Shortenings
Disinfectant	Latex paints	Soaps
Dry-cleaning agent	Leather	Solvents
Emollients	Margarines	Styptic pencils
Eye drops	Modeling clay	Suntan preparations
Fabric softeners	Mouthwashes	Textile finishes
Face masks	Oven cleaners	Tobacco
Fire retardant for textiles	Paper	Toothpastes
Flavorings	Perfume	Window cleaners
Food additives	Pharmaceuticals	

fection) because the aldehyde detoxification pathway is already overloaded.

❚❚ GLYCERINE

Glycerine—also called glycerol—is a clear, thick liquid about half as sweet as cane sugar. As the base of fat and oil molecules, it is a familiar chemical to our body, which uses glycerine as a source of energy or as a starting material for making more complex molecules. Many foods naturally contain glycerine. Any foods from which oil can be extracted, such as corn, peanuts, safflower, coconut, and animal fat, contain natural glycerine. It can also be processed from hydrocarbons.

Glycerine is used extensively in the food industry. Because it is a humectant (absorbs water from the air), manufacturers add it to foods to maintain a specific moisture content and to prevent foods from drying out and becoming hard. Glycerine is used as a humectant in tobacco, marshmallows, pastilles, and jelly-like candies. Glycerine is a solvent for oily chemicals, especially flavorings, which are not water-soluble. Glycerine serves as a bodying agent in combination with gelatins and edible gums and as a plas-

Forms of Petrochemicals

Solid	Plastics
	Synthetic fibers
	Wax coatings on fruits and vegetables
Liquid	Diesel oil
	Gasoline
	Other oil products
Gas	Natural and bottled gas
	Fumes from solids such as plastics
	Fumes from liquids such as gasoline
	Odors from soaps, perfumes, scented stationery, cleaning compounds, polishes, paints, and insecticides
	Oil evaporating from electric motors in household appliances
	Exhaust from automobiles and buses
	Fumes from chemicals used in copying or duplicating machines, inks, newspapers, typewriters, cosmetics, fabric softener sheets, medications, hair products, lipsticks

ticizer in edible meat and cheese coatings. Beverages, liqueurs, confections, baked goods, chewing gum, gelatin desserts, meat products, and fudge toppings all contain glycerine.

Glycerine is also used in the manufacture of nitroglycerine (dynamite); cosmetics; liquid soaps; blackening, printing, and copying inks; lubricants; elastic glues; and lead oxide. It helps to keep fabrics pliable, preserve printing on cotton, and to keep windshields frost-free. Glycerine is also found in automobile antifreeze, gas meters, hydraulic jacks, and shock-absorber fluid, and is used as a fermentation nutrient in antibiotic production.

In the cosmetics industry, glycerine is used in many products—read the labels! Glycerine is absorbed through the skin. Mixed with water or some other suitable liquid, glycerine acts as a moisturizing agent when applied to skin. However, rather than acting as a humectant, glycerine first draws whatever moisture it can from the skin's underlying tissues. As long as glycerine is applied, the external skin surface will have some semblance of elasticity and softness, but when the applications cease, the skin takes on a dry, raspy feel. Any preparation containing glycerine can be damaging to delicate skin tissues.

▌▌ PETROCHEMICALS

Petrochemicals are compounds produced by distilling crude oil. They may be solids, liquids, or gases.

Exposure to petrochemicals usually occurs through inhalation, skin contact, or ingestion of foods that contain them. Exposure can occur both in and away from the home. Odors from nearby gas stations, garages, storage tanks, refineries, and producing wells can affect sensitive people both indoors and outdoors. Driving a car or filling the gas tank is a petrochemical exposure that should be minimized as much as possible.

▮▮ ETHANOL (ALCOHOL)

In many petrochemical environmental exposures, ethanol is a common denominator. It is a clear, colorless liquid that has a pleasant odor and a burning taste. Industrial ethanol is synthetic, while "organic" ethanol, also called ethyl alcohol or grain alcohol, is made by fermenting such natural substances as grains (corn, barley, rice, rye), sugars (molasses, cane sugar, any sweet fruit juice), and potatoes. Ethanol makes up the alcohol content in liquors.

Whether organic or synthetic, ethanol can cause central nervous system depression, anesthesia, feelings of exhilaration and talkativeness, impaired motor coordination, dizziness, flushing, nausea, vomiting, drowsiness, headache, wheezing, vision problems, impaired perception, disorientation, stupor, coma, and death. Alcohol is rapidly absorbed through the gastric and intestinal mucosa, and it can magnify an allergic reaction four times. Ethanol forms naturally in the intestinal tract from the fermentation of sugar, alcohol, and simple carbohydrates. It is formed in excess in the lower bowel by the action of *Candida albicans*.

▮ SOURCES OF PETROCHEMICALS AND/OR ETHANOL

Because of their widespread use, it is impossible to provide a brand-name listing of all products containing petrochemicals and ethanol. Although reading labels helps, an ingredients label is not required on most of these products. When in doubt, consider a product to be of petrochemical origin until you can obtain more information from the manufacturer.

Ethanol neutralizing extracts are helpful both in preventing and alleviating symptoms caused by a petrochemical or ethanol exposure. Hands-on treatment for ethanol or petrochemicals is also helpful.

▮ GASOLINE EXHAUST

Emissions from automobiles (gasoline exhaust) have long been considered a prime source of pollutants involved in smog formation and ozone production. A large percentage of these emissions is composed of hydrocarbons. These hydrocarbon emissions can be divided into three classes, each class containing several compounds: paraffins; olefins; and aromatics.

Automobiles also emit some unburned fuel hydrocarbons, carbon, a small amount of sulfur (an impurity in gasoline), and tars (heavy, poor-burning components of gasoline and oils). The carbon combines with oxygen to form carbon monoxide. Similarly, the sulfur combines with oxygen to form sulfur dioxide, some of which is emitted from automobiles as an air pollutant. A larger percentage of sulfur dioxide is released by fossil-fuel burning plants.

Before lead was banned from gasoline in 1995, tiny specks of lead also floated out of exhaust systems along with lead bromide, which escaped as a gas. Lead can cause anemia, kidney disease, mental retardation, blindness, and death. Although enough lead

Sources of Petrochemicals

Air fresheners
Alcoholic beverages
Anesthetics
Baked goods
Bath oils
Beverages
Bubble bath
Butane
Candy
Catalytic heaters
Cigarette smoke
Cleaning agents containing
  naphtha
Coal heat
Colognes
Copy machines
Cosmetics
Deodorants
Detergents
Diesel oil
Dried fruits
Dyes derived from coal tar
Exhaust fumes
Explosives
Face creams
Facial tissue
Fireplaces
Flavoring agents
Frozen pizza crust
Fruits (all sprayed, even if
  scrubbed and peeled)
Fumes from:
  Any engine that burns
    petrochemicals
  Any motor lubricated
    with machine oil (electric
    mixers, sewing machines)
  Buses

Cars
Lawnmowers
Outboard motors
Trucks
Garage fumes
Gas appliances (propane
  and natural gas stoves,
  ranges, water heaters,
  refrigerators, dryers, oil
  or gas furnaces and
  space heaters, and the
  pilot light for any gas
  appliance)
Gasoline
Gelatin desserts
Glycerol
Hair care products
Hair pomades
Hand lotions
Ice cream
Ink
Insecticides
Kerosene
Lighter fluid
Lip balm
Lipstick
Liquors
Lotions
Machine oil
Meat (stored in the
  animal's fat cells)
Metal polish
Mineral oil
Mineral spirits
Motor oil
Nail polish and polish
  remover
Newsprint

Oil heat (furnaces)
Oil in electric appliances
Paints and stains
Paraffin
Perfume
Petroleum jelly
Photographic film
Pine scent
Plastics
Polyester
Preparation of:
  Essences
  Tinctures
  Extracts
Printers' ink (newsprint)
Propane gas
Rubber
Rubbing alcohol
Sauces
Soaps
Space heaters
Spray propellants
Stationery
Sterilization of medical
  instruments
Synthetic fibers
Tires
Toilet tissue
Varnish
Vaseline
Vegetables (all sprayed,
  especially the cabbage
  family)
Wax-coated fruits and
  vegetables
Wax-coated paper cups
Waxes
Wood-burning byproduct

was not emitted to kill anyone, its accumulation was a health hazard for urban children who put things that have touched the street into their mouths. Lead accumulations still exist in soil close to heavy traffic areas.

Ammonia, organic acids, and solids, including zinc and metallic oxides, are also found in gasoline exhaust. Gasolines also contain antioxidants, metal deactivators, anti-rust and anti-icing compounds, detergents, and lubricants. Fragments of these compounds are also found in exhaust.

Sensitivity to gasoline exhaust can cause sleepiness; mental confusion and loss of reasoning ability; loss of memory; headache; nausea; dizziness; paranoia; anger; irritation of eyes, nose, and throat; and wheezing and coughing. Many of the components of exhaust are fat-soluble and have a special affinity for the nervous system. The most important route into the body for the chemical composition of exhaust is through the nasal passages. The smell receptors of the brain are located directly behind the uppermost cavities in the nose.

▌ DIESEL EXHAUST

Diesel exhaust odors and irritants are generally considered to be nuisance pollutants. However, diesel exhaust is a potent allergen for many people. Symptoms caused by diesel exhaust exposure include nausea; headache; cough; disturbances of sleep, digestion, and appetite; irritation of eyes, nose, and throat; and mental confusion. Diesel oil is composed chiefly of aliphatic hydrocarbons, but amyl nitrate is added to raise octane and improve fuel ignition.

Operating conditions affect chemical emissions; for example, as a diesel engine goes from idle to high speed, full load emissions are reduced. There are two sources of odors in diesel engines: unburned fuel and its thermal breakdown products (hydrocarbons and some nitrogen compounds); and products of incomplete combustion.

Nitrogen dioxide, sulfuric acid, formaldehyde, acrolein, and phenol are also present in diesel exhaust and are known to act as irritants. Other aldehydes in addition to formaldehyde are also present. The total aldehyde level in diesel exhaust is frequently higher than levels known to produce irritation.

Wearing a charcoal mask is helpful in reducing exposures, as is using an automobile air cleaner. Auto hydrocarbon, ethanol, formaldehyde, and phenol extracts are available from some physicians and are effective in controlling symptoms to vehicular exhaust. The extracts should be used daily, and extra doses should be taken when one is exposed to heavy traffic conditions. Hands-on allergy treatments for hydrocarbons are also helpful.

▌ PHENOL

Phenol or carbolic acid is a colorless, crystalline solid that absorbs water from the air to become a liquid. It is poisonous and caustic, with a sharp burning taste. In weak solution, it has a mild, sweet taste and is a component of coal tar and wood odor.

Several phenols occur naturally. Natural phenol is part of the toxic agent in poison ivy and poison oak. It may also be present in spring water as a result of humus or natural coal around the spring.

Phenol is rapidly absorbed through the skin. It can cause skin eruptions, peeling,

Phenol Derivatives

Coal tar	Hexachlorophene	Pine tar
Creosote	Hexylresorcinol	Resorcinol
Cresols (ortho, meta, and para)	Juniper tar	Trinitrophenol (Picric acid)
	Parachlorophenol	

Sources of Phenol

Aftershave
Allergy extracts (some)
Aluminum foil (the plastic on the dull side outgases phenol when heated; put shiny side against foods)
Antiseptics
Aspirin and other medications
Bakelite (molded articles, such as telephones, toys)
Bronchial mists
Calamine lotion
Canned foods (the golden liner in the can contains phenol)
Carbolated vaseline
Chloraseptic (lozenges, mouthwash, spray)
Cleaning products
  Cosmetics (especially Revlon products):
  Cream blushes
  Liquid eyeliner
  Mascara
Deodorants, scented
Detergents
Dyes
Epoxy

Equal (sugar substitute— has a phenol ring in its chemical structure)
Explosives
Gasoline additives
Hair products:
  Dyes
  Hairsprays
  Setting lotions
  Shampoos
Hand lotion
Herbicides and pesticides
Laminated boards
Lysol, Lysol spray
Nasal sprays (Afrin, Neo-Synephrine)
Newsprint
NutraSweet (has a phenol ring in its chemical structure)
Nylon
Ointments (first aid cream, etc.)
Over-the-counter drugs:
  Antihistamines
  Aspirin
  Cold capsules
  Cough syrups
  Decongestants
  Eye drops

Perfumes (all):
  Aftershave
  Deodorants
  Hand lotion
  Powder
Pesticides
Phenolic resins (hard plastics that outgas phenol vapors when warmed— TV sets, computers, radios)
Photography solutions
Pine Sol
Plastic coatings on electric wires
Plastic dishes and wraps (when heated in microwave)
Polyurethane
Preservatives in medications
Refrigerator storage dishes
Scotch tape
Sunscreens and suntan lotions
Thermal insulation panels
Vaccines
Wallpaper (vinyl-coated)
Waterbeds

Chemically Similar Compounds

Benzene	latum, Vick's Vaporub,	Ethyl
Benzoic acid (widely used in	menthol cigarettes)	Methyl
foods and beverages)	p-dichlorobenzene (moth-	Propyl
Benzoin	balls, moth crystals)	Toluene
Camphor	Parabens:	Xylene (xylol)
Menthol (BenGay, Mentho-	Butyl	

swelling, hives, burning, numbness, nausea, vomiting, cold sweats, headache, irritability, and wheezing. More serious effects of phenol exposure include gangrene, circulatory collapse, respiratory failure, paralysis, convulsions, coma, and death. It is also a suspected carcinogen.

Half of the total production of phenol is used in the manufacture of plastics. One-quarter goes toward manufacturing medications of coal tar origin, such as aspirin and sulfa drugs. Phenol is often used as a preservative in many injectable medications, including some allergy extracts. It is also used in producing nylon. Thyme oil, a compound chemically similar to phenol, is used in producing menthol. Thyme oil is also used to flavor toothpastes and mouthwashes. Phenol-sensitive people may have to avoid these products.

Any product that has been manufactured with phenol will later outgas the chemical, which means that phenol is a major environmental exposure in our air, food, medications, and surroundings at home and work. Common phenol exposures include phenol emissions from computers, televisions, plastics, waterbeds, cleaning products, and newsprint.

Those who are allergic to phenol should also avoid phenol derivatives and chemically similar compounds. If you (or any member of your family) are phenol-sensitive, it is very important that no member of the family wear perfume, aftershave, or cologne. Avoid phenol exposures away from home as much as possible. A phenol neutralizing extract can provide relief from symptoms resulting from unavoidable phenol or phenol-derivative exposures, as can hands-on treatment.

■ SOURCES OF PHENOL

Usage is so widespread that it is impossible to list all brand-name products containing phenol, phenol derivatives, or chemically similar compounds. Read labels! Do not use products containing the chemically similiar compounds if you are sensitive to phenol. If you are not certain whether a product is phenol-free, do not use it. In some cases, you may need to write to the manufacturer for confirmation.

■■ BUILDING MATERIALS

Building a new home or remodeling an existing one can be an enormous problem for a chemically sensitive person. Most building materials are a chemical exposure, and many commonly used materials are a problem for some chemically sensitive people. However, with care and thorough investigation, finding safe building materials that will allow construction or remodeling of your home is possible. The following materials are a few examples of building materials that can be a toxic exposure for all people, including chemically sensitive people. (See chapter 12 for suggestions and alternatives.)

▮ LUMBER
Lumber can be treated with arsenic compounds and other preservatives. The common woods used—spruce, pine, and fir—can emit high levels of terpenes.

▮ PLYWOOD, PARTICLEBOARD, CHIPBOARD, AND PANELING
These wood products contain formaldehyde and phenolic compounds that will outgas for years. The glues holding these products together can also be toxic.

▮ INSULATION AND VAPOR BARRIERS
All insulation is toxic to a degree, and must be used with a vapor barrier. Fiberglass batts can contain fungicides and pesticides, and foam insulation can emit toxic chemicals when heated.

Vapor barriers are used over studs on sidewalls and ceiling joists. It protects indoor air from odors that could vaporize from wall cavities and attics. Some plastic vapor barriers emit toxic chemicals.

▮ WALL COVERINGS
The most widely used wall treatment is sheetrock, also called drywall or plasterboard. Although it is economical and generally well tolerated, some brands have been treated with fire retardant chemicals. Joint compound is used to tape and texture drywall. Many typical commercial joint compound products are toxic and will outgas

formaldehyde, as well as containing fungicides and preservatives.

Wallpaper (and all paper) is a formaldehyde exposure. In addition, vinyl wallpaper emits phenolic compounds. Many sensitive people do not tolerate Mylar-covered foil wallpaper.

Some wallpapers are self-adhesive. The wallpaper paste needed to apply other wallpapers may contain dextrin, animal glue, sodium bicarbonate, aluminum sulfate, bentonite, methyl alcohol or vinyl acetate. They may also contain fungicides and mildew killers.

▮ FLOORING
Carpets can contain formaldehyde, dyes, and stain repellents. Some carpets may emit toxic chemicals as they deteriorate. The typical foam padding used under most carpets emits toxic fumes.

Soft vinyl flooring can have high levels of odor that take several months to outgas. The grout used in laying tile floors is toxic to some people if it contains latex.

▮ PAINTS AND SEALANTS
Latex paints are lower in odor than sealants, but do not seal as well as may be needed for sensitive people. They contain fungicides and preservatives called biocides that can outgas for several years. Alkyd paints are toxic when first applied and can take three months or longer to air. However, they can seal surfaces and when cured form a hard and durable surface. Alcohol-based primers also seal surfaces. Their initial odor is quite strong, but it dissipates rapidly. Alcohol-based primers can take from six weeks to two months to outgas.

Clear sealants, such as silicones, urethanes, and acrylics, are useful, but are not tolerated by some people. Clear acrylic wood sealants are tolerated in some instances, and shellac is another possibility. However, alcohol-based shellac does not hold up well if washed. Urethane varnish is very toxic when applied, and can take nearly a year to outgas. Once cured, it makes a durable floor finish.

▮▮ JEWELRY AND METAL ALLERGY

A metal allergy is a special type of chemical allergy that usually manifests as contact dermatitis (a skin rash that develops after touching the metal). The metal itself may not be toxic, but a person may be hypersensitive to the metal. Metals that can cause reactions include chromium, cobalt, copper, iron, nickel, and mercury. Mercury is, of course, an extremely toxic metal. (See Dental Care for the Allergic Person section in chapter 22 for more information on mercury.)

Nickel is the most common metal cause of contact dermatitis. As our perspiration dissolves the metal, it attaches to our cells. Bonded to the cells, the nickel prompts symptoms long after the offending object has been removed.

One out of 10 women are nickel-sensitive, usually because they have had their ears pierced. Women with allergic tendencies should wear high-quality gold or stainless steel posts and wires. Stainless steel does contain nickel, but is tightly bound and perspiration cannot cause its release. Some women can wear sterling silver, but silver also tends to corrode in the presence of perspiration. There have been cases reported of women who developed dermatitis from the internal use of metal containing a minute amount of nickel (for example, stainless steel surgical sutures and copper-7 IUDs). Some nickel-sensitive women react to the metal hooks on their bras.

On some people, metal jewelry tends to turn dark or leave black marks on the skin. This is not an allergic reaction to the metal, but rather an indication that the person's pH (acid/base) levels are too acidic. This phenomenon can occur even with expensive gold jewelry if the person's system is extremely acidic. Such acidity can be a strong indication that the person has an allergy problem to other substances.

The following items are common causes of contact dermatitis:
• bra clips
• bracelets
• buckles
• buttons
• clips
• costume jewelry
• earrings
• frames for metal glasses
• garter clips
• necklaces
• rings
• snaps
• scissors
• thimbles
• watch bands
• watches
• zippers

▮▮ LATEX ALLERGY

Latex is natural rubber, a milky fluid obtained from tapping the rubber tree *Hevea brasiliensis*. More than five million tons of latex are produced each year. The elastic properties are utilized in many products, including tires, elastic clothing, erasers, gloves, and many other items. It is treated to prevent deterioration, forming a complex mixture with several new allergens in addition to latex. Latex products may contain a wide variety of petrochemicals, including organic solvents and polymers of chemicals, such as styrene and vinyl acetate. These chemicals can also cause allergic and chemical sensitivity reactions. Dipped latex materials such as balloons and gloves are more allergenic than molded latex products. The powder from latex gloves contains latex particles and can cause symptoms.

The development of latex allergy depends on genetics. In addition, people who have had surgery on the nervous system, spine, or genitourinary tract are more prone to latex allergy. Healthcare workers, medical housekeeping staff, or dental workers are at high risk to develop latex allergies because of their frequent exposure.

Latex allergy symptoms can vary from hives or itching from contact, to runny nose, red eyes, and fatal anaphylaxis. Healthcare workers with latex allergy may have to quit work because of their symptoms, or change tasks. Some employees continue at their jobs despite having symptoms. For sensitive employees to continue to work, both they and co-workers must use nonpowdered latex or nonlatex gloves made of plastic or vinyl, and other nonlatex products.

The most common exposure to latex is rubber gloves. Their use has increased dramatically in recent years, particularly for protection against communicable diseases. Even though glove manufacturers knew

Latex Cross-Reactivity

Latex allergies cross-react with certain foods, including avocados, bananas, chestnuts, kiwi, papaya, and pineapple. Researchers are now finding cross-reactions between latex and additional foods. The American College of Allergy has warned people with latex allergies to be wary of raw almonds, apples, apricots, carrots, celery, cherries, citrus fruits, coconuts, dill, figs, ginger, hazelnuts, mangos, melons, oregano, passion fruit, peaches, peanuts, pears, peppers, plums, potatoes, sage, and tomatoes.

about serious adverse reactions to gloves as early as 1991, they did not put warning labels on their products until 1998 when the Food and Drug Administration mandated that they do so. Not only do healthcare workers wear latex gloves, but restaurant workers and food handlers frequently wear gloves. Latex-sensitive people have had allergic reactions to food prepared by workers wearing latex gloves.

The second biggest latex exposure comes from environmental exposure to latex tire-wear fragments. Latex allergens can be demonstrated near highways, and the concentrations on highways are quite high during rush hour. Higher rates of asthma in people who live near busy streets may be due in part to the presence of large quantities of latex particles.

There are over 40,000 products made from latex. Many of them can cause problems for the latex sensitive. One three-

Sources of Latex

Adhesives	Elastic bands	Postage stamps
Balloons	Elasticized clothing	Rubber bands
Bandages	Ear syringes	Rubber boots
Band-Aids	Enema bags	Rubber dams for dental
Blood pressure cuffs	Erasers	work
Carpets (backing)	Face masks	Rubber stoppers
Catheters	Foam rubber	Shoe soles
Condoms	Gloves used by physicians,	Sports equipment
Diaphragms	dentists, and healthcare	Stethoscope tubing
Dishwashing gloves	workers	Swimsuits
Douche bags	Pacifiers	Tires

month-old baby had an unexplained chronic cough until her latex pacifier was changed to a silicon pacifier. Her cough then disappeared. Rubber chemicals are a common cause of foot dermatitis in children. Elastic in clothing can trigger rashes and urticaria (hives) in latex-sensitive people. Some people also react to chewing gum, which has a similar structure to latex.
Sources of Latex

▮▮ COSMETICS AND TOILETRIES

Cosmetics and toiletries have been used in some form throughout history. Early cosmetics and toiletries included simple unguents, and lotions made from flowers, fruits, vegetables and herbs. Some unlucky people even tried arsenic and lead, leading to their deaths.

Today's cosmetics and toiletries are formulated in chemical laboratories and contain harmful ingredients that have caused illnesses, injuries, and allergies. Despite their harsh contents, they are glamorized, advertised, and made irresistible so that the consumer ignores warnings that they may be unsafe. It was not until 1976 that the Food and Drug Administration (FDA) required the contents of cosmetics to be labeled. Even now, fragrances and trade secrets are exempt from this requirement.

Many chemically sensitive people have problems with cosmetics and toiletries. Personal care products, unless selected carefully, can be a constant source of chemical exposure. The scents as well as the skin contact pose problems for the chemically sensitive person. Some people must avoid cosmetics and toiletries totally; others are able to use some carefully selected products. Personal care products worn by others can also affect the chemically sensitive. Desensitizing extracts of ethanol, phenol, benzyl alcohol, and orris root provide prevention of and relief from allergic reactions to many cosmetics and toiletries, as do hands-on allergy treatments for specific chemicals and products.

■ PERFUMES

One reaction-causing substance, alone or as part of other products, is perfume, or fragrance. At one time perfumes were used to cover the smell of disease or the lack of personal hygiene. For centuries, only the rich could afford perfume. With the introduction of synthetic fragrance materials in the 1800s, more and more people began using perfumes.

Perfumery is considered an art, and much secrecy surrounds the industry. Formulas cannot be patented, and the "trade secrets" law protects them. Ingredients do not have to be listed—only the word "fragrance" needs to appear on the label. There are three basic types of perfumes:

- Essences or extracts, which are referred to as perfume, usually contain 10 to 20 percent perfume or essential oil dissolved in alcohol.
- Colognes contain 3 to 5 percent perfume oil dissolved in 80 to 90 percent alcohol, with the remainder being water.
- Toilet waters are 2 percent perfume oil in 60 to 80 percent alcohol, with the remainder being water.

Perfume oils or essential oils, used as the scents in perfumes, are obtained by a variety of processes from leaves, needles, roots, peels, whole flowers, petals, gums, and resins of plants. Essential oils usually carry the taste and smell of the original plant, and most of them are easily vaporized. A large number have antiseptic, germicidal, and preservative properties, but are used primarily for their scent.

Orris root, a highly allergenic substance,

No Such Thing As Nonallergenic

Hypoallergenic products are supposedly free of irritants and allergens, but they still contain potentially harmful chemicals. The FDA admits that there are no official standards for hypoallergenic products, other than that they must be less likely to cause adverse reactions than other similar products. While manufacturers of natural cosmetics genuinely try to make health and beauty products that are superior, due to individual sensitivities these products can still cause problems. There is no such thing as a nonallergenic cosmetic. Reading labels is as critical with cosmetics as with other products.

obtained from the root of the iris plant, is the oldest, most widely used, and most expensive ingredient used in perfumes.

Animal exudates, formerly used in perfumes, were obtained by slow evaporation of substances such as castor from the beaver, musk from the male musk deer, ambergris from the sperm whale, and civet from the civet cat. Synthetic chemicals that simulate natural aromas are now usually used in perfumes, and petrochemicals and coal tar are the source of raw materials for still other chemicals added to them.

Most perfumes are blends of flower oils, animal substances, synthetic chemicals, alcohol, and water. Alcohol is added to animal or plant substances and heated; water is used for dilution. Alcohols used include benzyl alcohol, methanol, and ethanol. Some perfumes have as many as 200 ingredients blended to create their "special" scent.

The substances found in a perfume relate to its usage. Expensive perfumes contain rare flower oils, whereas inexpensive perfumes and perfumes in soap come from artificial materials. Perfume aromas usually last longer than toilet waters and colognes, but there is no standard to dictate how much perfume oil must be used for a product to qualify as a perfume.

Synthetic materials and modern chemical analysis have made fragrances available at a fraction of their original cost. Fragrances are now found in products other than perfumes, colognes, and toilet waters. Shampoos, cream rinses, lotions, makeup, powders, soaps of all kinds, fabric softeners, detergents, deodorants, aftershaves, and many other products now contain fragrance.

Perfumes and fragrances are frequent allergens and are deleted from hypoallergenic products. Allergic symptoms from perfume exposure include headaches, dizziness, rash, hyperpigmentation, violent coughing, vomiting, skin irritation, and asthma. Perfumed ads in magazines can cause asthma and other symptoms.

■ LIPSTICKS

Lipsticks are a mixture of oil and wax in stick form with staining dyes, pigments, flavorings, and perfumes dispensed in oil. Typical lipstick formulas contain:

65 percent castor oil
15 percent beeswax
10 percent carnauba wax
5 percent lanolin
soluble dyes
insoluble pigments
perfume

Frosted lipsticks also include a pearlizing agent. Sheer lipsticks contain transparent coloring and no indelible dyes to create a more natural look. Medicated lipsticks, which treat or prevent chapping, usually contain petrolatum, mineral wax, and oils. Color-changing lipsticks contain iodine.

Many women suffer lip peeling caused by lipstick allergies. Sensitizing lipstick ingredients cause lips to react to the sun, become irritated, then crack and bleed. Even hypoallergenic lipsticks can cause these problems. Lipstick reactions reported to the FDA include burns, cracks, excessive dryness, lacerations, numbness, rash, and swollen gums.

Lip balms and gloss made from beeswax and vegetable or nut oils will prevent chapped lips and aid healing. Vitamin A and D ointment is also soothing and healing for chapped, peeling, or cracked lips.

■ FOUNDATION MAKEUP

Foundation makeup is used to cover blemishes, to control skin oiliness, to protect skin from wind and cold, and to give a healthy appearance to skin.

Pigmented foundation creams, which tint and cover the skin, are 50 percent water and contain:

• mineral oil
• stearic acid
• lanolin
• cetyl alcohol
• propylene glycol
• triethanolamine

- borax
- insoluble pigments

Foundation may also contain emulsifiers, detergents, humectants, lanolin derivatives, perfumes, preservatives, thickeners, and waxes.

Allergic symptoms caused by foundation makeup include rashes or itching on the face, arms, and chest; swollen eyes; inflammation; and skin swelling and eruptions.

▮ ROUGE

Rouge is one of the earliest types of makeup and is intended to give the wearer a rosy, healthy look. It usually contains synthetic ferric oxide, which occurs naturally as rust.

Cake rouge may contain:

- talc
- kaolin
- brilliant red pigment
- zinc oxide
- zinc stearate
- liquid petrolatum
- tragacanth (plant gum)
- mucilage
- perfume

Cream rouge contains:

- erythrosine for coloring
- stearic acid
- cetyl alcohol
- potassium hydroxide
- glycerine
- water
- sorbitol
- lanolin
- mineral oil
- color pigment
- perfume
- carnauba wax

- ozokerite (hydrocarbon mixture)
- isopropyl palmitate
- titanium dioxide
- talc
- petrolatum

Although consumer complaints about rouge are not common, eye irritation and fungal contamination have been reported.

▮ POWDERS

Face powder is applied at the end of the makeup process to remove shine. It may be loose or compacted. Talc is the principal ingredient, but face powders also contain:

- clay
- kaolin
- calcium carbonate
- zinc oxide
- zinc stearate
- magnesium carbonate
- pigments
- barium sulfate
- boric acid
- cetyl alcohol
- titanium dioxide
- rice starch or cornstarch
- perfume

Dusting powders, used after a bath or shower for absorbing moisture, contain talc, perfumes, and zinc stearate. Powders can cause irritation and breathing difficulties from prolonged inhalation and mechanical blocking of the pores.

▮ EYE SHADOW

Eye shadow is used to color the lid and area under the eyebrow. Eye shadows may contain:

- titanium dioxide
- petrolatum
- lanolin

- beeswax
- aluminum
- ceresin
- calcium carbonate
- mineral oil
- sorbitan oleate
- talc

Eye irritation is a common complaint arising from eyeshadow use. Eye shadows are easily contaminated by bacteria both in the factory and by the user.

▋ MASCARA

Mascara is used for coloring eyelashes, and it contains insoluble pigments, carnauba wax, triethanolamine stearate, paraffin, and lanolin. Other ingredients include:

- beeswax
- cetyl alcohol
- mineral oil
- glyceryl monostearate
- gums
- perfume
- vegetable oils
- preservatives
- isopropyl myristate

The newer lash extenders contain tiny fibers of rayon or nylon that make lashes appear longer and thicker.

Mascara may cause allergic reactions and is easily contaminated by bacteria, which may result in eye infections. Eye infections can be passed to another person when mascara is shared.

▋ HAIR SPRAY

Hair spray is used by both men and women to hold hair in place. In the past, hair spray contained insect shellac, alcohol, perfume, triethanolamine, and water. These sprays caused the hair to shine, but made it brittle.

Today's hair sprays contain polyvinyl-pyrrolidone (PVP) dissolved in glycerine with perfume, polyethylene glycol, cetyl alcohol, and lanolin. Pressurized hair sprays contain:

- PVP
- alcohol
- sorbitol
- water
- lanolin
- perfume
- shellac
- silicone
- sodium alginate
- gums
- freon

Hair sprays can cause headaches, dizziness, tinnitus, hair loss, rash, change in hair color, eye and lung damage, and throat irritation.

▋ SHAMPOO

Coconut, castille, and glycerine soaps were originally used to wash hair. Shampoos are relatively new, and today there are many different types. Liquid shampoo, the most popular, usually contains:

- sodium lauryl sulfate
- triethanolamine dodecylbenzene sulfonate
- Ethanolamide of lauric acid
- Perfume
- Water

Cream shampoo contains the same ingredients as liquid shampoo, but has added lanolin. Sequestering agents, finishing and conditioning agents, antiseptics and preservatives may also be added to shampoos.

Problems with shampoos include eye irritation; scalp irritation and itching; loss of hair; hardened hair; split and frizzy hair; shortness of breath; and swelling of the hands, face, and arms.

■ PERMANENT WAVE SOLUTIONS
Permanents bend or curl hair. At one time, permanents were available only at beauty shops, but home kits have been available for many years. Both at home and in beauty shops, a waving solution is applied that contains:
• thioglycolic acid
• ammonia
• water
• borax
• ethanolamine
• sodium lauryl sulfate

After the desired amount of curl is obtained, a neutralizing solution is applied. These solutions contain:
• sodium or potassium bromate
• sodium perborate
• hydrogen peroxide

Thioglycolates may cause skin irritation and low blood sugar. Other injuries reported from permanent wave use include hair damage; swelling of legs and feet; eye irritations; rash around the ears, neck, scalp, and forehead; and swelling of the eyelids.

■ HAIR COLORING
Permanent hair coloring changes the color of the hair and cannot be shampooed away. It remains until the hair grows out or is cut off. The roots must be retouched as the hair grows out. There are three types of these hair colors: natural organics, synthetics, and metallics.

Natural organic hair colorings include henna and chamomile. These dyes are more difficult to apply and are considered less reliable and less predictable for color than manufactured dyes. Some allergic reactions have been reported.

Synthetic dyes contain compounds such as para- or amino derivatives that work with the action of hydrogen peroxide or similar compounds to liberate oxygen. These dyes frequently cause skin rashes and allergic skin reactions. Patch testing is suggested to determine compatibility.

Metallic hair dyes contain a metal, usually lead, silver, or copper, and the color develops gradually with each use. They tend to dull the hair and must be used daily over a week or so to change the hair color. Men frequently use this type of dye for coloring hair, moustaches, and beards. However, they are not recommended for moustaches because of the danger of metal inhalation or ingestion, which can be toxic. Scalp irritation, hair breakage and loss, contact dermatitis, swelling of the face, and itching have been reported from the use of metallic hair dyes.

Temporary hair colorings are applied as rinses, gels, mousses, and sprays. They sit on the surface of the hair and wash out with subsequent shampooing.

These rinses contain:
• azo dyes
• citric or tartaric acid
• borax
• glycols
• amides
• isopropyl alcohol

They can cause allergic reactions and

swelling of the face and scalp, ear numbness, and headaches, as well as hair turning the wrong color. Eye damage is the greatest danger.

▌ HAND CREAMS AND LOTIONS

Hand creams and lotions are emollients that soften the skin. To increase consumer appeal, they must apply easily without being sticky, and have a pleasant odor. Most of them have a pH of 5 to 8. Hand creams contain:

    2 percent cetyl alcohol
    2 percent mineral oil
    1 percent lanolin
    13 percent stearic acid
    12 percent glycerine
    0.15 percent methylparaben
    1 percent potassium hydroxide
    68 percent water
    perfume

Hand lotions contain:

    0.5 percent cetyl alcohol
    1 percent lanolin
    3 percent stearic acid
    2 percent glycerine
    0.1 percent methylparaben
    0.75 percent triethanolamine
    85 percent water
    perfume

Rashes, blisters, peeling skin, and swollen hands and feet have resulted from the use of hand creams and lotions.

▌ NAIL POLISH AND REMOVERS

Nail products are used not only to color the nails, but also to give them a shiny surface and to keep them from breaking or chipping. The removers are used to take off the polish as desired.

Nail polishes contain:

- cellulose nitrate
- butyl acetate
- ethyl acetate
- toluene
- dibutyl phthalate
- alkyl esters
- dyes
- glycol derivatives
- gums
- hydrocarbons
- ketones
- pigments
- phosphoric acid
- D & C red #19 or #31 are commonly used for coloring.

Skin rashes of the eyelids and neck are common allergic symptoms to nail polish. Complaints to the FDA include reports of nail area irritation, discolored nails, nails permanently stained black, splitting and peeling of nails, cracking of the cuticle with subsequent infections, headaches, dizziness, and nausea.

Nail polish remover is highly volatile and is even more damaging. It contains:

- acetone
- toluene
- alcohol
- amyl acetate
- butyl acetate
- benzene
- ethyl acetate
- castor oil
- lanolin
- cetyl alcohol
- olive oil
- perfume
- synthetic oil

Many of these components are extremely

toxic and can cause central nervous system depression.

▌ ARTIFICIAL NAILS

Artificial nails are used to give natural nails the appearance of long, undamaged fingernails. In addition to improving the appearance of very short nails, they are also used to camouflage thickened and malformed nails. There are several types, the most common of which are made from materials used by dentists to fill teeth. They come in three types: press-on, preglued, and forms requiring glue application.

The basic ingredients of the nails include:
• methyl methacrylate
• catalysts
• plasticizers

The glues used are acrylic glues, usually a methacrylate-based glue. Stronger adhesives can provide better adhesion, but are difficult to separate from the nail bed and can cause it to split into layers.

Skin irritation, contact dermatitis, and nail damage can result from the use of artificial nails.

Another type of artificial nail is the sculptured nail. These nails are more natural-looking and are custom-made by sculpting on a template attached to the natural nail bed. The nails are formed from acrylic mixed with a number of substances. Nail damage can occur from allowing the acrylic to enter the nail fold and from fungal, viral, and bacterial infections caused by failure to sterilize the equipment and to apply antimicrobial solution to the nail bed.

Contact dermatitis is a possibility for both the operators applying the nails and the person getting the nails. When these nails are removed, the natural nails can be torn from the nail bed, and the natural nails will be broken, thinned, and yellow because they have been sealed off from the air.

▌ DEODORANTS AND ANTIPERSPIRANTS

The action of bacteria and chemicals on human sweat create the sometimes unpleasant smell of body odor. Deodorants control perspiration odors by inhibiting the growth of microorganisms. Antiperspirants retard the flow of perspiration. Deodorants may contain:
• hexachlorophene
• bithionol
• ammonium compounds
• aluminum chloride
• urea
• propylene glycol
• water
• sodium stearate
• sorbitol
• alcohol

Deodorant/antiperspirants may contain:
• aluminum chloride
• propylene chloride
• aluminum chlorhydroxide
• sorbitan monostearate
• poloxamers
• stearic acid
• boric acid
• urea
• water
• petrolatum
• perfume
• propylene glycol
• cetyl alcohol

There have been many side effects related to

using deodorants, including stinging, burning, itching, fatty cysts, enlarged sweat and lymph glands, pimples under the arms, and lung and throat irritation. Lung tumors, vision problems, and even death have been linked to inhalation of deodorant sprays.

AFTERSHAVES, PRESHAVES, AND SHAVING CREAMS

Aftershave lotions soothe skin irritated by shaving. Early aftershave preparations, such as bay rum and witch hazel, were merely substitutes for water. Today, aftershaves fall into two categories: alcoholic and nonalcoholic. Alcoholic aftershaves contain:

- alcohol
- glycerine
- water
- certified color
- perfume
- menthol antiseptics and alum may also be added.

Nonalcoholic aftershaves resemble hand lotions and may contain:

- stearic acid
- triethanolamine
- cetyl alcohol
- glycerine
- distilled water
- small amounts of lanolin
- preservatives

Other fats, waxes, perfumes, coloring, and emulsifying agents may also be added. All of the ingredients in both alcoholic and nonalcoholic aftershaves are potential allergens. Problems reported to the FDA include face irritation, burned or peeling skin, and eye irritation.

Because dry hair is difficult to cut with a razor, shaving creams are used to make beards softer and easier to shave. Some shaving creams are soaps which, when applied with a brush, form lather. The brushless preparations are emulsions of oil and water, and are creams rather than soaps. However, washing and rinsing the face with hot water a few minutes before shaving softens the beard as well as any type of shaving cream.

Men who use electric razors frequently use preshave to temporarily tighten the skin before cutting the beard. These products may contain:

- aluminum phenolsulfonate
- menthol
- camphor
- water
- perfume
- alcohol

Oily types of preshave may also contain:

- 75 percent alcohol
- isopropyl myristate or isopropyl palmitate
- water

Preshaves made for regular razors contain:

- coconut oil
- triethanolamine
- alkyl arylpolyethylene glycol ether
- fatty acids
- water
- perfume

INSECTS AND PESTICIDES

Pesticides are chemicals used to control insects, rodents, weeds, and other organisms considered by people to be pests. Pesticides include rodenticides, insecticides, herbicides, and fungicides. There are many chemical insecticides that are advertised as the answer to any insect problems. When these compounds are sprayed on insects, the animals supposedly die, but many insects are unaffected. Others reproduce so quickly that insecticides have little effect on the overall population of a particular species. Insects often become resistant to insecticides so that different, more potent chemicals are required to kill them.

Insecticides are more dangerous to us than to the insects—many contain neurotoxins that can cause permanent damage. Once used, insecticides can linger for many years. For example, chlordane has a half-life of 30 years. (Half-life is the length of time it takes half of the material to decompose. It takes another half-life for the "half of the half" to decompose, and so on.) Chlordane can cause cancer, nerve damage, and immune system damage. There is no safe level for this pesticide. Although the use of chlordane was banned in 1988, residues may still linger in the foundations of older homes.

In many areas of the continent, building codes require soil preparation with an insecticide before a foundation is laid. Many patios, sun rooms, and solar heat collection areas are floored with brick or flagstone on a bed of sand. The ground under these areas is often sprayed with insecticide before the sand is spread. Any immunocompromised person should ask in detail about prior use of insecticides in any dwelling where they intend to reside.

Pesticide exposure is not limited to attempts to control insects in the home. Pesticides used to control crop pests can get into the food chain. In the U.S., the agriculture industry uses 90 percent of the pesticides

> ## A World of Insects
>
> *Insects are the most plentiful life form on earth. The number of insect species is conservatively estimated at about 1.5 million. Insects like to inhabit our homes and eat our food, yet most of us are unwilling to share, and so we look for ways to get rid of these pests.*

applied. Unused pesticides may be poured down drains and sewers, and eventually enter our water supply. Pesticides from gardens, lawns, golf courses, and parks also find their way into the water supply.

Every North American is exposed to pesticides daily. Pesticides are used in paints, carpets, mattresses, paper, dentures, shampoos, hair wigs, disposable diapers, and contact lenses. Larger exposures occur in schools, offices, apartment buildings, churches, and factories.

Pets can represent a large pesticide exposure, both for the pet and for the owners. Insecticidal flea collars, sprays, dusts, shampoos, or dips are frequently used on pets. Residues from these pesticides will be in the family's bedding, carpeting, clothing, and food.

■ EFFECTS OF PESTICIDES ON PEOPLE

People can suffer severe health problems and permanent damage from exposure to numerous pesticides in food, water, and air, even though the exposure level for each is below the federally defined safe tolerance level. Pesticides are absorbed through the lungs, skin, and gut. Most insecticides are fat-soluble, and are deposited in the fat cells of exposed persons and animals.

Single pesticide exposures may not cause problems for some people, but combined exposures can. Many pesticides are broad-spectrum and can damage plants, birds, and humans. Pesticides may also interact synergistically, tripling or quadrupling the effect of each pesticide.

Pesticides contain active ingredients with lethal or toxic action against target pests. They also contain inert ingredients that include solvents, propellants, surfactants, emulsifiers, wetting agents, carriers, or diluents. These ingredients are inactive as far as pesticide action is concerned, but for humans may be the most toxic part of a pesticide. Inert ingredients are considered trade secrets, and the United States Federal Insecticide, Fungicide, and Rodenticide Act (FIFRA) does not require the inert ingredients to be listed.

Pesticides have two types of action, systemic and contact. Systemic pesticides are applied to the soil or leaves of a plant and are ingested when people eat the fruits, seeds, or nuts. These pesticides affect normal plant metabolism, preventing the plant from growing properly. Contact pesticides directly affect the target pest, killing very rapidly.

There are many different classes of pesticides, each with a different action on pests, and each causes numerous symptoms for people. For example, organophosphate pesticides affect the neuromuscular junction when they are absorbed through the skin, causing excess sweating, muscular twitching, extreme weakness, and paralysis. If they are inhaled, they affect the respiratory muscles, causing difficulty breathing. Ingestion causes the muscles of the GI tract and bladder to go into spasm, resulting in nausea and vomiting. Central nervous system symptoms can develop, including tremor, confusion, slurred speech, poor balance, and poor coordination. With large exposures, convulsions and death may result.

Safe pest control methods that avoid the use of pesticides are available. (See chapter 12, Living Safely, for safe alternatives.) Allergy extracts for pesticides and hands-on allergy treatment can help counter the symptoms of pesticide exposure.

People who have had numerous exposures to insecticides and pesticides carry a large toxic load in their fat cells, unless they go through detoxification. (See chapter 20, Detoxification.) Symptoms and damage will continue unless their bodies are cleansed of the pesticide. Immunotherapy for pesticides is also very helpful in the cleansing process.

Because of their toxicity, all pesticides must be tested *only* by EAV (Electroacupuncture According to Voll; see chapter 8) or muscle testing, and *only* homeopathic extracts can be used. These extracts help the body release the stored pesticides in the fat cells. An extract for the enzyme acetylocholinesterase is also beneficial for people who have had a pesticide exposure. Without cleansing, people with a high pesticide load may not respond well to immunotherapy, nutrient therapy, and exercise programs. Hands-on allergy treatment is helpful for pesticides, but again, detoxification procedures are also a must.

CHAPTER 12

Living Safely

How Can We Live Safely?

While there are many possible chemical exposures that can cause symptoms and health consequences for people who are chemically sensitive, there are many simple measures that can reduce problems. Even though exposures are numerous and can be frightening, it is possible to live safely with minimum health risks.

This chapter outlines ways for you to control your exposures. Implementing these measures requires some thought and effort, but they will allow you to create a "safe" haven and to reduce the toxic overload on your immune system.

Living with Chemical Sensitivities

You can avoid or reduce exposure to many chemicals by following these general guidelines. You must clean up your interior environment both at home and at work.

- Eat a diet of "clean" foods, uncontaminated by pesticides, fertilizers, or processing (see chapter 10).
- Drink only safe, uncontaminated water

(see The Importance of Water Quality, below).

- Use an air cleaner both at home and in your car (see The Importance of Clean Air, below).
- Provide nutritional support for your immune system (see chapter 19).
- Seek out testing and immunotherapy with chemical extracts, or have hands-on testing and treatment for chemicals (see chapters 8 and 11).
- Undergo detoxification procedures to lower your toxic body burden (see chapter 20).

If you are chemically sensitive, you need to "clean up" chemical exposures in your home as much as possible. Because there are many chemical exposures over which you have no control, it is important that you limit or eliminate all the possible exposures you can control. When you are not constantly reacting to chemical exposures at home, you will be better able to tolerate unavoidable exposures away from home.

To clean up your home, follow the guidelines in this chapter as closely as possible. While it would be overwhelming to accomplish all of these suggestions at once, you can incorporate a few at a time until your house is safe.

■ THE IMPORTANCE OF CLEAN AIR

Clean air is essential for chemically sensitive people. Some people must buy their air just as they buy clean water. There are many air cleaners on the market, in many price ranges. In general, the less expensive products remove particles such as dust, mold, bacteria, some viruses, cigarette smoke, and odors. These air cleaners do not contain enough activated charcoal to filter harmful chemicals.

You should purchase an air cleaner that:
- contains enough activated charcoal to remove chemicals, including formaldehyde. Charcoal that has been impregnated with potassium permanganate is available specifically for this purpose.
- contains an odor-removing charcoal filter in addition to the formaldehyde filter.
- contains a filter designed to remove dust, mold, bacteria, and viruses.
- has the fan motor located so that odors from the motor are filtered before the air leaves the cleaner.
- has a stainless steel or baked enamel finish.

Some people may have difficulty tolerating the filter materials; they will have to investigate their tolerance to charcoal from various sources. The material used in the HEPA (High Efficiency Particulate Accumulator) filter in air cleaners may also cause a problem for some. A cleaner with a final filter, containing glass beads, may reduce these problems.

Extremely sensitive people should use an air cleaner both in their homes and cars. Some air cleaners have electrical adaptors so they can be used in both places. Whole-house filtration systems are available that fit into central heating and cooling units. Specialized air cleaners are also available that fit over computers and printers to prevent their operating odors from filling the room.

For severely chemical sensitive people, it may be necessary to construct a box (with a glass front and vents to the outside) to hold the television set because chemicals released when the TV is in use can provoke symptoms. Reading boxes, vented to the outside, will eliminate problem fumes from paper and printers' inks.

Charcoal face masks, available in 100 percent cotton or 100 percent silk, have an activated charcoal filter. Using these masks makes trips outside possible for some very chemically sensitive people who otherwise could not tolerate the exposure. Wearing a silicone half mask is also helpful (see Recommended Sources and Organizations). Some people wear respirators, for which different types of filters are available. However, the rubber face mask on some brands of respirators is difficult to tolerate.

To keep the air in your home clean, run an air purifier continuously and change the filters frequently. Do not use any aerosol sprays, such as room or rug deodorants or spray starch, or insecticides, pesticides, or fungicides. Remove any existing aerosol products and containers of pesticides from the house, and as many rubber and plastic items as possible. Also remove all glues, adhesives, lighter fluids, shoe polish, mothballs and crystals, and canned or spray paints. If any members of the household have a hobby involving the use of glues, adhesives, paints, or chemicals of any kind, be sure that they never work on their hobby inside the house.

Do not allow any tobacco smoking in your home, and do not use a wood-burning stove or fireplace. Do not burn candles or incense. If a garage is attached to your house, use weather stripping to make sure any adjoining doors seal tightly. Never idle vehicle engines in the garage. Some very sensitive people may not be able to park their cars in their garages.

▪▪ THE IMPORTANCE OF WATER QUALITY

We do not usually consider water as a nutrient, but it provides our bodies with oxygen and hydrogen—two materials essential for proper metabolism. The average adult is made up of approximately 45 quarts of water, accounting for roughly two-thirds of body weight. Our body loses about three quarts of water each day through excretion and perspiration. Menstrual flow in women adds to the amount of water lost.

The rate of water loss depends on activity level and environmental conditions—it may range from less than a quart for a sedentary person in a mild or cold climate, to 10 quarts per day for a person in a desert. Body temperature is modulated as water evaporates from the skin and respiratory passages.

Water is involved in every body process, including digestion, absorption, circulation, and excretion. It is the primary transporter of nutrients to every cell in our body. It diffuses rapidly across membranes and also carries waste products out of the cells. Each cell not only contains fluid (intracellular), but is also bathed in fluid (extracellular). Water supplies the fluid for secretions and is a medium for chemical reactions in each cell.

Very little water is absorbed in the stomach, some is absorbed in the small intestine, and the greatest amount is absorbed in the large intestine. Water is excreted through the urine, feces, skin, and lungs. It is kept at an almost constant level in our body by precise regulatory mechanisms in the kidneys. However, continuous replacement is essential to prevent dehydration and salt depletion.

Organically grown fruits and vegetables are good sources of chemically pure water. About 500 cc of water is derived in the body from organic nutrients that we eat. This source of water is involved in energy and heat exchanges in the cells. Our water intake from food and fluids should be at least 2½ quarts daily.

▪ WATER SUPPLIES AND STANDARDS

Available water supplies differ greatly in different areas of the world. The most healthful water contains balanced amounts of minerals. Hard water is a good source of mineral nutrients needed by our body for proper cell metabolism; water that passes over rock or water from deep wells is usually hard water. Excessive hardness, however, can cause mineral imbalances, leading to poor health or sensitivity. Water that is too hard can be softened by using specific salts that react with minerals, causing a precipi-

Water and Allergies

Adequate water intake is very important for the allergic person. It keeps nutrients in solution, available for cell repair and nourishment. Positive and negative ions require sufficient fluid levels for electrical conduction and to help maintain a state of equilibrium in the body. Adequate water level is also required to flush chemical and biological toxins and waste products from cells. This flushing helps to reduce the total overload of the allergic person.

Water retention in extracellular spaces is referred to as edema, and is a problem for some allergic people. Edema can occur as a result of allergic reactions, stress, trauma,

disease, malfunction of certain organs (heart, lungs, kidneys, adrenal glands, and thyroid), and ingestion of drugs. As a result of the fluid buildup, nutrients cannot be transported as easily to the cells. Waste products begin to accumulate within cells, causing loss of function and cell damage. Early symptoms include swollen tissues in the hands, feet, ankles, or nasal membranes, or under the eyes. Later signs include swollen legs and abdomen, and headaches (caused by swelling of brain tissue). For edema treatment, see Natural Remedies for Common Complaints in chapter 22.

tate that is filtered out. Soft water (such as rain water) contains very few dissolved minerals.

In the past, most water sources were safe for drinking. As populations increased, however, drinking lake water, stream water, and water from common wells became increasingly hazardous. Epidemics of diseases, such as diphtheria and cholera, became more commonplace as water supplies became contaminated with human and animal waste. Attention had to be directed toward providing clean drinking water. Today, we continue to have problems finding safe sources of water. Water supplies on this continent may be relatively free of bacterial contamination, but many other hazardous materials and parasites may be present in the water you consume.

Water standards, regulated by public health departments, cover only the following:

- bacteriological quality (number of coliform organisms)
- physical characteristics (turbidity, color, odor)
- radioactivity
- chemical characteristics—maximum permissible limits are set for:

alkylbenzene sulfonate	manganese
arsenic	nitrates
cadmium	phenol
chlorides	selenium
chromium	silver
cyanide	sulfates
fluorides	total dissolved
iron	solids
lead	zinc

These standards fail to address other hazardous, human-created chemicals. Contamination of ground and surface water supplies may occur in many ways. Chemicals do not readily break down before they enter the groundwater supplies. For example, in England, recently dug wells were found to be severely contaminated by whale oil that was dumped in 1815.

■ SOURCES OF WATER CONTAMINATION

- Agricultural contamination from runoff containing residues of pesticides, herbicides, nitrites, chemical fertilizers, and animal wastes.
- Household contamination from detergents, phosphates, petroleum products, and hexachlorophene.
- Industrial contamination from the dumping of hazardous chemical wastes into surface water, seepage of chemicals into groundwater waste dumps, and brine from oil and gas drilling.
- Natural contamination from excess mineral deposits in the ground (such as molybdenum, lead, and copper).
- Leaching of excess minerals from old lead or copper water pipes.
- Plastic piping or containers, to which some people are sensitive.
- Chlorine added to public water supplies for bacterial contamination control, to which many people are sensitive.
- Fluorides added to water supplies to help control dental caries. Fluoride also liberates aluminum from cookware when heated, and poses a problem for some allergic people.
- Nitrates and bacteria from leaky septic tanks, or from community dumping of raw sewage into surface waterways.
- Old, inadequate water purification plants in many communities that are unable to handle increased populations and industrial contaminants.

■ SAFER WATER SOURCES

There are sources of water other than public supplies that may be considered safe, but even some of these may pose problems for the sensitive person. In the past, well water was considered to be relatively safe if the well was situated away from septic tanks or other human waste disposal systems. However, in some communities the deep ground water has begun to show chemical contamination. Some well water also contains high levels of minerals from the soil and is not tolerated by some sensitive people. Rain water, previously considered safe, can be contaminated with atmospheric pollution.

Some people elect to purchase their water. Bottled spring water and distilled water are available. Caution must be exercised when looking for a reputable supplier; a few companies have been known to bottle tap water and sell it as spring water. The sensitive person should inquire about the source of the spring water, since ground water in some areas is chemically contaminated. Some brands of mineral water are tolerated by some people with chemical sensitivities.

Boiling water will destroy bacteria and will remove chlorine and volatile chemicals in the steam. Heavy metals or nitrates, however, will remain in the water. Triple-distilled water may be safe for some sensitive people, but the distilling process removes minerals needed for proper metabolic function. Supplementing trace minerals and macrominerals is important for anyone using triple-distilled water.

Filtered water is relatively safe for many environmentally ill people. Many types of filters are available, from whole-house filters to portable filters or single-faucet filters. In choosing a filter, you must evaluate the severity of your illness, your finances, and the availability of various systems. In addition, some people are sensitive to the charcoal medium used in the filters.

If you use a filter, it is essential to clean your filter system regularly for effectiveness and to prevent mold growth. Mineral supplementation is wise when filter systems are used that remove minerals from the water. Store water in glass or ceramic bottles rather than plastic containers—soft plastic containers leak plastic components into the water.

To determine which water source causes the least problem, an environmentally sensitive person must test varieties of water. This can be done by rotating various waters, just as with food on a rotation diet. Safe water should be used for drinking and cooking, as well as for brushing teeth, and washing fresh foods. Some very sensitive people may also need filtered water for bathing if chlorine or fluoride is a severe problem.

For the extremely sensitive, whole-house filters are preferable since all water sources will be filtered. If you do not have a filter, let your drinking water stand in an uncovered glass jar for 24 hours to allow the chlorine to evaporate. The jar should be kept in a well-ventilated area to help prevent chlorine exposure.

▮ HOME WATER PURIFICATION SYSTEMS

(adapted with permission of Dr. William Rea)

▮ Distillation

These systems are somewhat noisy and give off heat. The units must have sediment and scale removed periodically.

Removes	*Does Not Remove*
Salts	Chlorine
Asbestos	All organic chemicals
Bacteria	
Viruses	
Fluorides	
Heavy metals	
Minerals	
Nitrates	

▮ Reverse Osmosis

These filters are arranged in a series (sediment filter, reverse osmosis filter, activated carbon cartridge).

Removes	*Does Not Remove*
Large particulate matter	Chlorine
Some organic chemicals	All chemicals
Some organic pesticides	All pesticides
Nitrates	All bacteria
Fluorides	All viruses
Asbestos	All minerals
Heavy metals	
Chlorine compounds	

▮ Carbon Block

The filters must be changed regularly in order to prevent breeding bacteria or molds in the carbon medium. Some people are sensitive to the carbon medium.

Removes	*Does Not Remove*
Chloroform	Heavy metals
Chlorine	Minerals

Pesticides   Salts
Organic chemicals   Nitrates
Bad taste and odor   All fluorides
Bacteria
Giardia

▋▋ PETROCHEMICALS

Within your home, eliminate all possible exposures to petrochemicals. Thoroughly air new plastics and paints for several weeks or longer before trying to live around them.

Although some petrochemical products may continue to outgas for two to three years, the older the product (car, plastic shower curtains, painted walls, carpets, furniture) the less toxic it will be. However, an extremely sensitive person may never be able to tolerate some products that contain petrochemicals.

▋▋ APPLIANCES AND HEATING SYSTEMS

Appliances, both large and small, are difficult to tolerate for some chemically sensitive people. The following guidelines will help you to select safe appliances.

Do not use gas appliances, as they are among the primary sources of chemical exposure in the home. A gas furnace, hot water heater, and clothes dryer can prevent a chemically sensitive person from being able to live in a house. If it is too costly to replace or move such appliances to an outbuilding, you should weather-strip the access doors with felt stripping to reduce exposure to combustion products. Unless you are electromagnetically sensitive, electric ranges, furnaces, hot water heaters, and clothes dryers are recommended.

Use appliances with the least amount of interior plastic. Avoid aluminum and Teflon coatings on all appliances. The following are "safe" appliances:

- *Blender:* Glass or stainless steel container
- *Broiler:* Stainless steel or porcelain
- *Crockpot:* Removable stoneware interior
- *Dishwasher:* Porcelain or stainless steel interior
- *Electric oven:* Porcelain-lined bake/broil section; ceramic top burners. Never use a continuous-cleaning oven. Self-cleaning ovens are also toxic. If you must use one, leave the house until the cycle is finished, the oven is cooled, and the house has been aired.
- *Iron:* Stainless steel sole plate. Use distilled water only.
- *Juicer:* Stainless steel interior
- *Refrigerator/freezer:* Porcelain interior and exterior
- *Vacuum cleaner:* Water-trap vacuum, double-filter vacuum, or built-in central vacuum system. Use disposable dust bags and wash the outer bag frequently.
- *Washer/dryer:* Porcelain and stainless steel interiors. Locate appliances in a room that can be closed off and vent your dryer to the outside.

▋▋ COOKING AND FOOD STORAGE

Cook in glass, china, or stainless steel. Some people are able to tolerate cooking with cast iron. However, food particles from previously cooked meals will be released from the porous iron surface. Do not use aluminum, copper, or Teflon cookware, and do not coat cookware with nonstick cooking sprays.

Chemicals can leach into foods stored in plastic containers. Do not use plastic wrapping or soft plastic containers. Store food in cellophane, in aluminum foil with the shiny side next to the food (the dull side may be coated with plastic), or in glassware.

▌ MICROWAVE COOKING

There is much controversy over preparing food in the microwave. Some scientists feel, and there is some scientific evidence to support their view, that all food prepared in the microwave is changed in ways that are harmful to us. Others feel that microwaves are safe for rewarming food, but not for cooking raw foods, especially meats and protein. Microwaving particularly changes milk products, and baby bottles should never be warmed in the microwave.

People who use a microwave oven should have it checked yearly for leakage using a well-calibrated meter. If the door gasket is damaged, replace it before using the oven again. Because the dose and time of microwave exposure that can cause problems are unknown, never stand in front of microwave ovens while they are in operation. Stay four feet or more away from the oven.

▌▌ CLEANING AND LAUNDRY SUPPLIES

Most commercial cleaning supplies are toxic and can contaminate a home. Clean the house with *safe* cleaning products only. See Safe Household Cleaning and Deodorizing, later in this chapter. Stop using and remove all nonsafe cleaning products, such as furniture polish, ammonia, and dishwashing detergents, from all areas of the home—including the kitchen, laundry room, and bathroom. Even if the lids are on the containers, molecules of these substances can escape. These items are all chemical exposures; offending items *must* be removed from the house.

Laundry products can pollute your house, as well as providing a constant chemical exposure when you wear your clothes. Stop using bleach, scented laundry soap, and fabric softener. Fabric softeners and dryer sheets, both scented and unscented, contain carcinogenic and neurotoxic chemicals. Remove these items from the house. Substitute $1/2$ to 1 cup baking soda in the rinse water for softness. For static cling, use $1/4$ cup vinegar in the wash cycle.

▌▌ CLOTHING

Do not wear dry-cleaned clothes or leather garments. Freshly dry-cleaned garments can contaminate your whole closet as they outgas. Wearing them will also be a chemical exposure if you do not allow them time to outgas. If you have garments that must be dry-cleaned, allow them to outgas outside the house for two weeks to a month.

The dyes in leather clothing and the tannins used to cure the leather can be a long-term chemical exposure. As much as possible wear natural fiber clothing that can be washed. Remember that new clothes are a formaldehyde exposure and they should always be washed before wearing or storing in your closet.

▌▌ PERSONAL CARE PRODUCTS

Stop using and remove all standard commercial, scented personal care products

from the house. Even when sealed in plastic bags, the following items are sources of chemical exposure:
- aftershaves
- bar soaps
- body lotions
- body powder
- colognes
- cosmetics
- deodorants
- hair oils, sprays, and tonics
- hand creams and lotions
- makeup
- mousse
- mouthwash
- nail polish and removers
- perfumes
- setting gels
- shampoos and conditioners
- shaving cream
- toothpaste

Use only toiletries that are prepared without petrochemicals and that are fragrance-free. Remember that many products have a masking fragrance to hide chemical smells and need not be labeled except as "other ingredients." Many safe products are available at health food stores. However, be certain to read labels even at the health food store; not all products sold at health food stores are safe for everyone.

Use baking soda both as toothpaste and underarm deodorant. Unless you are sensitive to olives, extra virgin cold-pressed olive oil can be used as a makeup remover and moisturizer for dry skin. Some people use the oil of the day from their rotation diet as a moisturizer.

A safe shampoo can be made by simply

Safe R & R: Rest and Repair

Extremely sensitive people will need a virtually allergen-free place to allow their immune system to rest and repair. Dr. William Rea of the Environmental Health Center in Dallas, Texas, suggests creating an environmentally safe "oasis." Because we spend the majority of our time at home in the bedroom, it is best to make this the oasis—free of chemical, inhalant, and food exposures.

dissolving baking soda in water. Make hair gel for use by men or women by dissolving one packet of unflavored gelatin in about 3 cups of hot water. When cool, apply to dry or wet hair and blow dry. Your hair will hold the position in which it dries. Diluted further it will serve as a hair spray.

■■ MAKING A BEDROOM OASIS

To prepare a bedroom oasis, follow these guidelines carefully.

Always keep the bedroom door closed. If the door does not seal tightly enough, put felt weather stripping around it. Do not eat or bring food into this room.

■ AIR/INHALANTS
- You should not allow anyone to smoke in your home, but it is critical to prohibit smoking in this room!
- Use an air purifier; run it continuously and change the filters regularly.
- Remove all plants, which can be a source of terpenes and mold.
- Remove books, magazines, and other

printed materials from the room. The ink and paper are phenol and formaldehyde exposures.

- Remove candles from the room. Many candles are scented and can release acetone, benzene, lead, soot, and other harmful particles when they are burned.
- Do not use any insecticides, pesticides, or fungicides.
- Do not allow pets in the room. Pet dander and saliva is allergenic for many people, and pets also bring in dust, mold, and pollen from outdoors.

See also the sections on dust and molds in chapter 14, Breathing Safely, for information about controlling inhalant allergens and exposures.

▌ FLOORING

- Hardwood floors with a urethane finish are acceptable; however, allow sufficient time for the finish to outgas before the using the room for a sleeping area.
- Use sanded wood for flooring, but do not use pine, cedar, or spruce wood, as they have a high terpene (hydrocarbon) content. Harder woods are better tolerated.
- If the floor absolutely cannot be replaced, cover it with a foil barrier and use cotton or jute carpeting to cover the foil.

▌ FURNITURE

- Do not use a waterbed; the plastic covering is a phenol exposure and the electric components are a problem for electrically sensitive people.
- Some extremely sensitive people may not tolerate conventional beds. One option is to use a metal cot and many folded blankets for a mattress. If you tolerate cotton, you can buy an all-cotton futon mattress, but you must ask your physician to write a letter to the manufacturer saying that you cannot tolerate the flame retardants, which are otherwise required by law.

- Remove all particleboard furniture, including bookcases.
- Older, solid wood furniture is usually tolerated unless it has been treated with insecticide. If there is any mildew odor, it can be removed with a citrus cleaner, if it is tolerated, and cleaned with Murphy's Oil Soap.
- Unless you are electrically sensitive, metal dressers are also a possibility.
- Remove all synthetic materials (carpeting, drapery, and bedding.) Use only natural fabrics, such as linen, cotton, silk, or wool (if tolerated).
- Do not use sponge or foam rubber pillows. Pillows may be made of cotton, kapok, or feathers (if tolerated). You can make a pillow by folding cotton batting, a cotton blanket, or clean cotton diapers and covering them with a pillowcase.

▌ CLOSETS

- Clean out closets. Remove any possible contaminants (such as mothballs, old books, shoes, boots, and clothes with scents on them).
- If there is an access door to a crawlspace in the bottom of the closet, seal it with weather stripping in order to prevent mold exposure from the soil under the house.

▌ CLOTHING

- Do not keep freshly polished shoes in the bedroom until all of the polish odor has dissipated, or store shoes outside of the bedroom if possible. Remove any leather clothing, which is processed with tannin, a potent allergen.

- Wash new clothing before storing in the closet, drawers, or shelves.
- Dry-cleaned clothes should not be stored in the bedroom.

▌ CLEANING AND PERSONAL CARE

- Clean the room with *safe* cleaning products only (See Safe Household Cleaning and Deodorizing, below).
- Remove *all* scented cosmetic items—perfumes, colognes, hand and body lotions, powders, deodorants, hair sprays, hair products, nail polish and remover, after-shave lotions, or astringents.

▌ ELECTROMAGNETIC

- Because of the electromagnetic polarity of the earth, it is important to position the head of the bed facing north. For more information, see chapter 4, Our Body Electric.
- Determine where the main electric source enters the house and do not use this room as a bedroom.
- Do not use electric blankets, as the heated wires give off chemical fumes. The current in the wires can also cause electromagnetic problems. Even when unplugged, these blankets are not safe because of their wire configuration.
- Do not use clock radios, TVs, hairdryers, computers, or any other electric appliances in the room. Use a wind-up clock.

▌ HEATING SYSTEM

- Block the air vents from forced-air heaters with aluminum foil.
- Portable electric heaters may be used in cold rooms. (Electrically sensitive people may have problems with this heat source.)

▌▌ SAFE HOUSEHOLD CLEANING AND DEODORIZING

Always wear gloves while cleaning with any product to prevent absorption of the substance through your hands. The skin is our largest organ and it absorbs any substance with which it comes in contact. Extremely sensitive people may also need to wear masks.

▌ LEMON

Fresh-cut lemon, lemon peel, or lemon juice may be substituted for commercial household cleaning and polishing products. This is important for chemically sensitive people who cannot tolerate chemically loaded products. However, as with any substance, some people will react to lemon; the only way to know whether you can tolerate this use of lemon is to try it.

Note: Anyone who is already aware of a lemon sensitivity should not use these cleaning procedures, but use vinegar or baking soda instead.

Commercially bottled lemon juice can be substituted for fresh lemon, but it will not clean as well as the fresh fruit.

- *Appliances:* Remove soap film from the interiors of ovens and refrigerators by adding fresh lemon juice to the rinse water after cleaning.
- *Baby bottles:* Add lemon juice to the water when boiling bottles to remove mineral deposits.
- *Brass and copper:* Rub with lemon juice or a slice of lemon sprinkled with baking soda. Rinse with clear water and dry with a soft cloth. For heavy corrosion, rub with a paste made of lemon juice and salt. Rinse with

clear water and dry with a soft cloth. You can also use a paste made of lemon juice and cream of tartar. Rub the paste on gently and leave it for five minutes. Rinse in warm water and dry with a soft cloth.

- *Chinaware:* To restore the original shine, scour chinaware with lemon juice and salt. To clean inside a china decanter, use one part salt and two parts lemon juice.
- *Chrome:* Rub with lemon peel and rinse with clear water. Polish with a soft cloth.
- *Faucets (kitchen and bath):* To remove spots and shine faucets, rub them with lemon peel and wash with a soft cloth. Then polish with a dry, soft cloth.
- *Furniture polish:* Use a solution of one part lemon juice and two parts of any vegetable oil.
- *Garbage disposal:* Put used lemons in the garbage disposal to help keep it clean and deodorized.
- *Glass:* Soak glass in lemon juice and water or rub it with cut lemon juice to clean and remove spots. Dry with a lint-free cloth. Shake a small piece of freshly cut lemon and a small amount of water inside glass decanters to renew their sparkle.
- *Glass surfaces:* Clean glass surfaces as above with lemon juice or cut lemon to remove dirt and spots. To remove dried paint, apply hot lemon juice with a soft cloth and leave it on until it is almost dry, then wipe it off with a soft cloth.
- *Ivory (piano keys):* Rub ivory with half a lemon or a paste made of lemon juice and salt. Wipe with a clean, wet cloth to rinse. Dry with a clean, dry cloth.
- *Leather (picture frames, book bindings, furniture):* Apply a mixture of equal amounts

lemon juice and warm water. Wipe clean with a dry cloth.

- *Lipstick stains on fabric:* For white, washable fabrics, use full-strength lemon juice to remove lipstick stains. Use diluted lemon juice for colored, washable fabrics.
- *Mildew stain on fabrics:* Rub salt and then lemon juice on the mildew stain. Place the fabric in the sun to dry.
- *Paintbrushes (hardened):* Dip hardened paintbrushes into boiling lemon juice and immediately lower heat. Leave brushes in the juice for 15 minutes before washing in soapy water.
- *Pastry boards and rolling pins:* Rub occasionally with a freshly cut lemon half to bleach out stains.
- *Refrigerators:* Place a freshly cut lemon half on the refrigerator shelf to absorb odors.
- *Rust spots on fabrics:* Cover the spot with a paste of lemon juice and salt. Let it dry in the sun or hold the fabric over steam until the spot is gone.
- *Silverware:* Rub with lemon juice or a slice of lemon. Rinse with hot water and polish dry. For heavy oxidation, soak the silverware in lemon juice for five minutes before rinsing and polishing.
- *Tile:* Rub tile with a cloth soaked in lemon juice. Polish tile with a dry, soft cloth or chamois.
- *White marble:* To clean, rub with half a lemon or a paste made of lemon juice and salt. Wipe with a wet cloth and dry with a soft, dry cloth.
- *Wine stains on fabrics:* For washable fabrics only, spread a paste of lemon juice and salt on the wine stain. Rinse. Wash in soapy water.

- *Wooden furniture (scratches)* Mix equal amounts of lemon juice and any vegetable oil. Apply this mixture to the scratches on wooden furniture and rub gently with a soft cloth until they are no longer visible.
- *Woodwork* Will keep its gloss if the juice of one lemon is added to one quart of water for the last rinse after cleaning. This also works for any painted, enameled, or linoleum surface.

▎ BAKING SODA

Simple baking soda and hot water will clean almost anything. In fact, many people use baking soda as their toothpaste, deodorant, shampoo, and clothes-washing detergent. Use 1 Tbsp. baking soda per quart of hot water for a cleaning solution.

- *Kitchen cleaner:* For cleaning the kitchen, apply baking soda to a sponge, scrub, wipe, and rinse. This will scrub away grease and soils without scratching surfaces. You can clean sinks, counters, microwaves, pots, pans, refrigerators, cutting boards, coffee and tea pots, silverware, and food containers this way. Rinse with warm or hot water.
- *Deodorizing:* Baking soda is also an excellent deodorizer. Special containers of baking soda for use in the refrigerator and freezer are available at most grocery stores. Loose baking soda in the bottom of the garbage can keeps odor to a miminum.
- *Bathroom cleaner:* To clean in the bathroom, apply baking soda to a damp sponge, wipe, and rinse. This removes soil, dirt, and soap scum. Use on sinks, counters, tubs, shower, toilets, tile, and cabinets.
- *Laundry:* If you use a laundry detergent, 1/2 cup baking soda added to the usual amount of liquid detergent will boost enzyme action and neutralize odors. For bleach boosting power, add 1/2 cup baking soda to liquid chlorine bleach. (People who do not tolerate bleach will not be able to use this tip.)
- *Stain removal:* To remove wine or grape juice stains in fabric, pour boiling water over the fabric first and rinse with soda water.

▌▌ REMODELING OR BUILDING A HOME

The need to remodel or build a home can be a serious problem for chemically sensitive people, because many building materials are a serious chemical exposure. However, if building materials are selected with care, a safe home can be created. Remember that there are no materials that are safe for everyone. Individual sensitivities vary, and if possible, you should have all building materials tested by a healthcare professional before you use them in your project.

The contractor you choose to do the work is of equal importance. The person must have concern for you and your safety. Make sure it is clearly understood that work must stop if there is a problem. Also have it clearly understood that no one is permitted to smoke on the job. Air the new construction for at least a month before you move in.

As a general rule of thumb, avoid any building materials containing asphalt, tar, flame-retardants, fungicides, insecticides, mold retardants or mold on materials, glues, particleboard, styrofoam, and vinyl products. The suggestions below are a few of many safe alternatives. To speed up gasing of all building materials, do a "bakeout." Close the house or new construction area and turn up the furnace to 80°F for 12 hours. Have someone turn off the furnace and open the house to air. Allow it to air for at least 6 to 12 hours before using the area.

■ LUMBER

Use only untreated lumber. You may have to trace your local source back to the processing mill to be certain it is truly untreated. Kiln-dried fir is the most tolerated wood. If you need lumber for decks, railings, and steps, use untreated redwood or red cedar in these areas.

■ PLYWOOD, PARTICLEBOARD, CHIPBOARD, AND PANELING

Plywood, particleboard, chipboard, and paneling must all be sealed with a tolerated sealant if they are to be used. These products will outgas for years without sealant. Remember that each coat of sealant seals out 50 percent of the vapors, and six coats will be required to obtain a 98 percent seal. If painting on a sealant is not an option, wrap the object with aluminum foil.

■ INSULATION AND VAPOR BARRIERS

Yellow, unfaced insulation batts are usually tolerated when used with an appropriate vapor barrier. Investigate safer, less odorous vinyl vapor barrier. Some people tolerate aluminum foil products for a vapor barrier. However, people with electromagnet problems may not tolerate this product in large amounts.

■ WALL COVERINGS

Most drywall is well tolerated if it has not been treated with a fire retardant. Use joint compound to which no fungicides or preservatives have been added.

Should you elect to use wallpaper, you will probably have to seal it to make it safe. Also, you will have to select a wallpaper paste that contains all-natural ingredients.

■ FLOORING

Hardwood floors, particularly oak, are well tolerated. Avoid wood flooring that must be installed with an adhesive.

If you use vinyl flooring, use a "brittle" vinyl that cracks easily or a commercial-grade vinyl composition. These types of vinyl have lower odor emissions.

Ceramic tile floors are quite safe if installed with the proper latex-free grout. Portland-based commercial thinsets and grouts without latex are safe for most people.

Some carpets are available today that are less toxic. Investigate these special carpet mills, but be aware than even the safest carpets collect dirt, dust, dust mites, and mold. Take a carpet sample home with you to live with for several days before making a decision regarding carpet to see whether you react to it. Use felt underlay instead of foam.

■ PAINTS AND SEALANTS

The choices for safe paints increase every year. Thoroughly investigate the possibilities available to you, and have them tested if at all possible. If testing is not available to you, paint a sample board with the desired paint. Bring it into the house and live with it for a few days to see how you tolerate it. Always paint in a well-ventilated area.

Most latex paint slowly releases petrochemical gases. To speed up this dispersion process, add baking soda to the paint before applying it. Some paints will become gluey when soda is added, so experiment with a small amount of paint first (1 Tbsp. baking soda to 1 cup paint). Then paint a small board with this mixture, letting it dry outdoors for several days before bringing it inside to determine whether you will experience symptoms.

Use the following guide to add baking soda to the paint:
One gallon of paint: Add 1 cup baking soda.
One quart of paint: Add 1/4 cup baking soda.
One pint of paint: Add 1/8 cup baking soda.
Mix the paint outdoors while wearing a mask (and if possible, paint during the summer months for better ventilation). Blend the baking soda in thoroughly. The paint will bubble and cause rapid dispersion of the petrochemicals.

In recent years, many companies have developed low VOC paints. Some of these new paints are advertised as having no VOCs. Volatile organic chemicals (VOCs) are the chemicals in paint that give them their odor and speed up drying time. It takes these new paints longer to dry, but they dry to a durable surface, and they have virtually no odor.

Some people do not tolerate any type of sealant. In these cases, it may be preferable to use an olive oil/lemon juice and beeswax finish, or sodium silicate. Several coats of the olive oil/lemon juice mixture must be applied, followed by wax; however, beeswax is difficult to apply. Sodium silicate prevents unsealed concrete from releasing dust, but limits the application of future sealants, as other chemicals will not adhere to the sodium silicate.

▌▌ CONTROLLING HOUSEHOLD INSECTS

While there are useful, helpful insects, such as the ladybug and the praying mantis, we tend to focus on those that are a problem for us. Many insects are disease vectors (they carry disease-causing organisms). Their bites and stings can cause swelling, itching, and systemic reactions. (See Natural Remedies for Common Complaints in chapter 21.) Insects can kill either through their toxic venom or through causing severe allergic reactions to venom and other substances injected through a sting or bite. Insects cause more deaths each year than poisonous snakes.

The first step in insect control is keeping your home in good repair. Most insects need only a fraction of an inch to crawl through and enter a house. Cracks in walls, openings around plumbing pipes, broken window screens and sills, loose flashing around grilles and vents, and rusted-out floor drains all provide doorways for insects to enter your home. Sliding glass doors allow garden crawlers to get in the house.

Be sure your yard is not attracting insects because of the landscaping around your home. Plants should not hug outside walls. A clear strip of concrete or sand against your house's foundation will act as a barrier for crawling insects.

Try to prevent dampness next to the foundation of the house. Moisture both outside and inside the house draws insects; they

Home Maintenance Is the Key

Insects in the home must be controlled in the most nontoxic way possible, but this takes hard work and the understanding that there are no magic solutions. Careful home maintenance is the most important factor in pest control. You will not get instant results or 100 percent success, but you can have a home with very few insects.

feed on the mold that may grow in hollow wall construction or in moist areas on slab foundations. Lush foliage and damp crawlspaces also draw moisture-loving insects.

Cleanliness is the most important factor in indoor insect control. Adult insects, larvae, and eggs can be removed by vacuuming, which also eliminates food crumbs that might serve as their food. Spring cleaning disturbs and rids the home of insects, while clutter attracts both insects and rodents. Move your furniture from time to time and remember to clean under it frequently.

Proper food storage is also extremely important. Food should be stored in glass and metal containers to keep insects out. Separate older food from new food so that any infestation will not be spread, and avoid storing food for long periods of time. Do not purchase food in dirty or stained packages, or with breaks or tears in the packaging. Buy only fresh-looking packages and look for signs of insect infestation.

▌ FOOD PESTS

There are four categories of kitchen pests that get into stored food:

- *Beetles:* Eat flours, dried soups, herbs and spices, cereals, cake, cookie and pancake mixes, and cured meats.
- *Weevils:* Eat grains and dried beans of all kinds.
- *Moths:* Adults do not feed on food, but larvae eat cornmeal, grains, dried fruit, and nuts.
- *Mites:* Eat cornmeal, grains, dried fruit, and nuts, as well as barley, caramel, cheese, rotting potatoes, sugar, and wine.

The following measures will help eradicate these insects:

- Do not buy damaged packages at the grocery store.
- Keep your kitchen cool and dry.
- Rotate your food stocks; eat older foods first.
- Store foods properly and discard any food with holes in the containers.
- Put a bay leaf in flour and cereal boxes or containers.
- Heat or freeze foods suspected of infestation.
- Keep your kitchen and pantry scrupulously clean.

▌ COCKROACHES

Cockroaches are a common household pest. They are immune to insecticides, and while they prefer carbohydrates, they will eat almost anything. Cockroaches will nest anywhere, including in refrigerator insulation. While they prefer the kitchen and bathroom, they will spread to all parts of the house.

Roaches are known carriers of the organism that causes boils, and of dysentery, plague, polio, hepatitis, salmonella, typhus, and toxoplasmosis (a disease affecting the central nervous system). Roach feces and body parts can be allergenic and will trigger asthma in sensitive people.

The following measures will help fight cockroaches:

- Store food in glass or metal containers.
- Do not leave dishes unwashed.
- Cover pet food and water overnight.
- Sweep up crumbs and spills promptly.
- Wipe off containers before returning them to cupboards.
- Put your garbage out every night.
- Do not save grocery sacks or cardboard boxes.
- Do not buy any packaged foods or drinks with spilled beverages or food on them.
- Use commercial- or technical-grade boric acid to kill roaches. It penetrates the insects' outer covering, and can be picked up on their feet and swallowed while the roaches preen themselves. Sprinkle boric acid with a small amount of sugar added on surfaces where roaches are likely to crawl, such as behind appliances and under the sink. The sugar attracts the insects so they will walk across the boric acid. Wear a mask and gloves while distributing the boric acid, and do not sprinkle the mixture where you store food. Keep the mixture out of reach of children and pets.
- Mix equal parts of oatmeal with plaster of Paris. Spread on the floor of infested areas. Or, sift and mix together 1 ounce trisodium phosphate (TSP), 6 ounces borax, and 4 ounces flour. Spread where needed. Another fatal roach food is a mixture of 2 Tbsp. flour, 1 Tbsp. cocoa, and 4 Tbsp. borax. Spread in roach traffic areas. Repeat these treatments in four days and again in two weeks in order to kill newly hatched cockroaches.
- Use roach traps. Wrap the outside of a jar with masking tape, and fill the jar half-full with beer or a few boiled raisins. Smear a band of petroleum jelly 1 or 2 inches below the rim inside the jar so the roaches cannot crawl out. Drown the trapped roaches in hot, sudsy water. Be sure to wash your hands thoroughly afterward.
- Heat kills roaches—temperatures of 130°F will kill any insects in heating system ducts. Roaches will also die when temperatures dip below 23°F. Open the windows on a freezing day and wipe out cockroaches, silverfish, and clothes moths.

▌ SILVERFISH

Silverfish eat paper, textiles of vegetable origin (linen, rayon, and cotton), and cereals. They enter the house on secondhand books and cardboard boxes. Damaged papers and books signal their presence.

The following measures will help with silverfish control:

- Fill in holes around pipes entering the house and repair any plumbing leaks.
- Vacuum your bookshelves and books frequently.
- Check your books periodically by opening and shaking them.
- Carefully inspect any secondhand books and old papers before bringing them into the house.

- Check lined draperies for silverfish between the drapery and the lining.
- Make a trap for silverfish by covering a jar with masking tape to provide a good foothold for the insects and baiting the jar with flour. Smear a band of petroleum jelly 1 or 2 inches below the rim of the jar so the silverfish cannot crawl out.
- Sprinkle boric acid, flour, and sugar on a piece of paper and place it in a corner or on a window ledge. Keep the mixture out of the reach of children and pets.

■ HOUSEFLIES

Flies have caused more human and animal deaths than any other insect. They are carriers of bacterial, parasitic, and viral disease. Flies eat and lay their eggs in filth, and when they get into our houses, they bring larvae, bacteria, and excreta. Flies very rapidly become immune to chemicals.

The following measures will aid in controlling houseflies:

- Sanitation is vital, since flies have a keen sense of smell. Keep all dishes clean, and rinse containers before putting them in the trash. Keep your garbage covered and dispose of it at the end of each day.
- Use proper lawn-care methods, such as spreading manure thinly so that maggots and eggs will die. Do not leave lawn clippings to decompose on the lawn. Pick up animal droppings and dispose of them properly.
- Use fly swatters to kill flies in the house. Since flies are drawn to light, darken a room and open a screened door or window. The flies will alight on the screen. At night, cover all windows, but leave an open slit at one of them so the flies can escape into the cool night air. Flies will collect on the windowsill and on the grass just outside during the night. They will be easy to kill with a flyswatter in the morning.
- Be sure that all screens on your house fit well.
- Some herbs will repel flies—clove, tansy, and pine oil are helpful. Camphor trees close to the kitchen door repel flies.

■ MOSQUITOES

Mosquitoes also cause many human diseases. They are carriers of malaria, yellow fever, dengue fever, and encephalitis. There is no effective treatment for the latter two illnesses. Mosquitoes are able to develop immunity to almost all pesticides.

The life cycle of the mosquito has four stages: egg, larvae, pupa, and adult. The males never bite, but females require a blood meal in order to lay fertile eggs. All eggs are laid on still water. If the water dries up before the eggs hatch, the larvae will hatch the next time water accumulates, even if the interim is as long as five or six years. Water management is the most important aspect of mosquito control.

The following measures will help in mosquito control:

- Eliminate all objects around your house that will hold water.
- Fill any holes, cavities, or pools that can hold water.
- Be sure flat roofs drain well.
- Be certain you have no leaky faucets.
- Help your community control all breeding sources for mosquitoes.
- Be certain your screens fit well and have no holes.

- Use natural mosquito repellents: oil of citronella, garlic, pennyroyal mint, tansy, and basil.
- If you have a pond, keep minnows for mosquito control.
- If you are particularly prone to mosquito bites, wear long sleeves and keep your pant legs tucked in. Try taking vitamin B_1 (thiamine) before going outdoors. This works to stop mosquitoes from biting for about half the people who use it.
- Bug control lights are effective if they are hung about 100 feet from the house or outdoor living area.
- If you live in an area that supports blue martins or swallows, erect a habitat that will attract these birds. They will devour a large number of mosquitoes.

▌ CLOTHES MOTHS

Moths are notorious for destroying clothes of animal origin, particularly wool. These moths are found mainly in warmer areas, and signal their presence by making holes in your clothes and upholstery. The larvae, which cause the damage, will eat straw, rayon, cotton, paper, fur, tobacco, hemp, and felt. The adults of one species will even eat mothproofed fabric.

To prevent clothes moth infestation:
- Seal all small openings into the house and attic.
- Clean closets and stored clothes regularly. Vacuum in all the cracks, backs of furniture, and under the furniture.
- Sun, air, and brush your clothing regularly.
- Freezing clothing, pressing with a steam iron, dry-cleaning, and heating your clothes in an oven at 140°F will kill all stages of insect life.

- Store clothing carefully, sealing it in plastic bags or clean cardboard boxes.
- Mint, tansy, bay leaves, rosemary, lavender, cloves, spearmint, and cedar will repel moths.

▌ TICKS

Ticks do not normally pose a problem for city dwellers, unless your home is close to a forest or wilderness area. Some species of ticks are dangerous carrying Rocky Mountain spotted fever, tularemia (a disease caused by bacteria), relapsing fever, and Lyme's disease.

The following measures will aid in controlling ticks:
- Make your home rodent-proof to keep out tick-carrying animals.
- Check your dogs and cats regularly and remove any ticks.
- Remove ticks with tweezers. Be careful that you do not crush the body, and be certain not to leave the insect's head in the wound. Place the ends of the tweezers as close as possible to the skin before pulling out the tick.

▌ FLEAS

Fleas are remarkable insects, capable of pulling 400 times their weight and lifting objects 150 times their mass. They have incredible jumping ability and many hiding places. Although not as dangerous as mosquitoes, fleas can spread plague (bubonic, pneumonic, and septicemic), typhus, tularemia, and tapeworm. Flea bites can also provoke allergic reactions.

Fleas are very difficult to eradicate. They are able to survive for long periods without food and can move from one host to another. Four species are important to humans: the human flea, the dog flea, the cat flea, and the rat flea, which is the plague carrier. Flea eggs cannot hatch if the temperature is lower than 40°F or the humidity less than 40 percent. Wet winter and spring seasons increase flea populations.

Fleas may live in upholstery, carpets, cracks in wooden floors, attics, basements, and walls, as well as in the yard. Even if you do not have pets, it is possible to have a flea infestation.

Anti-flea sprays, flea powders, and flea collars are toxic to both humans and animals. Many people are allergic to these chemicals, though it is doubtful whether flea insecticides bother fleas significantly.

The following measures will help to control fleas.

- Prevention is most important. Keep dogs outside and do not let them roam around the neighborhood. Cats that go outdoors will have flea problems, so comb them daily for fleas. Drop any fleas that you find in very hot water to kill them.
- Take precautions outdoors. Destroy all rodent nests, making sure the outside of your house is in good repair. Overwater or dry out the yard to kill fleas. Do not allow stray animals on your property.
- Vacuum your house frequently and empty the dust from the vacuum, being careful to bag and burn it, or bake it in the sun.
- Have your upholstery and carpets steam cleaned.
- Wash pet beds every two days (eggs take two days to hatch).
- Use repellents—brewer's yeast in pet food seems to help protect some animals. Some herbs that help repel fleas are citronella,

eucalyptus, pennyroyal mint, and rosemary. Use these in your animal's collars.
- Washing your dog's fur with lemon infusions helps to keep them free of fleas. To make the treatment, cut four lemons into eighths. Cover with water and bring to a boil, then simmer for 45 minutes. Cool, strain, and store in a glass container. Brush the infusion into the fur; allow to dry and brush again.
- Frequent bathing of animals can help to control fleas.
- Light and water traps may be helpful. Make one by filling a shallow dish with water and detergent. For one month, place a lamp over the dish and leave the light on all night.

▌ANTS

Ants are found everywhere on earth, in all types of climates. They live in structured societies and eat everything that humans eat. Ants are beneficial to us because they prey on other insects, including cockroaches, mealy bugs, cone nose bugs, larvae of filth flies, termite queens, and scale insects. They also enrich the soil and eat mosquito eggs.

Ants are most likely to invade a home after their nests have been flooded. It is easier to keep ants out than to try to get rid of them once they are established inside your house. However, if you see them around your house's foundation, you may want to leave them alone—they will help protect your home from termites.

The following measures will help to control ants:

- To prevent their entry, cut plants away from the house. Do not overwater the garden.
- Seal entry holes with petrolatum, putty, or caulking.

- Wipe up spilled foods and rinse dishes before putting them in the dishwater. Store foods and leftovers properly, and sweep the kitchen floor daily.
- Use mint or tansy to temporarily repel ants. Honey and boric acid on small pieces of paper placed in the path of ants will help control them. Keep the mixture out of the reach of children and pets.
- Destroy ant nests outdoors by pouring boiling water or hot paraffin into the nests.

■ TERMITES

Termites are divided into two groups: those that live in the earth and those that live above it. Subterranean termites live in colonies under the ground but feed above it. Drywood termites nest in the wood they eat and do not need ground contact. Those that live in the earth cause more damage. The termite problem is getting worse in North America—the only region free of termites is the far north.

Although most insects can be handled by nontoxic methods, most eradication companies still use chemicals. Drywood termites are treated using a "drill and treat" method if the infestation is local; chemicals are injected into drilled holes. Electroguns are a more recent and effective method, sending a current of electricity through the galleries in the wood and killing the termites. This procedure is much safer for people than the use of chemicals.

Subterranean termite infestations were treated primarily with chlordane until 1988, when its use was banned. However, dursban, which is more immediately toxic to humans, is still in use. It is an organophosphate and many people, including exterminators, react to it. Many companies now use

> ## Termite Signs
>
> *All houses, including brick houses, are vulnerable to termite infestation. Homes over 35 years old are likely to have termites. Signs include shelter tubes or fecal pellets, and wood flooring with dark or blistered areas.*

either Tribute or Dragnet, which are pyrethrin compounds. Pyrethrin is a compound (found naturally in some flowers, such as chrysanthemums) that has insecticidal properties. It appears to be effective in both killing and controlling termites. While it is considerably less toxic than dursban and chlordane, the pyrethrin compound can cause allergic reactions and symptoms in some individuals exposed to it. Its long-term exposure effects are not yet known.

To prevent subterranean termites:
- Keep your home as dry as possible. Be sure the lot drains adequately away from the house. Check that doors and windows are adequately flashed. Attics and crawlspaces should be adequately ventilated, and walls should be fitted with vapor barriers.
- Be sure all wood debris is cleared away from the house, particularly from the fill dirt under porches and steps.

To prevent drywood termites:
- Silica aerogel dust in wall spaces will kill insects that crawl over it.
- Arrange an annual termite inspection of your home.

To keep houses termite-free:
- Keep plumbing in good repair.
- Make sure there is a foundation of concrete

or concrete-filled block under all wood portions of your house.

• Avoid wetting stucco and wood siding.

• Fill all cracks in and around the house. Keep gutters and downspouts in good repair.

Ants pose the greatest threat to the termite. If you see them around your house's foundation, let them be—they will help protect your home.

■ FINDING AN EXTERMINATOR

Should you need the help of a professional exterminator, be certain you find a competent pest control company. Find out how well the employees are trained. Ask whether they receive continuing education and whether they will be supervised when they apply the pesticide. Find out what kind of insurance the company carries, as coverage against errors and omissions is important.

Ask whether the company is familiar with new, nonchemical controls, such as the Electrogun for killing termites. If chemicals are needed, find out what types of chemicals the company will use and ask for information on the toxicity of any of the chemicals. Double-check this information at a library. If you are chemically sensitive, ask your physician for information about the chemical ingredients of the materials to be used. If fumigation is necessary, find out:

• How will foods, plants, photographic equipment, artwork, leather, and rubber items be affected and protected?

• How will weather affect the fumigation?

• How long will the fumigant last?

• How will it be determined when the house is safe to reoccupy?

• How will your home be secured to prevent burglary?

Beware of a company that tries to pressure you into doing something quickly. Check the reputation of the company you choose with a consumer protection agency. When the company employees arrive at your home, check whether the workers, their clothing, and their truck are clean.

CHAPTER 13

The Allergens We Inhale

What is Inhalant Allergy?

We breathe in more than two tablespoons of solid particles every day. Inhalants (substances that are inhaled when breathing) include: pollens from trees, grasses, and weeds; mold; animal danders (dog, cat, horse, rabbit); mold; dust and dust mite; fibers such as cotton linters (the short fibers left on the seed), kapok, jute; feathers and down; orris root; tobacco; and other substances. Sensitive people can develop allergic responses to these inhalants.

Inhalant allergy symptoms include sneezing; hoarseness; increased mucus production; scratchy throat; runny nose; hay fever; itchy, red, watery eyes; and sinus symptoms of headache, pressure behind the eyeballs, pain in the frontal area, tenderness over the cheekbones, and aching teeth. Those affected have allergic shiners (dark circles under the eyes), and many, particularly children, will show signs of the "allergic salute." The allergic salute produces a horizontal crease across the nose from wiping a runny nose upwards with the palm of the hand. However, both allergic shiners and the allergic salute crease can also be from sensitivity to foods and chemicals.

Allergic responses to inhalants can also appear as multiple systemic symptoms, such as eczema, cold and flu-like symptoms, insomnia, asthma, fatigue, depression, cramps and diarrhea, headaches, hives, swollen lymph glands, flushing, skipped heartbeats, panic attacks, and many others. Some women experience irregular periods, vaginal itch, toxemia of pregnancy, or uterine hemorrhaging during pollen season, particularly when ragweed is pollinating. The same processes that cause symptoms in response to pollen can affect any organ of the body.

Most inhalant reactions of our bodies are IgE mediated and many people with severe inhalant allergies will have high IgE antibody levels in their blood. IgE molecules attach to various tissues, including lung and nasal passage tissues. When the allergen attaches to two adjacent IgE molecules on a mast cell or a basophil, chemicals are released, which cause the symptoms of an inhalant allergy. These released substances include histamine, heparin, kinins, enzymes, and leukotrienes. Small amounts of serotonin and acetylcholine are also released.

Some people have low IgE levels in their blood, but experience significant inhalant symptoms. Their reactions may be IgG mediated. These people must be tested by a different method (provocative neutralization) than the high IgE people in order for them to receive relief with allergy extracts. They will also receive relief from hands-on allergy treatment. Testing methods for IgE-mediated allergies include the scratch test and serial endpoint dilution titration for skin tests, and RAST, ALCAT, and ELISA for blood tests. (See chapter 8, Allergy Testing and Treatment, for more information on tests.)

▋ PHARMACEUTICAL TREATMENT FOR INHALANT ALLERGIES

Unfortunately, most inhalants cannot be totally avoided (especially pollens, mold, dust, dust mites, and tobacco), and lessening sensitivities to these substances depends on making environmental changes, as well as treatment. Some physicians treat only with drugs. Using antihistamines or oral steroids to treat allergic symptoms is only palliative, as these substances treat just the symptoms and do not decrease sensitivity to the allergen. In fact, sensitivity to allergens may actually increase, even though symptoms are being lessened with medications. These medications can be hazardous, and can produce serious side effects in some people.

Most antihistamines cause drowsiness, so that someone who is already fatigued from allergic reactions becomes more tired. Three new antihistamines, Allegra, Zyrtec, and Claritin, cause far less drowsiness than over-the-counter antihistamines but, as with other such medications, afford only symptom relief. Of these three antihistamines, Zyrtec is more likely to cause drowsiness. Allegra is less likely to cause driving impairment. Orally administered steroids (cortisone) taken over a long period of time can lead to cataracts, high blood pressure, ulcers, diabetes, edema, and suppression of adrenal gland function.

Steroid nasal sprays and Nasalcrom (cromolyn sodium) are two relatively new types of medications that may be helpful, and that do not cause the side effects seen with antihistamines and oral steroids. It can take up to two weeks for them to become effective, though. Nasalcrom is thought to stabilize mast cell membranes, thus inhibiting the allergic response. Inhaled steroids decrease both inflammation and the late phase of the allergic reaction. They are not absorbed into the bloodstream and cause fewer side effects than steroid pills. However, repeated use of inhaled steroids can cause perforation of the nasal septum, the mucous membrane-covered bone and cartilage partition dividing the nostrils.

Allergy testing for inhalant allergies and treatment with extracts affords safe relief of symptoms while decreasing sensitivity to the substance over a period of time. Hands-on allergy treatments for inhalant allergies are helpful, as are supportive treatments for the immune system. (See chapter 8, Allergy Testing and Treatment, for more information on these measures.)

Seasonal Allergies

Pollen allergies are referred to as seasonal allergies. Symptoms come and go as the seasons change.

▐▌ POLLEN

All seed-bearing plants product pollen (analogous to human sperm) as part of their reproductive cycle. Pollen can cause problems for humans; however, not all pollen-producing plants cause allergic symptoms. There are about 100 plant species that produce pollen that can be significant in human sensitivities.

Plants that cause pollen problems in humans must:

• be abundant and widely distributed
• produce pollen in large quantities
• produce pollen that is windborne
• produce pollen light enough to be carried some distance
• produce pollen containing specific antigens for hypersensitivity

Generally, plants that display brightly colored, perfumed flowers do not affect the allergic person. (There are some exceptions, such as goldenrod.) These plants have heavy pollen that is spread by insects and birds, and if the pollen does fall it will stay on the ground because of its weight and will not become airborne.

Trees, grasses, and weeds are the wind-pollinated plants that cause allergy problems. These plants have small, unattractive flowers that lack odor or nectar and they produce pollen grains that are "dry," containing no fats, pigments, or waxes. They also have a mechanism to arrest pollen release so that it occurs only as a result of the shaking motion of the wind.

To be airborne, pollen must be between 15 and 50 microns in diameter. When inhaled, these small grains enter the nose and pass into the small ducts of the bronchi, causing mild to severe problems, depending on the nature of the pollen and the person's sensitivity. Eighty-five percent of the pollen inhaled ends up in the stomach. Some pollens contain as many as 15 allergenic compounds, while others contain only one or two. People who are sensitive to all 15 of these compounds will be severely affected by pollen.

Plants producing windborne pollen fill the air with literally tons of pollen, most of which is composed of protein. This large production ensures that the pollen will be spread by sporadic breezes. In addition to being lightweight, different types of pollen grains frequently have efficient structures that aid in their dispersal, so that the wind can carry them for many miles. Fortunately, most pollen travels only a few feet from the parent plant.

Several factors affect the amount of pollen in the air. Heavy rains prevent distribution and help destroy pollen more quickly. Since most pollen is released between 6:00 and 9:00 A.M., afternoon rains do not help. However, high humidity weighs down the pollen and slows its movement. On dry, sunny days the slightest breeze can send it

Ragweed

Ragweed is a rascal. It grows all over North America except in the extremely cold regions. Its pollen contains at least three different allergens, and many people are allergic to it. One plant can produce 2 trillion pollen grains during its lifetime, which extrapolates to one acre of ragweed being able to produce 60 pounds of pollen during its late summer to early fall season. Its seeds are capable of germinating years after they have been sown. Disturbing the soil for farming or building homes, highways, or shopping centers causes ragweed to flourish.

Ragweed can also cause other problems. Some people develop contact dermatitis to the pollen, and for others, the ragweed plant can trigger a photosensitivity reaction when the plant touches their skin and they are subsequently exposed to the sun. The incidence of miscarriages is higher during ragweed season.

far and wide. Even after a frost, which stops plants from pollinating, existing pollens can still be spread by wind for a short period of time. This existing pollen will continue to be allergenic until it deteriorates.

■ RECOGNIZING POLLEN ALLERGIES
You should suspect a pollen problem if you experience symptoms, or if the symptoms are worst:

• in the early spring when trees pollinate
• in the late spring and early summer when grasses and weeds pollinate
• in the autumn when weeds are a continuing factor

When symptoms occur from spring to first frost with a peak in the fall, mold often is the prime offender. If you experience symptoms during the winter, suspect allergy to house-dust, dust mites, pets, and/or the gas furnace. Combustion products and airborne allergens are circulated by the forced air.

Symptoms of a pollen sensitivity are:
• itching of eyes or nose with thin, watery nasal discharge

• worse outdoors from 8:00 A.M. to 12:00 noon
• worse on clear, windy days
• improved on rainy days
• improved indoors with the house closed and air conditioning and filtration on
• worse when going from an air-conditioned room to open air when the pollen count is high
• worse at peaks of specific pollen seasons
• improved after the first light frost

If the whole eye itches, pollen allergy is likely to blame. However, if the inner canthus (inside corner of the eye) is itchy, this suggests a food allergy, even though it may be pollen season.

If you experience any of the above symptoms you should suspect a pollen allergy. Because pollens are difficult to avoid, you should consider some form of testing and treatment for pollen sensitivity. It is not necessary to test and treat for every allergenic pollen. There is cross-reactivity between pollens of plants in the same family, so that an extract containing one member of the family will help desensitize the person to other members of that family.

Some pollen will always be present in our homes. It enters the house through open windows and doors, as well as on shoes, clothing, and pet fur. Air cleaners help to create a pollen-free environment in the home and are a must for the extremely sensitive person. Filters in air cleaners should be changed or cleaned as needed. Wearing a mask when outdoors will also filter out pollens. (See The Importance of Air Quality in chapter 12.)

▌ POLLEN ACTIVITY DATES

Pollination dates vary slightly from year to year, depending on weather conditions. The timing of the first and last freeze will affect the dates. However, pollination dates usually fall within a given time span, making it possible to predict, within limits, when a particular plant will pollinate. The amount of rainfall and the temperature will also affect the amount of pollen produced.

The Regional Zone Map on the following page shows the different pollinating zones within the continental United States and Canada. Spring-flowering plants bloom and pollinate from south to north, and fall-flowering plants bloom and pollinate from north to south. In most areas, trees pollinate from late winter until spring, grasses pollinate from spring until early summer, and weeds pollinate from summer until early fall.

Below the map are listed the general pollinating times for each zone. These are broad time frames; pollination times within a particular zone will vary between states or provinces, and within the states or provinces

Juniper Terpenes

Many people come into our office in the middle of December complaining that their juniper pollen allergies are "killing" them. This could be a mystery, because there is not a grain of juniper pollen in the air until the middle of January. However, when we take into account the fact that the level of juniper terpenes increases about a month before the trees pollinate, the source of their symptoms is obvious. They are reacting to the terpenes. Many people require treatment for both pollens and terpenes to obtain complete relief.

themselves. The variation depends on the size of the area, the type of terrain, and the plant species in each state or province. Varying altitudes and proximity to sea coasts also affect the length of the pollen season. More detailed information should be available from your environmental medicine physician, county agent, or appropriate government agency.

▌▌ TERPENES

Terpenes are types of unsaturated hydrocarbons occurring in both animals and plants. They are most widely distributed in plants, particularly in the essential oils and resins, and are responsible for the plant's odor and taste. There are many classes of terpenes, which depend on their chemical structures. Turpentine, rubber latex, and vitamin A are examples of plant terpenes. Cholesterol is a type of animal terpene.

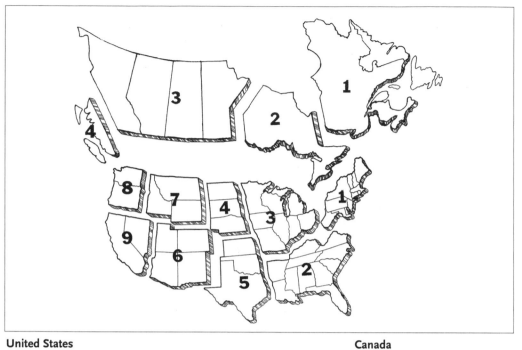

United States

ZONE 1
Trees	February–July
Grasses	February–September
Weeds	April-October

ZONE 2
Trees	December–October
Grasses	January–October
Weeds	April–October

ZONE 3
Trees	December–July
Grasses	February–September
Weeds	April–October

ZONE 4
Trees	February–July
Grasses	February–October
Weeds	April–October

ZONE 5
Trees	January–October
Grasses	January–October
Weeds	April–October

ZONE 6
Trees	January–October
Grasses	January–October
Weeds	March–October

ZONE 7
Trees	February–July
Grasses	March–September
Weeds	April–September

ZONE 8
Trees	February–September
Grasses	February–August
Weeds	March–November

ZONE 9
Trees	Year-round (some trees pollinate every month)
Grasses	January–October
Weeds	March–November

ALASKA
Trees	March–July
Grasses	April–August
Weeds	May–September

HAWAII

The pollen season in Hawaii is less easily defined than it is in the continental United States. At lower elevations, Hawaii's growing season is essentially continuous, with a few peak periods for grasses and weeds.

Canada

ZONE 1
Trees	February–June
Grasses	April–September
Weeds	May–September

ZONE 2
Trees	March–May
Grasses	April–August
Weeds	May–October

ZONE 3
Trees	April–June
Grasses	April–September
Weeds	April–October

ZONE 4
Trees	February–April
Grasses	May–September
Weeds	May–October

Terpenes are found in all parts of the plant—the pollen, stems, leaves, and flowers—but terpene concentration is highest in the stems, leaves, and flowers. Although they are present year-round, terpene production increases before flowering and then decreases rapidly. Terpenes are responsible for some of the blue haze seen over mountains, for the smell of freshly cut grass, for the pine scent of all conifers, and for the sweet smell of lilacs. The unique taste of meat broiled over mesquite wood charcoal comes from the mesquite terpene. People who cannot tolerate live Christmas trees are sensitive to conifer terpenes. Terpenes give the spices used in cooking their flavor. Chemically sensitive people are always sensitive to terpenes and may have difficulty eating spicy or smoked foods.

Many sensitive people experience adverse reactions to both terpenes and pollens. This is evident in those who develop pollen symptoms long before pollen appears. These symptoms coincide with the rise in terpenes that occurs just before trees, grasses, and weeds flower. Some of these people will receive symptom relief or control using only pollen extracts, while others require testing and treatment with allergy extracts for both terpenes and pollens. Hands-on allergy treatment can give relief from both terpene and pollen sensitivity.

Perennial Allergies

Perennial allergies include allergies to molds, animal danders, dust mites, and other substances. These allergies—and allergens—are present year-round.

Windspread Molds

Winds, including hurricanes, gales, and tornadoes, spread mold spores far and wide, even into the atmosphere. Mold spores have been found at altitudes of 16,000 feet. On windless days, it takes several hours for mold spores to drop 100 feet, which guarantees their being in the air for many hours after a weather disturbance. Sometimes pollen allergy is blamed for what is actually a reaction to mold spores in the air.

▌▌ MOLDS

Molds are the primary fungi that cause inhalant reactions in people. (See chapter 17, Fungi, Yeast, and Mold, for fungi that cause infections.) These organisms are widespread, found in great numbers in soil and in the air. Molds are not restricted by season, but are present all year, except when there is snow on the ground. They require abundant moisture for growth and spore dispersion. They also need a supply of organic matter and oxygen. Molds are hardy, thriving at 70° to 90°F, but some are able to endure subfreezing temperatures. They remain dormant until thawed, when they will start to grow again. In general, molds grow best at room temperature, since intense heat and excessive dryness are both detrimental to them.

Mold growth can take place in any part of the continent. Molds send their spores into the air when it rains and when snow thaws. In many areas, spore production peaks in late summer or early fall, but some molds continue to produce spores for many months. After the first hard freeze, spore production becomes minimal.

Environments containing sugar are conducive to mold growth, as well as acidic conditions in which bacteria cannot grow. These properties enable mold to develop on the surfaces of foods such as jellies, jam, and pickles.

Molds can be found in homes, schools, factories, hospitals, farms, and outdoors. No environment is devoid of molds. They can grow on food, plants, soil, paint, wallpaper paste, wood, leather, hay, animal waste, paper, and many other fibers. Mold can contaminate food, such as bread, or it can be an essential added ingredient, as in the production of some cheeses. Roquefort, Camembert, and blue are examples of mold-ripened cheese.

One of the best-known mold products is the antibiotic penicillin, which is produced by *Penicillium notatum*.

Molds can be highly destructive agents. They damage the substrate on which they are growing in an attempt to turn it into nutrients. They are one of the chief causes of disease in cultivated plants, causing considerable loss of stored seeds. Molds cause deterioration of many products, such as wood, leather goods, rubber articles, paper, fabrics, and even glass lenses.

▮ HOUSEHOLD MOLD

When mold spores are plentiful outside, they dominate the indoors also. Molds originating indoors are more obvious when buildings are closed to the outside; a musty smell signals the presence of mold. Indoor mold levels are in proportion to the relative humidity. Ventilation is extremely important in controlling household mold.

In the home, mold is frequently found in the basement, because this area is usually somewhat damp. Basement mold can send spores throughout the house. Mold production is also high in bathrooms and kitchens. In the bathroom, mold will grow on the caulking between the tub and the tile, on the shower curtain, and on the floor behind the toilet. In the kitchen, mold frequently develops at the sink-wall junction and around the bottom of the cold-water pipe. The surplus water tray on self-defrosting refrigerators is a particularly notable mold source.

Sunrooms, atriums, or other areas of the house that contain houseplants are major sources of mold from the soil. The rugs and flooring beneath water beds are also a prime spot for mold growth if the bed has even a minuscule leak. Hot tubs that are not properly maintained or that have small leaks may also be a mold source.

Walls in adobe houses that have been built directly on soil rather than on concrete foundations frequently have a great deal of mold caused by upward seepage from the ground. Flat-roofed houses also have mold problems because of leakage into ceilings and walls. Insulation and wallboard can be moldy long before it is possible to detect any mold on the painted surface.

Outdoors, mowing the grass and raking leaves constitutes a mold exposure. In farming areas where there are grain crops, harvesting the grains is an enormous exposure, not only for the harvesters but for the surrounding communities. Mold spores can be spread by winds, insects, and humans. Because they are microscopically small, spores can be carried by the wind for 15 to 20 miles.

For a typical mold-sensitive person, symptoms will be:

- worse outside between 5:00 and 9:00 P.M., in the cool evening air
- worse in damp places (woods, or particular rooms in a house, especially the basement and bathroom)
- worse when mowing or playing on grass, or when raking leaves
- worse when exposed to hay (fields, haystacks, barns)
- distinctly worse from August until heavy frost
- ongoing after the ragweed season
- improved inside a closed house when the air conditioning or furnace is on
- improved when temperatures drop below freezing and snow covers the ground. (Snow covers outdoor sources of mold such as decayed vegetation, dry leaves, and grass.)
- worse when eating foods made by fermentation: beer, wine, sharp cheese, sauerkraut, pickles, and vinegar
- worse following ingestion of mushrooms, other fungi, and seaweed
- worse after exposure to a number of days of damp weather in succession

With mold allergies there is no itching of the eyes and nose; those symptoms strictly relate to pollens or foods. Allergy extracts are very useful in controlling a mold allergy, as are hands-on allergy treatments for mold.

▮ COMMON AIRBORNE MOLDS

▮ *Alternaria*

This mold grows on organic debris in the soil; on the leaves, stems, flowers, and fruits of many vegetables; on cereal grains; and on ornamental plants (such as tomatoes, beans, chrysanthemums, and cabbage). Its spores easily become airborne and are very common from late spring until fall, especially between noon and 3:00 P.M.

In September, symptoms caused by *Alternaria* are frequently mistaken for ragweed symptoms. *Alternaria* is one of the two major widespread molds that produce allergic symptoms, and it is probably the most clinically reactive airborne mold allergen.

▮ *Aspergillus*

A common soil mold, *Aspergillus* also grows on stored food products under damp conditions. One species is common on wet surfaces in bathrooms and in drip pans of refrigerators and other appliances. *Aspergillus* also grows on damp hay, grain, fruits, and sausage. Indoor and occupational exposures are common.

▮ *Aureobasidium (Pullularia)*

The spores of this mold are most plentiful in the air during the afternoon (1:00 to 5:00 P.M.). When they germinate, these mold colonies have a slimy, yeastlike appearance, due to the numerous spores that bud off the mold growth. *Aureobasidium* is found in soil, but also grows on decaying vegetation and plants. It frequently occurs in large numbers.

▮ *Cladosporium (Hormodendrum)*

The spores of this mold are very plentiful in the air, sometimes making up half of the total spore count. These spores are released in large numbers after rain and damp weather. The highest levels occur from mid-summer until December, and spore counts peak between 11:00 A.M. and 3:00 P.M.

This mold grows on decomposing plants, leather, rubber, cloth, paper, and wood products. It may also be a parasite on the living leaves of some plants. *Cladosporium* and *Alternaria* are the primary widespread molds that produce allergic symptoms.

❙ *Fusarium*

The spores of this mold are often produced in a slimy mass, and the mold colonies are usually a prominent salmon color. They need water-splashing to be dispersed, and so may be especially common in the air after a rain.

Many *Fusarium* species are parasitic on vegetable and field crops, such as peas, beans, tomatoes, corn, sweet potatoes, rice, and cotton. *Fusarium* is also found on decaying plants. Its spores may be released from infected grasses and cereals, and from stored fruits and vegetables such as cucumbers, tomatoes, and potatoes.

❙ *Helminthosporium*

Found on cereal grain plants, such as corn, wheat, oats, and rye, *Helminthosporium* spores are fairly common in the air, and are also dispersed by grain-threshing operations. The daily peak of *Helminthosporium* production is at about 2:00 P.M.

❙ *Mucor*

A soil inhabitant, *Mucor* is found around barns and barnyards growing on animal waste. It also grows on food residue and leaf litter. While this mold is plentiful in the soil,

its level in the air is usually low. Because of ground water seepage and dirt tracked into the house, *Mucor* can flourish indoors and contribute to inhalant allergies.

❙ *Penicillium*

Normally a soil inhabitant, *Penicillium* can grow on breads, cheese, citrus fruits, jams, apples, other foods, leather, and organic materials. Colonies of this mold are often blue or green. Its spores are plentiful inside houses during the winter, and peak at about 2:00 P.M. (Mutant strains are used to produce the antibiotic penicillin.)

❙ *Phoma*

This mold grows on paper products, such as books and magazines, and also on some paints and plants. *Phoma* spores arise in flask-shaped organs and are extruded in mucinous masses of slime spores. The spores are dispersed by dew and raindrop washout. *Phoma* reactivity is common and is similar to *Alternaria* allergy.

❙ *Rhizopus*

This mold grows on bread, cured meats, harvested root vegetables, and sugary, stored food products (bakery goods, fruit, and sweet potatoes). It also grows on a variety of plants and is widespread in nature.

▮▮ ANIMAL DANDERS

All animals, including humans, shed dander into the air. Dander is composed of skin scales and scurf (dandruff). It is light, airy, and floats about freely, and it may remain in an area for days after the animal has been removed. People may be allergic to both animal and human dander, as well as to animal serum or saliva. Reactions to animal dander or saliva can include hives, difficulty breathing (asthma), headaches, loss of voice, itching or watering eyes, and sneezing.

You should suspect an animal dander sensitivity if your symptoms occur or worsen when:
- you are exposed to animals, such as cats, dogs, or horses
- you are exposed to animal hair (rabbit, mohair, wool) in blended form (sweaters, gloves, liners, blankets), rug padding, or furniture stuffing
- you are licked by an animal

The degree of animal sensitivity varies from person to person. For some people, animals must be removed from the home environment. For others, reducing contact (by keeping animals outside) may be sufficient. Regardless of the intensity of your sensitivity, animals should never be allowed in the bedroom or on the bed. Animal dander can be spread throughout the house by a forced heating or cooling system. Even after an animal has been removed from your house, it may take years to completely remove all traces of hair and dander from carpeting and furniture.

Cat dander and saliva are both extremely potent allergens, but the saliva is most allergenic. Many people develop symptoms after being licked by a cat, and saliva can cause a reaction even when it has dried on the cat's fur.

The dander is very lightweight and difficult to remove from an area. Cat dander has been found in homes that have never housed cats, and in houses under construction. Cat dander and saliva have been detected in living quarters of permanent settlements in the antarctic where there are no cats. It migrated there by "passive transfer," probably on human clothing. School classrooms are a cat exposure because of the dander and cat hair brought in on the students' clothing.

Cat-sensitive people can be affected by more than just housecats, and should avoid clothing or furnishings, such as rugs, made from leopard, tiger, or other feline skins, as well as the wild cat cages at the zoo. Although no longer common, cat fur was at one time used in toys, gloves, slippers, imitation fur, upholstered furniture, bathrobes, and caps. Dry-cleaning these items can reduce the potency of the dander or saliva, but avoiding them is best.

Dogs are the second most common source of animal dander, hair, or saliva allergies. All species of dog, short- or long-haired, can cause sensitivities. Many sensitive people also react to licks from dogs. All dogs share common allergens, as well as having special, breed-specific antigens. Because of this, some people may tolerate one breed better than another. As well, some dog breeds shed very little, and if the animals are kept clean and trimmed, these breeds cause fewer problems. Dog hair was formerly used to make fur coats, rugs, and robes.

Horse dander can also be a potent allergen, but it is less of a problem today because there are few horses in our cities. However, exposures are likely in rural areas. Horse hair is also found in manure, posing a problem for those who use it to fertilize gardens and lawns.

Because horse dander is antigenically similar to horse serum, people allergic to horse dander should be careful about receiving horse antisera shots, such as snake venom antiserum, antivenom for black widow spider bites, and tetanus antitoxin.

Horse hair is no longer used as often in upholstered furniture, mattresses, mattings, padding, and felt. However, rugs, upholstered furniture, carpet padding, blankets, pillow stuffing, mattress stuffing, clothing, drapery, and some toys may still contain horsehair.

Rabbit dander and fur may also cause allergic reactions. Rabbit fur coats and hats, fur trimmings, fur pillows, toy animals, fabrics, linings of gloves and slippers, angora yarn, the sounding hammers of pianos, and some felts constitute exposure to rabbit fur or dander.

Sensitivities to cattle, pig, and goat hair and dander, sheep wool, sheep dander, and lanolin are also possible. The hair and wool from these animals may be found in clothing, cloth, cushions, bedding, carpets, and wigs.

∎ DUST

Outside dirt is basically inorganic, composed of rock and mineral dust. Housedust, on the other hand, is considered organic dirt because it is so laden with organic matter. Housedust is a very complex mixture, composed of the breakdown products of the following items:

Plant
- cellulose: cotton, jute, kapok, linen, wood
- food remnants
- mold spores
- pollen

Animal
- felt (made from wool)
- fragments: ants, beetles, cockroaches, cocoons, feathers, fleas, flies, mosquitoes, moths, silverfish, spiders, webs
- furs (of all types)
- hair (camel, goat (mohair), horse)
- housedust mites
- human dander
- insect feces
- pet dander
- silk
- wool

Inorganic
- acrilan
- dacron
- fireplace soot
- nylon
- paint
- plastic
- rubber
- cigarette smoke
- fiberglass
- lycra
- orlon
- paper
- rayon
- spandex

The mold spores in housedust are a bigger problem in damp climates than in drier areas. When molds release their spores, they are sent throughout the house and into the air we breathe. (See Molds, above.)

Another major component of housedust is the housedust mite. This is a microscopic insect (arthropod) which, in damp climates, is found in abundance in the dust of homes. (See Dust Mites, below.)

No matter how well we clean our houses, we will be surrounded by some dust and we breathe it continually. An average six-room house accumulates 40 pounds of dust in a year. Dust is formed as materials that make up household articles, furniture, and clothing age and deteriorate. It also collects in stored articles and furniture. Housedust could be considered an occupational hazard for the homemaker, as housecleaning stirs up enormous quantities of dust.

Housedust can produce year-round symptoms, but they occur principally during the months when the house is closed and the furnace is operating. The harder the furnace works—and the drier the house—the greater the problem of housedust allergy.

The following are possible indicators of a dust sensitivity. Symptoms occur or worsen:

- indoors, and improve outdoors
- when the heating season starts (symptoms improve in the spring)
- when the house is swept or dusted
- when the bed is being made
- when sitting on upholstered furniture
- in a library
- in the bedroom
- when you arise in the morning, improving during the day
- when you have been in bed for 30 to 60 minutes

▮▮ DUST MITES

Dust mites, which are related to ticks and spiders, make up a microscopic insect component of housedust. There are 15 species living around the world. They eat the 50 million skin scales that people shed every day. They cannot survive on living skin.

Mites are harmful only to people who are allergic to them. Mites and their excrement induce bronchial inflammation and hyperreactivity, leading to asthma and other forms of breathing difficulty. Other symptoms caused by dust mites include rhinitis, sneezing, congestion, and itchy, watery eyes. Al-

Asthma-Dust Mite Link

The Institute of Medicine (IOM) in Washington, D.C. has found strong, causal evidence that indoor substances contribute to the development or worsening of asthma. Dust mites, dust, and allergens produced by cats and cockroaches can aggravate symptoms in some asthmatics, as can exposure to second-hand tobacco smoke. A combination of factors, both genetic and environmental, seems to determine whether an individual will develop asthma. Controlling indoor allergens, removing pets from the household, eliminating chemical pollution, and controlling indoor humidity are important factors in helping to control asthma.

lergy extracts for dust mites are helpful in controlling these symptoms, as are hands-on allergy treatments.

Dust mites do not live in dry climates or at high altitudes; they proliferate in warm, humid environments. Dust mite allergy is as high as 25 percent in humid areas. However, even in the cold, dry antarctic where the humidity rarely exceeds 20 percent, dust mite antigens accumulate. They migrate there by "passive transfer," most likely on human clothing. In damp climates, mites are found in abundance in dust, and colonize mattresses, comforters, carpets, and upholstered furniture. They also live in stuffed toys. A typical double bed can harbor more than 2 million dust mites and can double its weight in 10 years as a result of being filled with dead dust mites and their feces.

Dust mite carcasses and excrement float about, entering our lungs. Live mites are not inhaled, as they have sticky feet that cling to surfaces. The average dust mite produces about 20 highly allergenic fecal pellets per day, enough to equal its own weight in just a few days. The pellets are so light that they stay in the air for 10 minutes after being disturbed. They are covered by a membrane so strong that soaking for 16 hours does not affect it.

Signs of dust mite allergy include:
- persistently stuffy nose or ears
- repeated sneezing on awakening
- worsening of symptoms when beds are made
- improving symptoms outside the house

■■ FEATHERS AND FIBERS

■ FEATHERS

Many people are sensitive to chicken, goose, and duck feathers. The feathers of canaries, parakeets, parrots, pigeons, turkeys, and sparrows rarely produce reactions. Pillows, comforters, quilts, jackets, sleeping bags, and beds are common sources of feather exposure. Because feather allergies are usually products of decomposition, most feather-sensitive people are able to eat the meat and eggs of fowls without problems. They also do not usually experience allergic reactions from egg-containing vaccines.

You should suspect a feather allergy if your symptoms occur or worsen when you are:
- exposed to feathers (in pillows, down sleeping bags, comforters, and jackets)
- exposed to chicken, geese, or ducks
- exposed to someone working with fowl

■ COTTON LINTERS

Cotton linters are not the same fibers used in cotton cloth, which is usually safe for people with health problems. Linters are the short fibers that cling to the seed after longer fibers have been removed, and they contain fragments of the seeds. These short fibers, when inhaled, can cause local irritation in the nasal passages.

Cotton linters are used to make cotton wadding or batting in pads, cushions, comforters, some mattresses, and upholstery. Linters may also be found in stuffed toys, some carpets, and rope. The type of varnish used to coat metals and artificial leather and for water-proofing may contain ingredients made from cotton linters.

■ JUTE

In this age of synthetic fibers, allergies to natural fibers are frequently overlooked. Jute is a natural, tropical fiber that may trigger asthma in some people. Jute is found in burlap, carpet padding, grassplace mats, hula skirts, and braided rugs.

■ KAPOK

Kapok is another natural fiber that can be a potent allergen. Its silky fiber, obtained from the Indonesian silk-cotton tree, is used as stuffing for cushions, mattresses, pillows, life jackets, and toys. Exposure to kapok can cause asthma, sneezing, itching of the skin, and itchy, watery eyes.

■ ORRIS ROOT

Orris root comes from the iris plant. The roots are washed, dried, then stored for three years, during which time they acquire their fragrance. The fragrance is faintly violet with a fruity undertone. After drying, the roots are pulverized and distilled to extract their yellow, semisolid oil. The majority of orris root production takes place in Italy, with the distillation process done mostly in France. It is one of the oldest, most expensive, and most widely used perfume ingredient.

Orris root is also used in cosmetic powders and toiletries because its oil and fine starch granules hold perfumes. Many manufacturers have stopped using orris root powder in cosmetics because of its high allergenicity. However, even if orris root powder is not listed on the label, a cosmetic may contain tincture of orris root.

Reactions can include infantile eczema, hay fever, stuffy nose, red eyes, headaches, nausea, and asthma. Orris root extracts or hands-on allergy treatment help to control these symptoms.

Orris root may be found in bakery goods, dusting powder, face powder and creams, gin factories, hair tonic, lipstick, lotions, perfumes, rouges, sachets, scented soaps or shampoos, shaving creams, sunburn lotions, teething rings, and toothpaste or tooth powder.

▮▮ TOBACCO

Tobacco smoke is a major contributor to indoor pollution. About one-third of the adult North American population smokes tobacco, and everyone is exposed to tobacco smoke in varying degrees. A major irritant for both smokers and nonsmokers, tobacco smoke causes burning eyes, nasal congestion and drainage (rhinitis), sore throat, cough, headache, and nausea. Even those who enjoy smoking find the irritating "side-stream" smoke from smoldering tobacco to be unpleasant. Smoking one cigarette releases three mg of carbon monoxide and 70 mg of dry particulate matter.

Cigar and pipe smoke is even more irritating to the eyes, nose, throat, and bronchial passages.

There are two types of smoke: mainstream smoke, which is the smoke drawn through the tobacco during inhalation (active smoking), and sidestream smoke, which arises from burning tobacco (passive smoking). Ninety-six percent of the gases and particulates (small solid particles) produced when cigarettes burn become sidestream smoke. Higher concentrations of these compounds are found in the sidestream smoke inhaled by the nonsmoker than in the mainstream smoke inhaled by the smoker.

Results from studies show that compared to mainstream smoke, sidestream smoke contains:

- twice as much tar and nicotine
- three times as much 3, 4 Benzo[a]pyrene (a carcinogen)
- five times as much carbon monoxide
- five times as much ammonia

▮ GASES AND VAPORS PRESENT IN SIDESTREAM SMOKE

▮ *Acetaldehyde*

Acetaldehyde damages the cilia, which line the upper respiratory tract. This damage lessens our body's ability to protect itself against infection, because the capacity to remove particulates from the respiratory tract is impaired. Coughing and wheezing result. Acetaldehyde can also depress and disrupt the central nervous system.

❚ *Ammonia*

Ammonia vapors are present in sidestream smoke, irritating the eyes and mucous membranes.

❚ *Carbon Monoxide*

The National Ambient Air Quality Standard for carbon monoxide is 9 ppm (parts per million); the allowable concentration in industry is 50 ppm. In rooms and vehicles where cigarettes are being smoked, carbon monoxide concentrations may range from 12 to 90 ppm. One study shows that if seven cigarettes are smoked in one hour, even in an average-sized ventilated room, the carbon monoxide level goes up to 20 ppm. In the seat next to the smoker this level will be 90 ppm, almost twice the maximum allowable level set for industry.

Carbon monoxide, even in small amounts, can cause:

• diminished ability to distinguish relative brightness
• diminished ability to judge time intervals
• diminished attention to sounds
• difficulty with hand-eye coordination
• headaches, dizziness, fatigue, and nausea

(See chapter 11, Chemical Sensitivities, for more information on the effects of carbon monoxide at higher levels.)

Ventilation helps lower the carbon monoxide level, but not right next to the smoker. A carbon monoxide "hangover" lasts for three to four hours after leaving a smoky area.

❚ *Formaldehyde*

Formaldehyde is found in sidestream smoke, as are other aldehyde compounds resulting from chemicals sprayed on the to-bacco. Formaldehyde causes coughing; eye, nose, and throat irritations; fatigue; headaches; nausea; skin reactions; wheezing; and other symptoms. (See chapter 11 for more information on formaldehyde.)

❚ *Hydrogen Cyanide*

Hydrogen cyanide is a poisonous gas that attacks respiratory enzymes. Levels above 10 ppm are considered dangerous. The concentration of hydrogen cyanide in cigarette smoke is 1,600 ppm.

❚ *Nitrogen Dioxide*

Nitrogen dioxide concentrations in sidestream cigarette smoke are 250 ppm; 5 parts per million is considered a dangerous level. Nitrogen dioxide causes irritation, inflammation, and fluid retention in the air passages in the lungs, triggering "tightness" in the chest, coughing, and wheezing. It destroys cellular and subcellular structures in the lungs and induces emphysema in laboratory animals.

❚ PARTICULATES PRESENT IN SIDESTREAM SMOKE

❚ *Benzo[a]pyrene and Dimethylnitrosamine*

These substances are carcinogens that are measurable in small amounts in sidestream smoke. Cigar and pipe smoke contains even more of these compounds than does cigarette smoke.

❚ *Cadmium*

Cadmium is toxic to humans and is measurable in sidestream smoke. In high concentrations, cadmium is a poisonous metal. Only minute amounts are inhaled in smoke, but the metal builds up in the body in direct proportion to the amount of smoke inhaled. Cadmium accumulates in the liver, kidneys,

studies show that they are starting to smoke at earlier and earlier ages, the FDA is focusing on preventing this addiction. It is trying to limit the access to and appeal of cigarettes and smokeless tobacco to children and adolescents.

It is now a federal violation to sell cigarettes and smokeless tobacco to anyone younger than 18 years of age. Manufacturers, distributors, and retailers must comply with certain conditions regarding the sale, distribution, and promotion of tobacco products. Free samples are prohibited, and vending machines and self-service displays are prohibited except in facilities where the retailer or operator ensures that no person younger than 18 is present or permitted to enter at any time.

Billboards and other outdoor advertising is prohibited within 1,000 feet of schools and public playgrounds. Advertising is generally limited to a black-and-white, text-only format. The sale and distribution of non-tobacco items, such as hats and T-shirts that carry cigarette logos, is prohibited. Sponsorship of sporting and other events is limited to the use of the corporate name only.

CHAPTER 14

Breathing Safely

How Can We Breathe Safely?

Even when we are in our own homes, we cannot totally control our exposure to inhalants. Plants will pollinate and release their pollen into the air regardless of our allergies. Molds grow everywhere and under almost any condition. Our pets lick us to show their affection, and their dander is inevitable. We do have a greater measure of control over fibers, feathers, and tobacco exposures.

In spite of the inevitability of inhalant exposures, there are environmental controls you can exert that will minimize your exposures. This chapter will show you measures you can use to reduce and control your exposures to inhalants. Most are very simple ways to decrease your allergic reactions, dramatically increasing your comfort. Allergy extracts or hands-on treatments for inhalants will also help control your reactions.

■ CONTROLLING POLLEN EXPOSURES AND ALLERGIES

In addition to taking pollen and terpene extracts or having hands-on allergy treatment,

there are other methods that will aid in controlling your pollen and terpene allergies. One important step to take in controlling your pollen allergies is to prevent pollen from getting into your house. You cannot prevent pollen exposures outdoors, but you can lower the levels in your home.

Keep your windows and doors closed, and run an air cleaner that removes particles 24 hours a day, particularly in your bedroom. If you have air conditioning, use a filter on the air conditioner also. When you travel in your car, keep the air conditioner on and the windows up.

Pollen can enter a house on the fur of pets, and it can be tracked in on clothing and shoes. Wash your house pets regularly, and minimize their trips out of the house. If the pet is an outdoor animal, do not let it in the house.

If you have been outdoors for more than just a trip from the house to your car, change your clothes and rinse or wipe off the soles of your shoes. If pollen counts are high, you may need to leave your shoes at the door.

Rinse your nose with sterile saline (avail-

Pollen Report

Monitor the daily pollen count. Avoid being outdoors on the days it is high, and particularly avoid being outside on windy days. Remember that plants release most pollen in the morning, some of it before sunrise. If you must go outside, wear a dust mask or a mask that filters out particles, and limit your outdoor activities in the morning.

able at pharmacies) each time you come in from outdoors. This will remove the pollen in your nose and prevent it attaching to the mucous membranes. You can make your own saline solution by using ¼ tsp. salt in 1 cup of warm water. Wash your bedding weekly and dry it in a dryer. Pollen clings to fabric dried outdoors.

Wash your face every morning and evening in warm water to which the solution for High Performance Hygiene System has been added (See Recommended Sources and Organizations). This solution contains hydrogen peroxide, iodine, potassium, magnesium, zinc, and manganese. Submerge your whole face, blink a few times, and blow air out your nose. This cleans out your tear ducts and stimulates your nose and bronchi to eliminate pollen and allergens.

People with long hair should cover it when they go outdoors. Pollen-sensitive people should take a bath and wash their hair at night to reduce pollen in the bedding.

Do not have high levels of vegetation in your yard. Select low-pollinating plants and plant female trees to avoid pollen from male

trees. You will still have terpenes, but you will have less pollen. Do not plant trees such as elm and cypress that are monoecious, containing both male and female characteristics. Do not work in the yard, but be certain that your grass is mowed regularly so that it does not have a chance to produce its seedheads and pollen. Also remove weeds before they pollinate. If you must work in the yard, wear a pollen mask. Change clothes, take a bath, and wash your hair when you have finished. Do not go in and out of the house while you are working as this will track pollen into the house.

Many people who are pollen sensitive are also terpene sensitive. Avoid exposure to terpenes by not having scented live plants in the house. Do not use a live Christmas tree or fresh evergreen decorations. Spices and grilled foods are also high in terpenes and you will need to avoid them if you are terpene sensitive.

Be certain your food and chemical allergies are under control. Many people who are suffering from pollen allergies and are finding them difficult to control are laboring under a large allergic overload. Taking care of food and chemical allergies will significantly reduce pollen symptoms. Diet and environmental control are essential for pollen symptom control.

Be aware of concomitant foods, those to which people react in the presence of a pollen, dust, or mold. Many people have to avoid their concomitant foods during pollen season. The relationships between pollens and food are discussed in chapter 9, Food Allergies.

Take quercetin, a potent bioflavonoid

with antihistamine action. Take 400 to 500 mg between meals twice a day. (See chapter 20 for more details on quercetin.) In addition, take the herb stinging nettle (*Urtica drocia*) to help control symptoms.

Because physical activity can reduce respiratory congestion, maintain a regular exercise program. Exercising indoors is preferable during pollen season.

■ CONTROLLING MOLD EXPOSURES AND ALLERGIES

The difficulty and efficacy of mold control varies dramatically with the climate. It will be very difficult in damp, humid climates, and relatively easy in dry climates. When some items, such as carpet, upholstered furniture, fabrics, gypsumboard walls, wallpaper, wood, or any porous material stays wet for more than 24 hours, they will mold. No amount of cleaning will get rid of the mold permanently. However, many common-sense measures will reduce exposure to molds and help control allergic reactions to molds, in addition to mold extracts or hands-on allergy treatment for mold.

Avoid eating mold-laden foods: cheeses, fermented beverages, cider, vinegar, pickles, mayonnaise, sauerkraut, dried and candied fruits, mushrooms, sour cream, buttermilk, smoked meats, and spices (which may become moldy during processing and drying). Also, do not eat foods that have molded in your refrigerator or pantry.

Car air conditioners can also be a potent source of mold, sending spores throughout the car each time they are turned on. In addition, the interior of a car can become moldy if it gets wet. To prevent mold growth, be certain that any items stored in a car or truck are not damp. A bowl of white vinegar in a vehicle will completely neutralize the smell of mildew in a car interior in a few hours.

Avoid old dust (which is full of mold) found in attics and unoccupied buildings. Also avoid anything that smells musty, as mold produces this odor. Do not use mildewed items, as mildew is caused by mold.

■ INDOORS

Avoiding mold is the best strategy for those who are sensitive to it. Controlling dampness and increasing air circulation are basic steps in preventing mold growth.

It is important to determine the mold population of your home, particularly in rooms in which you spend long periods of time, or which are notorious for the presence of mold. The bedroom and bathroom are important, as well as the den or family room. Mold counts can be determined by using mold diagnostic plates (see Recommended Sources and Organizations). The results can help you determine which parts of your house require more attention for mold control.

■ BASEMENT

Unfortunately, many basements tend to be damp, which is supportive of mold growth. In addition, many basements are unheated. Heaters will help keep them dry. Keep your basement clean and check regularly it for mold. Take care with items that support mold growth. These items should never be stored in damp places, particularly the basement.

Use a dehumidifier if the basement humidity exceeds 50 percent. Correct and clean up after any flooding or seepage problems.

■ BATHROOM

Most bathrooms are a major source of mold in homes. It is essential to ventilate all bathrooms well. Use an exhaust fan to reduce moisture and mold in the bathroom. Do not use carpeting in bathrooms. When it gets wet, it cannot dry properly and will mildew.

Dry off the shower walls, floor, and fixtures after bathing to decrease the amount of standing water. Pick up bath mats and dry them after use. Never put damp clothing or towels into a hamper or closet. Allow these items to dry thoroughly before putting them away. Discard shower curtains if they cannot be cleaned thoroughly.

Check wallpaper frequently for mildew. Also check for dampness accumulating from condensation at the base of the toilet.

■ KITCHENS AND LAUNDRY ROOMS

Kitchens and laundry rooms are the next most important source of mold in a home. Clean the drip pan of self-defrosting refrigerators regularly. Check for mildew on refrigerator seals. Do not allow molded fruits, vegetables, or leftovers to remain in the refrigerator.

Wash dirty dishes after each meal to avoid mold growth on the food remains. Clean garbage cans frequently to prevent mold growth. Regularly check the area underneath both the kitchen and laundry room sinks for mold growth.

In damp climates, soiled clothes in hampers or baskets sometimes produce mold, as do clothes that have been washed and not yet dried. Do not leave wet clothes in the washing machine. Keep the lid of the washing machine open when not in use in order to provide air circulation and prevent mold growth. Vent your clothes dryer to the outside.

■ BEDROOMS

Discard items that have molded, with no exceptions. These may include old newspapers, books, or magazines; old furniture; bedding; carpet; clothing; and pillows. Cover furniture and bedding made of latex rubber or urethane with barrier cloth to prevent harboring of mold. (Barrier cloth is cotton cloth that has an increased number of threads per inch. Its dense construction forms an effective "barrier.")

Use stringent dust control procedures as they also help prevent mold growth. (See Controlling Dust Exposures, below.) Do not use carpeting with foam-rubber backing or padding, which can foster mold growth.

■ MISCELLANEOUS

Houseplants may harbor mold, both on the plant and in the soil. Watering plants causes them to releases mold spores into the air. In cases of severe mold allergies, plants must be removed from the house. Even dried flowers may sometimes become moldy, particularly in a damp climate. If so, they must be discarded.

Do not use a humidifier unless absolutely necessary. Humidifiers frequently grow mold and then disperse spores into the air. If you do use them, clean them frequently. Most manufacturers include a compound to prevent mold growth, but a chemically sensitive person may not be able to tolerate these chemicals.

Air conditioners, particularly "swamp coolers" (evaporative coolers) may be sites of mold growth because of their dampness. Change the pads frequently to avoid operating the cooler with moldy pads. Some chemically sensitive people may not tolerate the use of a swamp cooler because of the mold retardants on the pads.

Mold grows on tree bark. Do not keep fireplace logs inside the house. Avoid live Christmas trees and evergreen decorations.

Air sleeping bags thoroughly after each use. Before using them, air out cabins or houses that have been closed for the winter season. Avoid storing mattresses, pillows, upholstered couches, and bedding in unheated cabins.

A family member who works where there are large numbers of mold spores must change work clothes and leave them outside the house when returning home from work. This includes the following occupations and activities: sawmills, dusty factories, mattress or furniture factories, breweries, cheese factories, floral shops/nurseries, farmers, botanists, lumberjacks, hikers, or gardeners.

▌ OUTDOORS

Mold grows in the soil, and activities outdoors can constitute a large mold exposure. An acutely mold-sensitive person should avoid raking, burning, or jumping in leaves. Mold grows rapidly on damp leaves. Do not do cleanup chores in the yard or mow the grass. Avoid exposure to peat moss, compost, and greenhouses. Mold-sensitive children should not play under shrubbery or climb trees.

Keep the exterior of the home free of leaves and debris and remove vines on outside walls of the house. Remove shrubs resting against the walls of the house and clean leaves and debris from gutters on and around the house. Avoid stacking or playing on fireplace logs.

Avoid sweeping porches, basements, and garages (approximately one-third of cement dust is mold). Eliminate areas of standing water, and remove obstacles that cause constant shade.

Hay, straw, and combining, shoveling, or storing grains can be a massive mold exposure. Do not walk through weedy fields or vacant lots, and avoid deep woods and caves.

▌ MOLD CLEAN-UP AND CONTROL

A mold-sensitive person should avoid cleaning chores associated with mold clean-up. If this is not possible, wear a mask and gloves during the clean-up, keep the area well ventilated. Wash your clothing immediately, and take a shower (including hair washing) when you are finished.

• Use soap and water and wash molded items thoroughly, scrubbing with a brush if possible.
• Bleach will kill mold, but people sensitive to chlorine/chemicals should not use it.
• Zephiran (17 percent aqueous solution) diluted 1 ounce per gallon of distilled water will kill mold. It has no odor when diluted, and it is available at drugstores.
• Borax sprinkled in moldy places will retard mold growth. Do not use borax where children or pets might come into contact with it. Mix borax and water in a spray bottle and wash the walls of your shower or bathroom. Let it dry on the walls to prevent mold growth.
• Keep all areas dry and well lit. Allow space for air circulation behind furniture to keep the walls dry.
• Heat will kill mold, drying it into a powder

that can be brushed off. You can use a hair dryer or a portable electric heater to destroy mold. However, the spores remain viable unless the temperature is extremely high, and the dead mold spores are still allergenic. Always wear a mask while using this method of cleaning.

- Air cleaners will remove mold spores from the air. Be sure to change or clean the filters as needed.
- Ozone generators can be used to kill mold. These can be rented from some physicians, cleaning companies, or fire departments. They produce ozone gas, which penetrates all parts of the room while the generator is producing ozone; exercise caution and follow directions carefully when using an ozone generator.
- Adding Impregnon, a fungal retardant, or Taheebo tea to houseplant water will retard mold in the potting soil. Both are available at health stores.
- To kill mold in the dirt under the house (pillar and post foundation), spread copper sulfate or borax crystals.

▌▌ CONTROLLING DUST EXPOSURES AND ALLERGIES

While all of us could probably benefit from some dust-control measures in our homes, the acutely sensitive person may have to take extreme measures. These procedures should be used all over the house; however, the bedroom should receive the most attention. Cleaning should be done while the extremely sensitive person is out of the house. (If a sensitive person does any housecleaning, wearing a mask is imperative.) Consider investing in a double-filtered or water-filtered vacuum cleaner in order to reduce recirculating dust particles.

▌ PREPARING A DUST-FREE BEDROOM

To prepare a dust-free bedroom, empty the room of furniture and clean it thoroughly to eliminate all traces of dust. Wash the walls, and scrub the woodwork, baseboards, and floors. Clean each item of furniture thoroughly before returning it to the bedroom. Empty and clean drawers with a damp cloth. Use drawers only for storing laundered clothes. Upholstered furniture and an upholstered headboard are taboo!

Take the bed mattress outside the room and clean it thoroughly. Vacuum, then wipe with a damp cloth. For extreme sensitivity problems, cover the mattress and pillows with barrier cloth. Eliminate under-the-bed storage and use only freshly laundered linens. Blankets and bedspreads should be washed at least once a month; avoid blankets that have not been washed. Avoid fuzzy blankets and chenille bedspreads, and do not use any bedding or pillows that cannot be washed, including comforters.

Clean out the closets. Remove all items and clean the closet and its contents thoroughly before returning appropriate items. Keep all clothes in the closet with the doors shut at all times. Use closets only for storing laundered clothes. If you are extremely sensitive, you may have to store clothes outside the bedroom.

Eliminate carpeting and padding. Remove books and bookshelves unless the shelves are covered, or install covers on all open shelves. Eliminate drapes and blinds; use washable curtains instead. Remove dust catchers, such as pennants, pictures, trophies, books, models, and dried or silk flower arrangements.

Dust the bedroom once a day with a damp cloth, and vacuum frequently. Open the windows to blow away the dust you raise, particularly when vacuuming. (In winter, wear a coat if you have to.) Close the windows after you have finished cleaning, and keep them closed.

Use an air cleaner with a dust filter and change the filters or clean them as needed. (See chapter 12, Living Safely, for more information on air cleaners.)

Never allow pets in the bedroom, and keep the bedroom door closed at all times.

▎ DUST CONTROL MEASURES FOR THE HOUSE

If possible, remove carpeting, especially wall to wall. Vacuum upholstered furniture and rugs daily for acute cases, and one to two times per week for mild cases. Avoid knickknacks. Do not use brooms or feather dusters. Dust with rags dampened with water or a safe cleaning product. Do not use commercial dusting oils or other scented preparations.

Replace furnace air filters at least twice a year. Have the furnace ducts cleaned regularly by professionals.

Do not sit on upholstered furniture or use feather pillows. If you have severe allergies, it may be necessary to replace these items. Be sure anything that has been stored is thoroughly cleaned and aired before using. Dust-sensitive children should not play with stuffed toys. They should play in their clean rooms with clean toys.

Avoid wearing clothing made from lint-producing materials. New sweaters, fleece-lined fabric, and chenille garments should be washed several times before wearing, as should new bath and kitchen towels.

Do not allow any animals, including birds and reptiles, in the house.

Dust-sensitive people should avoid attics, closets, basements, or storerooms and spend most of their time in the cleanest, barest rooms—the bedroom and the kitchen. They should not rummage in drawers, handle dusty items, or handle items that have been stored for a long period of time.

Live Christmas trees are a source of dust, terpenes, and molds and should not be used in the homes of dust-sensitive people. Exercise care when using Christmas and other decorations also, as these items are usually stored in dusty attics or storerooms. Clean and seal all decorations in plastic bags before placing them in storage boxes. When unpacking the decorations for the next season, open the storage boxes outside and bring only the clean decorations into your house.

The severity of your dust sensitivity will determine how many of these measures you must use. Dust extracts are also beneficial, as are hands-on allergy treatments for dust. Anything you can do to minimize your allergic load contributes positively to your health.

▮▮ CONTROLLING DUST MITES

If you live at a high altitude, in a cold climate, or in a very dry climate, you will not have as much difficulty controlling dust mites as someone living at a lower altitude and in a humid climate. It is almost impossible to rid a house of dust mites—vacuuming removes

Humidity Breeds Dust Mites

Controlling humidity is the single most important in curbing dust mites. They thrive in 70 percent humidity and tend to hit their population peak in late summer. When home heating systems come on, the numbers of mite colonies drop off, hitting their lowest in January. Their numbers increase again in the spring when the heat goes off and the humidity rises.

only dead ones. Heat and low moisture appear to be the best ways of prevention, although hot washing will destroy mites in bedding. A 1999 study at the University of Sydney in Australia showed that washing wool blankets with eucalyptus oil in addition to laundry detergent after soaking them in the mixture for 60 minutes killed 99 percent of the dust mites. The blankets were soaked and washed in 6 Tbsp. eucalyptus oil, 1¼ Tbsp. liquid laundry detergent, and 13 gallons of warm and cool water.

Chemical measures to control dust mites have not been practical. They are hazardous to people and the mites are resistant to most chemicals. However, there are now two chemicals available to aid in mite control. Tannic acid neutralizes protein in dust mite allergen, and benzyl benzoate powder kills mites. It is not yet clear which product is best for repeated use in the home. Chemically sensitive individuals may not be able to tolerate either of these products. Even if they are tolerated, people other than the sensitive person should apply both products.

Extracts or hands-on allergy treatment for dust mites and other types of environmental control are more effective for controlling allergy symptoms to dust mites.

Regularly washing bedding in hot water (140°F) and drying it in a hot dryer is the most important control method for dust mites in the bed. Dry-cleaning is not as effective for killing dust mites.

Other general control measures include washing drapes regularly, vacuuming carpets and upholstery once a week, and disposing of the vacuum cleaner bag immediately. Consider replacing upholstered furniture with wood or leather.

Cover bedroom air vents with several layers of cheesecloth or special vent covers to minimize dust blowing into the room.

Remove carpets from the bedroom and put down tile or wood flooring. Shampooing carpets has only a temporary effect. Use area rugs and remove them for the summer, which is the peak dust mite season. Beat them to remove the residues in which mites hide, and return them to the floor in the fall. If the rugs are washable, wash them before returning them to the floor. Protect mattresses and pillows with barrier cloth, and do not use foam rubber pillows.

Clothes can harbor dust mites, particularly in humid climates. Store out-of-season clothes in plastic, and launder clothing before wearing if storage has been lengthy.

▌▌ CONTROLLING ANIMAL DANDER EXPOSURES AND ALLERGIES

If you are extremely allergic to animal dander, you may have to forego having a pet with fur or feathers. Keeping the animal outside will be somewhat helpful, but you will still have some exposure to the animal dander and saliva.

Regular bathing of cats and dogs helps decrease their allergenicity. Plain water is effective; it is not necessary to use soap. However, to comfortably bathe cats, you must begin regular baths when they are very young kittens. Animals should never be groomed in the house, and certainly never by the person who is allergic to animal danders. The person allergic to animal dander also should not empty litter boxes.

For the very sensitive person, animal hairs or dander on the clothing of another person can trigger symptoms. Animals in the classroom can pose a problem for the sensitive child. Allergy extracts and hands-on allergy treatment for animal danders can afford relief and protection.

■ CONTROLLING FEATHER EXPOSURES AND ALLERGIES

Down pillows, comforters, and sleeping bags should not be stored in a sensitive person's bedroom nor used by them, and they may not be able to wear down jackets. Sensitive people should not keep any type of bird for a pet, and if they live in a rural setting, they should not keep chickens, ducks, or turkeys. Feather extracts and hands-on allergy treatments help to prevent and control allergy symptoms from feathers.

Rubella vaccine cultured on duck embryo tissue can produce an allergic response in people sensitive to feathers. Skin testing before measles, mumps, and rubella (MMR) vaccines can be done if the person is ex-tremely feather- or egg-sensitive, although recent studies do not show a need for skin testing.

■ PROTECTING YOURSELF FROM TOBACCO SMOKE

Exposure to tobacco smoke is an extremely serious exposure both for smokers and nonsmokers. It is imperative for your health and longevity that you avoid and protect yourself from tobacco smoke of all kinds, including cigarette, cigar, and pipe.

To protect yourself from the harmful effects of tobacco smoke, consider the following.

- If you are a smoker, stop smoking *immediately*. The risk of lung cancer mortality is reduced when smoking is stopped. Former smokers who quit 15 or more years ago have lung cancer mortality rates only slightly above those for nonsmokers.
- Your smoking also endangers the health of the nonsmokers around you, including your spouse, children, relatives, friends, and others. The sidestream smoke from your tobacco can cause many health problems and even death for these people.
- Smokers who have quit are less likely to backslide if surrounded by spouses and friends who do not smoke.
- For most people, quitting smoking "cold turkey" seems to work better than gradually tapering off.
- Smokers of low-tar and low-nicotine cigarettes find it easier to quit than do smokers of high-tar and high-nicotine cigarettes.
- Only one-third of smokers who quit gain weight. One-third lose weight when com-

bining a general fitness program with their efforts to stop smoking.

If you continue to smoke, in consideration to nonsmokers:

- Smoke only in designated areas.
- Smoke only in well-ventilated areas.
- Put out your cigarettes quickly and completely. Do not let them smolder in ashtrays.
- Use smokeless ashtrays.
- Do not smoke in the presence of children or nonsmokers.
- For the sake of your health and that of your family, try to quit smoking.

If you are a nonsmoker, you should:

- Never allow smoking in your home or car.
- Dine only in restaurants with a nonsmoking section.
- Stay only in motels or hotels with nonsmoking rooms or floors.
- Insist on high air quality at your workplace.
- In social situations, politely insist that no one smoke in your presence.
- Extracts or hands-on allergy treatment for tobacco and tobacco smoke will help control allergic reactions to these substances.

CHAPTER 15

Do Your Own Home Survey

THE FOLLOWING FORM is a modified version of the one used by our staff when determining the allergenic safety of a person's home. By applying the material in chapter 11, Common Chemical Sensitivities, and chapter 13, The Allergens We Inhale, along with the information on this questionnaire, you can do your own house call and determine what should be changed to make your home an environmentally safer place to live.

If you live in an apartment or townhouse rather than a single-family dwelling, there will still be positive changes you can make. Complete the survey in relation to your own unit and the entire building. You will have less control over the building than over your own unit. Remember that any changes you can make will be helpful.

General Information

- Age of home _____ How long have you lived here? _____
- Did you have allergies before moving into this home? _____

  Did your allergies begin after moving into this home? _____
- In which part of the home do you feel best? _____ worst?_____
- In which part of the home do you spend the most time? _____
- Do you feel better: Inside _____ Outside? _____
- In which season do you feel the best? _____ worst?_____

Do Your Own Home Survey

CONSTRUCTION OF HOME

- Foundation: Slab _____ Pillar and post _____

  Outside walls: Stucco _____ Wood _____ Masonite _____ Aluminum siding _____

  Brick _____ Adobe _____ Vinyl siding _____ Paint _____

  Stain _____ Other _____

- Insulation in home: Batting _____ Foam _____ Spray-in _____ Other _____

- Roof: Flat _____ Pitched _____ Attic _____

- Storm windows made of: Glass _____ Plastic _____ None _____

- Basement? _____ If yes, is it dry or damp? _____

  What is stored there? _____ Are stored items moldy? _____

- Garage: Attached _____ Detached _____ None _____

  Location: _____

  Do you park cars in the garage? _____

- Greenhouse: Attached _____ Detached _____ None _____ Location: _____

PESTICIDE HISTORY

- Termite-proofing: Yes _____ No _____ Date: _____

  Part of house treated: _____

  Ground pretreated before construction of house? _____ Material used: _____

- Sprays with which your yard is treated: _____ How often? _____

- Has your home been treated with pesticides indoors? _____

  Most recent date _____ How often? _____

  Materials used? _____

RENOVATION HISTORY

- Renovations to your house since you moved in (include dates of renovations):

  Additions _____

  Paint _____

Insulation_____

Stain_____

Appliances_____

Floor coverings _____

Carpeting_____

Paneling_____

Wallpaper_____

CHEMICAL EXPOSURE INVENTORY

	Frequency Used?	Where Used or Stored?
Insect strips	_____	_____
Room deodorizers	_____	_____
Furniture oils	_____	_____
Spray or other waxes	_____	_____
Floor cleaner	_____	_____
Oven cleaner	_____	_____
Cleansers	_____	_____
Glass cleaner	_____	_____
Ammonia	_____	_____
Rug shampoo	_____	_____
Disinfectants	_____	_____
Scratch remover	_____	_____
Lye	_____	_____
Plastic glasses/plates	_____	_____
Plastic tablecloth	_____	_____
Air cleaners (type, location) _____		_____
Space heaters	_____	_____

Plants (check for molds and note number of waterings per week) _____

Mothballs _____   _____

Do Your Own Home Survey

Sachets (hangers, etc.) _____   _____

Shoe polish _____   _____

Nail polish/remover _____   _____

Scented soaps _____   _____

Scented deodorant _____   _____

Scented makeup/aftershave _____   _____

Electric rollers _____   _____

Curling brush/iron _____   _____

Perfume _____   _____

Hair spray _____   _____

Clothing fabrics _____   _____

Dry-cleaning _____   _____

Leather clothing/accessories _____   _____

New clothes/shoes _____   _____

Kerosene _____   _____

Gasoline _____   _____

Solvents _____   _____

Pesticides _____   _____

Weedkillers _____   _____

Fertilizers _____   _____

Oil (used, new) _____   _____

Paint (stored) _____   _____

Changes needed: _____   _____

_____   _____

_____   _____

PETS

- Pets in house _____ _____
- Pets sleep with anyone? _____ _____
- In bedroom? _____ _____
- Kitty/pet litter (location)_____ _____
- Dog bed (material, location) _____ _____
- Any other pets? Bird _____ If so, where kept? _____

  Snakes or lizards?_____ If so, where kept? _____

  Aquariums? _____ If so, where kept? _____

GAS AND ELECTRICAL INFORMATION

- Gas meter _____ Propane tank _____ Location _____

  Specific information _____

- House heated with: Electricity _____ Gas _____ Solar power _____

  If solar, materials used: _____

- Wood-burning stove/furnace _____ Forced hot air _____ Water-circulated_____

  Furnace location(s): _____

- Humidifier: Built-in _____ Portable _____ Hot _____ Cold _____ None _____

- Air conditioner _____ Type _____ If window, in which rooms? _____

- Water heated with: Electricity _____ Gas _____ Solar power _____

  Heater location(s): _____

- Note where the main electrical current enters the house: _____

- Distance _____ to nearest building _____

  to nearest power line _____ to nearest ponds/water _____

  to nearest transformer _____ to nearest antennae _____

  to nearest wire fence _____ to nearest electric meter/pole _____

Do Your Own Home Survey

LIVING ROOM

- Note type and age of: Floor covering _____

  Furniture _____

  Curtains _____

  Wall covering _____

  Is this room dusty? _____ How often does it need to be dusted? _____

- Wood fireplace? _____ Natural gas? _____ Electric? _____

  Fireplace used: Never _____ Sometimes (how often?) _____

  Location: _____

  Wood-burning or pellet stove used: Never _____ Sometimes (how often?) _____

  Location: _____

  Airtight? _____ Fuel burned _____

- Ceiling fan: Yes _____ No _____ Location: _____

- Wood stored for fireplace use _____ Type of wood _____ Location: _____

- List other living room items not covered above (include age of item): _____

  _____

  _____

- Closets (made of cedar?) _____

  Unusual contents: _____

  _____

- Changes needed: _____

  _____

  _____

KITCHEN

- Appliances (note if gas or electric):

  Stove _____ Fan _____ Refrigerator _____ Dishwasher _____

  Exhaust fan _____ Ceiling fan _____ Garbage disposal _____

  Microwave _____ Microwavable plastic dishes _____ Television _____

Note type and age of: Floor covering _____

- Curtains: _____

- Wall covering: _____

- Food storage containers and wraps:

  Soft plastic _____ Glass _____ Foil _____ Plastic wrap _____ Wax paper _____

- Mold (check under sink, dishwasher, refrigerator): _____

  Can you smell mold anywhere in the kitchen? _____

- List other kitchen items not covered above (plants, deodorizers, insect strips, cleaning

  agents): _____

  _____

  _____

- Pantry and cupboards: _____ Unusual contents: _____

  _____

  Broom closet? _____ Contents _____

- Changes needed: _____

  _____

LAUNDRY ROOM

- Location of laundry room in house: _____

- Dryer: Gas _____ Electric _____ Vented to outside _____

- Type and frequency of use:

  Detergent _____

  Fabric softener (liquid or sheet) _____

  Bleaches _____

  Spot remover _____

  Rinses _____

  Sprays _____

  Other _____

Do Your Own Home Survey

- Ironing board cover: _____
- Spill (indicate what and when): _____
- Mold: Does this room smell of mold? _____ Is there mold inside the washer? _____

  Has there been a leak in this room? _____ When? _____
- Closets and cupboards: _____

  Unusual contents:_____

  _____

  Does the bathroom smell moldy? _____
- List other laundry room items not covered above:_____
- Changes needed:_____

  _____

BATHROOM

- For each bathroom, note type and age of:

  Floor covering _____

  Wall covering_____

  Shower/tub walls _____

  Shower door/curtain_____
- Note presence of: Toothpaste _____ Soap _____ Shampoo _____

  Conditioners _____ Mouthwash _____ Air freshener _____ Bowl deodorizer _____

  Scented toilet paper or tissues _____
- Location of bathrooms in house:_____

  Makeup _____ Other personal care products _____ Cleaners _____
- Check for mold: Around the tub _____ On shower curtain/door _____

  Under sink _____ Around toilet _____ Under wall covering _____

  Under floor covering _____ Ceiling _____ Does the bathroom smell moldy?_____
- List bathroom items not covered above:_____

  _____

- Dirty clothes hamper? _____
- Closets and cupboards: _____

  Unusual contents: _____

  _____

- Changes needed: _____

  _____

BEDROOM

- For each bedroom, note type and age of:

  Floor covering _____

  Wall covering _____

  Curtains/drapes _____

  Mattresses _____

  Mattress cover (foam back?) _____

  Sheets and pillowcases _____

  Blankets _____

  Bedspread _____

  Pillows _____

  Furniture _____

- Location in house: _____
- Direction of head of bed: _____
- Scented items in room? _____
- Is this room dusty? _____ How often does it need to be dusted? _____
- Closets: _____

  Unusual contents: _____

- Television _____ Radio _____ Home office _____

  Computer and printer _____ Fax _____ Telephone _____

- Note items not listed above (pets, plants, bookcases, items under bed): _____

  _____

- Changes needed:

  _____

  _____

OTHER ROOMS
(Den, Family Room, or Home Office)

- Note type and age of: Floor covering _____

  Furniture _____

  Curtains _____

  Wall covering _____

  Is this room dusty? _____ How often does it need to be dusted? _____

- Wood fireplace? _____ Natural gas? _____ Electric? _____

  Location: _____

  Fireplace used: Never _____ Sometimes (how often?) _____

  Wood-burning or pellet stove used: Never _____ Sometimes (how often?) _____

  Location: _____

  Airtight? _____ Fuel burned _____

- Ceiling fan: Yes _____ No _____ Location: _____

- Wood stored for fireplace use _____ Type of wood _____ Location: _____

- Television _____ Radio _____ Home office _____

  Computer and printer _____ Fax _____ Telephone _____

- List other room items not covered above (include age of item): _____

  _____

  _____

- Closets: _____

  Unusual contents: _____

- Changes needed: _____

  _____

PART III

Infections and Allergies

WE COEXIST IN OUR WORLD with millions of organisms and microorganisms. Usually the relationship is peaceful. Most organisms live out their lives with little or no interaction with us and some are helpful to us: molds are used in cheese and antibiotics; "good" bacteria in the gastrointestinal tract aid digestion, help control disease, and produce vitamins; and yeasts ferment wine and cause bread to rise. If all microorganisms were eliminated, life on earth would cease to exist. However, sometimes the coexistence is not peaceful, and disease results.

Organisms and microorganisms are able to grow and multiply only in tissue that provides conditions in which they can survive. Organisms that infect humans do not usually infect animals such as cats, dogs, horses, and sheep. Organisms that infect other animals do not usually infect humans, but there are exceptions. Plant pathogens do not infect animals. Because of this tissue specificity, humans are resistant to many organisms that are pathogenic to plants and animals.

When disease results from interaction with microorganisms, the effects on our bodies can cause serious health problems and crisis. The chapters in Part III describe the disease processes caused by bacteria, viruses, parasites, fungi, yeasts, or molds. We will also look closely at the role these organisms play in the development and treatment of allergies. In addition, less toxic, more natural treatment methods for infections are discussed.

Bacteria, Viruses, and Parasites

Bacteria

Bacteria are single-celled organisms that occur as spheres (cocci), rods (bacilli), curved cells (vibrios), or spiral-shaped cells (spirochetes or spirilla). A special bacterial form, rickettsiae, are coccobacilli. These organisms reproduce by simple division, called binary fission. Some bacteria are motile (able to move by themselves), and have one or more flagella (appendages) for this purpose. Others have creeping mobility, enabled by contraction within the cell.

A few rod-shaped bacteria form spores, also called endospores. The spore is formed within the bacterial cell and is capable of producing one new bacterium. Spore formation is not a part of the usual reproductive cycle of these bacteria. These spores, probably the most resistant form of life known, help the bacteria survive adverse conditions. Some spores can survive an exposure to steam for more than an hour, and they are highly resistant to chemicals. The endospore will remain in spore form until conditions are favorable for bacterial growth, at which time it

will germinate. Some spores can remain viable for many years, complicating sterilization procedures. True bacteria can grow on nonliving as well as living matter. Rickettsiae are the exception and grow only in the cells of their hosts.

Bacteria are divided into species on the basis of:
- size, shape, mode of movement, and resting stage
- biochemical and nutritional traits
- response to oxygen, temperature, pH, and medications
- genetic composition
- ecological traits

Our concern with bacteria lies primarily in the diseases they cause. Pathogenicity refers to an organism's ability to cause disease; any organism pathogenic to humans causes disease in humans. However, different strains of the same organism may affect us in different degrees. This difference in pathogenicity is called virulence. The same organism may be highly virulent or nonvirulent, depending on the strain.

The virulence of a bacterial strain is partially determined by its invasiveness. Invasiveness refers to an organism's ability to multiply in the body of the host. Bacteria generally reach our bodies in small numbers. Contact usually takes place on the skin or mucous membranes, where a primary focus of infection is formed. The host's defense mechanisms then attempt to deal with the invading bacteria. The bacteria release substances called aggressins to aid in resisting the defense mechanisms. Some aggressins prevent destruction of foreign matter by our body's phagocytic cells, some defy the efforts of those cleanup cells, and some aggressins actually kill phagocytes. If the strain of bacteria is a virulent one or if the body's immune system is weak, the body's defense mechanisms will be overcome and a serious infection can result.

Toxicity also contributes to the virulence of bacteria. A number of pathogenic bacteria produce toxins. One type is called an exotoxin. Exotoxins are heat-liable (destroyed by heat) proteins and are excreted into the fluid around the bacteria. They are also released when the bacteria is destroyed.

Endotoxins are heat-stable complexes containing protein, lipid (fats), and polysaccharide complex carbohydrates, occurring in the cell wall of the most pathogenic bacteria. When injected into experimental animals, endotoxins all produce the same symptoms, regardless of the bacteria of origin. In the bloodstream, endotoxins may cause rapid and irreversible shock. This occurs when massive numbers of bacteria are present in the blood or when contaminated materials are injected intravenously.

▮ TRANSMISSION OF BACTERIA

Bacterial diseases may be transmitted in several ways.

- *Fecal contamination:* Bacterial diseases may be spread by fecal contamination of food and drink by persons practicing poor hygiene, by healthy carriers, or by houseflies. Diseases transmitted in this manner include typhoid fever, enteric fevers (bacterial food poisonings), cholera, and bacterial dysentery.
- *Droplet infection:* Diphtheria, tuberculosis, plague, meningococcal meningitis, streptococcal infections, pneumococcal pneumonia, and other respiratory infections are spread by a method called droplet infection. Organisms are spread in drops of saliva released when a person sneezes, coughs, or speaks. Sneezes can propel water droplets six feet into the air at speeds of up to 100 miles per hour.
- *Direct contact:* Diseases spread by direct contact include anthrax, tularemia, brucellosis, gonorrhea, and syphilis. Organisms causing these diseases cannot survive outside their host and require direct mucous membrane contact for transmission.
- *Vector transmission:* Some bacteria and rickettsiae are able to live in two or more hosts. Transmission involves a vector (a species that transmits the pathogen, such as fleas, ticks, and mosquitoes) and a reservoir of infection, from which the vector receives the infection. Some vectors receive the infection from their parents. For ticks, fleas, and mosquitoes, the reservoir is humans or animals. Disease is spread when the vector bites a human. Plague, tularemia, endemic and epidemic typhus, scrub typhus,

spotted fevers, rickettsial pox, Lyme disease, and Q fever are transmitted this way.

• *Wound infection:* Whenever nonsterile foreign material enters a wound, wound infections from bacteria can result. Tetanus, gas gangrene, pseudomonas, streptococcus, and staphylococcus are other common causes of wound infections.

• *Ingestion of toxins:* Ingesting bacterial toxins in contaminated food may also cause diseases. Food poisoning can develop from the toxins of *Clostridium botulism* or *Staphylococcus aureus.* Only people who ingest the toxin are affected. The disease cannot be spread from person to person, but occurs in clusters because of people ingesting food from the same source.

▐▌ BACTERIA IDENTIFICATION

In human infections, rapidly isolating and accurately identifying the bacterial organism is very important so that effective treatment can be initiated. Specimens for identification may be taken from blood, spinal fluid, stool, sputum, skin, body orifices, and abscesses. Identification of the bacteria in the samples taken is made by first producing a slide, staining the organism, and examining the slide under a microscope for stained organisms. Bacteria are difficult to see under a light microscope without staining, because they appear colorless. The specimens are also cultured to further confirm identification of the bacteria.

The Gram stain is the most important stain used in bacteriology. Developed by Christian Gram in the early 1800s, it is usually the initial step in identifying bacteria. This staining technique divides bacteria into two groups. Gram-positive organisms stain blue, whereas Gram-negative organisms stain red. One half of the bacilli, one third of the cocci, and all of the spiral organisms are Gram-negative.

Another important stain in bacteriology is the acid-fast stain, also called the Ziehl-Neelsen stain. It is used to stain bacteria that have lipid (fats) in their cell wall, and is used specifically to identify *Mycobacteria.* Although there are nonpathogenic (non–disease causing) organisms in this group of bacteria, the tuberculosis and leprosy organisms are in this group.

Many additional stains allow specific parts of bacteria to visualized. The capsule (a protective layer around the bacteria), cell walls, nuclei, flagella, endospores, and other structures can all be stained using two or more dyes. None of these additional stains are used routinely.

Material from the specimens is cultured to further identify or confirm identification of the bacteria involved. In some cases, pure cultures may be obtained. In others, a mixture of organisms is obtained and a subculture must be done to isolate the pathogenic organism. In most cases, identification can be made in 12 to 48 hours. However, some organisms, such as the tubercle bacillus responsible for tuberculosis, may require two to eight weeks of incubation before the organism appears on the growth media.

Tests utilizing metabolic characteristics of the organisms are common, since over 60 percent of human pathogens can be identified by this method. By using specialized culture media that demonstrate various metabolic traits, precious hours can be saved in identifying which pathogen is present. The ability of a bacteria to utilize a particular sugar in the growth media can help to identify it. For example, *Salmonella typhi,* the organism that causes typhoid fever, does not produce gas from glucose whereas other similar organisms do so.

■■ COMMON BACTERIAL INFECTIONS

At one time bacterial infections were very prevalent, but became less common with improved hygiene and sanitation practices. The advent of antibiotics and other treatment methods also reduced their frequency. However, bacterial infections still occur and are on the rise as many strains of bacteria are developing antibiotic resistance. This is rapidly becoming a serious problem, as some strains do not respond to any therapeutic agent. The indiscriminate use and overuse of antibiotics is the primary cause of this problem.

■ STREPTOCOCCAL INFECTIONS

Streptococcus, a Gram-positive cocci, can cause a variety of diseases, including pharyngitis with and without scarlet fever, puerperal sepsis (uterine infection), cellulitis of the skin (tissue infection), and impetigo (skin rash). The most common infection that affects many of us from time to time is strep throat. It is primarily treated with antibiotics to which the strep bacteria are sensitive. Some people suffer from recurrent strep throat that is difficult to treat. A strep extract or hands-on allergy treatment is very helpful in treating acute and chronic recurrent strep throats, as well as other diseases caused by the strep organism. A homeopathic remedy, *Belladonna,* is also helpful in treating strep throat.

A very virulent species of strep, the "flesh-eating" organism, has received much publicity in recent years. It grows very rapidly and tends to be resistant to most antibiotics. It is a new strain of the same strep that causes strep throat, but it produces a toxin that poisons the skin. This virulent species can spread an inch an hour. It enters the body through a cut, scrape, or other break in the skin. Antibiotics can combat this strep if it is in tissue that still has circulation, and many times new, powerful antibiotics must be given. Surgical removal of skin, large muscle groups, and even amputation must sometimes be done to save the patient's life. About half of those infected have a condition that hinders their immune system function. If the toxin from the strep enters the bloodstream, the body goes into shock and the victim dies. This organism can kill within two days and is fatal to 25 percent of its victims.

Bacteria can be the cause of pneumonia, as can viruses and fungi. *Streptococcus pneumoniae* is the most common cause of bacterial pneumonia. It has 84 distinct serotypes (can be distinguished by surface antigens), is pathogenic for humans and animals, and is the leading cause of morbidity and mortality for all ages. It can also cause meningitis, sinusitis, otitis media (ear infections), endocarditis, arthritis, and peritonitis (infection of the abdominal wall). This illness is usually treated with antibiotics to which the organism is sensitive.

■ MYCOPLASMA PNEUMONIAE

Approximately 20 percent of all cases of pneumonia are caused by *Mycoplasma pneu-*

moniae, a polymorphic organism that may appear as coccoid bodies, filaments, and large forms with multiple nuclei. Because they have no cell wall, the *Mycoplasma* organisms stain very poorly with the Gram stain and most other stains. Their lack of cell wall also makes them insensitive to penicillins and cephalosporins (antibiotics produced from a fungus). The pneumonia is less severe than that caused by other bacteria, and most cases do not require hospitalization. Most people experience fever, headache, and malaise for two to four days before the onset of the respiratory symptoms of pneumonia. However, a tracheobronchitis with fever, cough, headache, and malaise is the most common symptom caused by *Mycoplasma pneumoniae.* Some people may have a sore throat, and these symptoms are indistinguishable from those caused by some viruses and strep. Ear problems may also occur.

Infection with *Mycoplasma pneumoniae* occurs throughout the year, is worldwide, and is more common in children and young adults. In these age groups the disease is relatively mild, but increases in severity with age. This suggests an allergic component to the disease. Attack rates in families approach 60 percent, and prolonged shedding of the organism in the nasal secretions may cause infection to spread over a period of time. Because immunity is not complete, repeated infections of *Mycoplasma pneumoniae* are common. Treatment is with tetracycline or erythromycin.

▌ WHOOPING COUGH

The childhood disease whooping cough is bacterial. It is caused by *Bordetella pertussis,* a Gram-positive coccobacillus, and in spite of vaccination still occurs throughout the world. The "P" in the DTP immunization stands for pertussis. Whooping cough is highly contagious and outbreaks occur every few years in North America. In 1999 a whooping cough epidemic occurred in Los Alamos, in which 95 percent of those ill had been vaccinated. Mild whooping cough requires no treatment, but is usually treated to prevent spread. More severe cases are treated with the antibiotics erythromycin or tetracycline. An extract for *Bordetella pertussis* helps to lessen the severity of symptoms and speed recovery. Anyone who has ever had whooping cough will improve with a *Bordetella pertussis* extract or with hands-on allergy treatment for *Bordetella pertussis.* Homeopathic remedies for cough also help.

▌ LEGIONNAIRES' DISEASE

Even more publicity has been generated by Legionnaires' disease, an illness caused by *Legionella pneumophila,* a Gram-negative rod. Malaise, headache, myalgia, fever, and cough characterize Legionnaires' disease. Twenty-five to seventy-five percent of patients develop mental changes, and complications include renal failure, lung abscess, and infection outside the lung. The large outbreak of Legionnaires' disease that generated publicity in the United States in 1976 was spread by infected water in the air cooling towers of a hotel.

▌ DIPHTHERIA

Although it is no longer a common infection, diphtheria bears mentioning because of its presence in the DTP vaccine. This disease is caused by *Corynebacterium diphthe-*

riae, a Gram-positive rod. Its exotoxin is responsible for the severity of diphtheria, causing degenerative lesions in the heart, nervous system, and kidneys when it is absorbed into the body's general circulation. The disease presents as a sore throat or tonsillitis, but the identifying characteristic is the white-gray membrane produced at the site of infection. It causes mechanical obstruction to the airway, along with edema and hemorrhage.

In the past, it was spread by infected droplets from healthy carriers. This organism can survive for periods of time outside the human body. Diphtheria is now rare in North America.

▌ HELICOBACTER PYLORI

Chronic infections of *Helicobacter pylori*, a Gram-negative, curved rod, may result in peptic ulcers and gastric cancer. These infections are accompanied by dyspepsia (upset stomach, heartburn, and nausea) and abdominal pain. The mode of transmission, incubation period, and communicability is unknown. Treatment is with antibiotics.

▌ TUBERCULOSIS AND LEPROSY

Tuberculosis and leprosy are caused by different species of *Mycobacteria* bacilli. Because of the lipid content of their cell walls, these organisms do not stain well with the Gram stain. Instead, the acid-fast stain is used to make these organisms visible and identifiable. Leprosy, or Hansen's disease, occurs in two forms. Tuberculoid leprosy, in which there are lesions on the face, trunk, and limbs, is the less serious of the two forms. Lepromatous leprosy causes extensive skin lesions and severe damage with loss of nasal bones and septum, loss of dig-

its, and testicular atrophy. The incidence of leprosy is very low in North America, but does occur in Texas, California, Louisiana, Florida, New York City, and Hawaii. Most of these cases are found in immigrants. About 50 percent of people with leprosy have a history of either prolonged or intimate contact with an infected person, usually a household member.

Eight million people annually develop tuberculosis, and three million die from it. Tuberculosis is extremely contagious and is spread by airborne droplets either coughed or sneezed. These droplets can remain suspended in air for up to two hours. The bacteria thrive in a high oxygen environment and those breathed into the lungs will begin to multiply. The bacteria can survive in moist or dry sputum for up to six weeks, but die very quickly in direct sunlight.

Both tuberculosis and leprosy have historically been difficult to treat, but modern drugs have made them somewhat easier to control and cure. Both must be treated with multi-drug therapy, and patient compliance with therapy is imperative. Drug-resistant strains of both of these diseases have become a serious problem. Tuberculosis has become more common in recent years because of the infections that occur in immunocompromised AIDS patients. People with normal immune systems have contracted drug-resistant TB and have died from it.

▌ PROTEUS MIRABILIS

Proteus mirabilis is the second leading cause of urinary tract infections. It is a Gram-negative bacilli. *Proteus* is also a major cause of nosocomial infections (infections received while in hospital). It can cause wound infection, pneumonia, and septicemia (blood infections), and can be fatal to debilitated people. Although bladder infections are normally treated with antibiotics to which the organisms are sensitive, several homeopathic preparations offer very effective treatment.

▋ GONORRHEA AND SYPHILIS

Bacteria cause the venereal diseases of gonorrhea and syphilis. Gonorrhea is caused by *Neisseria gonorrhoeae*, a Gram-negative rod. (Bacterial meningitis is caused by another species of *Neisseria*.) *Treponema pallidum*, a Gram-negative spirochete, causes syphilis. Both of these diseases are sexually transmitted and are treated with antibiotics. However, drug-resistant strains are now developing.

Without proper treatment, gonorrhea can cause blindness in infants born to mothers with active disease. Gonorrhea can also cause infertility because of scarring to the fallopian tubes. Syphilis organisms can pass through the placenta and a mother in any stage of her clinical disease can transmit the organism to her baby. Many of these babies are stillborn or survive only a short time.

The incidence of venereal disease in North America had decreased over the past 40 to 50 decades with the advent of antibiotics, but is on the rise again, partially due to antibiotic resistance.

▋ CHLAMYDIA

Chlamydia trachomatis, an intracellular bacteria, is the most common cause of sexually transmitted disease in North America. Four million people are infected with it each year. In women the vaginal infection causes a yel-

Armadillo Link?

In some areas of the southwest U.S., armadillos may be a link for leprosy, as animals infected with the leprosy bacteria are found in the wild.

low-green discharge and can result in scarring of the fallopian tubes, infertility, and chronic pain. Men have an infection of the urethra and epididymis with a discharge from the penis, accompanied by changes in urination. Also known as nongonococcal urethritis, the period of communicability is unknown. *C. trachomatis* can be responsible for chlamydial conjunctivitis passed from the mother to her baby, for which eyedrops must be given at birth. Oral antibiotics are the recommended treatment for chlamydia.

Another species, *Chlamydia pneumoniae,* has been implicated in heart disease. Evidence suggests that it can linger in the lining of blood vessels for years, and could fuel the inflammation that causes heart attacks and strokes. It never appears in truly healthy tissue.

▋ GARDNERELLA

Gardnerella vaginitis, a Gram-variable coccobacillus, causes a form of vaginitis that is often called nonspecific vaginitis, because it is not caused by trichomonas, gonorrhea, or candida. The second most common cause of infectious vaginitis, it causes a discharge that is described by some as "fishy." It has been associated with septic abortion (a spontaneous abortion caused from an infection) and puerperal fever with bacteremia (fever with a bacterial infection resulting after childbirth). Gardnerella is normally treated with the antibacterial vaginal gels Cleocin or Metrogel.

▌ CLOSTRIDIUM INFECTIONS

Food poisoning can be caused by several different species of bacteria. A very serious form that can be fatal without immediate and proper treatment is caused by *Clostridium botulism,* a Gram-positive rod. It is not an infection, but an intoxication caused by ingesting food that contains the toxin produced by this organism. (Staphylococcal food poisoning is caused by this same mechanism). Botulism can be fatal without immediate and proper treatment, as it paralyzes the eye, throat, laryngeal, and respiratory muscles. *C. botulism* grows in anaerobic, low-acid food preparations, usually during storage. It causes no change in the color or taste of the food, and home-canned foods, smoked fish, and occasionally faulty commercially canned foods have caused outbreaks of botulism. Some infants have developed botulism from honey. Children under one year should not be fed honey.

Gas gangrene and tetanus are caused by other species of *Clostridium.* Gas gangrene is caused by *Clostridium perfringens* and is a serious wound infection. It develops in traumatic, open lesions, such as bullet wounds or compound fractures, if they become contaminated with dirt or other foreign material. This condition is usually seen in war wounds, and the growing bacteria produce gas that can be heard and felt on palpation. If the toxins reach the bloodstream, it can be fatal unless treated promptly.

Clostridium tetani produces a toxin that interferes with the neurotransmitter acetyl-choline, causing tetanus or lockjaw. The "T" in the DTP immunization stands for tetanus. The spores of this bacteria exist in many soils, particularly if manure is present. Tetanus results when these spores enter the body through puncture wounds contaminated with soil or foreign objects. Treatment involves neutralization of any unbound toxin (one that has not yet attached to the cells) with large doses of human tetanus immune globulin, along with nonspecific supportive measures such as a quiet, dark room and the provision of an adequate airway. Penicillin therapy is used as a prophylactic adjunct in serious or neglected wounds.

▌ SALMONELLA

An infection of *Salmonella,* a Gram-negative rod, causes food poisoning characterized by headache, chills, and abdominal pain followed by nausea, vomiting, diarrhea, and fever. Infections of *Salmonella enteritidis* and *S. choleraesuis* are acquired from contaminated food and, less often, water. Symptoms begin 4 to 24 hours after ingestion and are usually self-limiting, without extension beyond the gastrointestinal tract. In infants, the aged, and the sick, this infection is more common, severe, and prolonged.

Another *Salmonella* species, *S. typhi,* causes typhoid fever, and sanitary control of food, water, and sewage have contributed to its decline. Human carriers can spread the disease and are difficult to treat. In typhoid fever, the organism multiplies in the small intestine causing prolonged fever. A rash known as rose spots may appear on the abdomen for a few days in the second or third week. If typhoid fever and its toxic symptoms are not treated with antibiotics, it can last for three to four weeks. It is usually not fatal, but an oral vaccine is available.

▌ ESCHERICHIA COLI

Some strains of *Escherichia coli*, a Gram-negative rod, cause food poisoning. A particularly virulent mutant strain of *E. coli* has caused deaths from food poisoning. In 1993, this strain of *E. coli* caused an outbreak of illness from contaminated beef that was undercooked in hamburgers. The beef was contaminated at the slaughterhouse by cattle feces, and the undercooking allowed consumption of live organisms. This affected more than 500 people in Washington, Idaho, California, and Nevada with bloody diarrhea, severe abdominal cramps, occasional vomiting, and low-grade or no fever. Four children died from the infection.

E. coli is normally a beneficial bacteria in the bowel, but when it gets into the bladder, cystitis (a bladder infection) results. Antibiotics are the usual method of treatment.

▌ CHOLERA

Cholera, caused by *Vibrio cholera*, a slim, short, curved Gram-negative rod, is an emerging infection that has been rising in frequency in recent years. In the past, it caused epidemics, and Samuel Hahnemann, the founder of homeopathy, received the Medal of Honor from the French government for his work during cholera epidemics in the 1800s.

Cholera is spread through contaminated food and water, and colonizes in the small intestine. The El Tor strain produces a potent enterotoxin (a toxin that particularly affects the gastrointestinal tract), which causes the symptoms of cholera. This toxin causes a diarrhea referred to as "rice water,"

with fluid loss so severe that it can cause death within a few hours. Aggressive intravenous rehydration is required for treatment, as a person can purge 100 percent of his weight in diarrhea over four to seven days. Although some antibiotic-resistant strains are developing, penicillin is the drug of choice.

▌ PSEUDOMONAS INFECTIONS

Hot tubs have called attention to *Pseudomonas* infections. *Pseudomonas aeruginosa* is a Gram-negative rod that is free-living in moist environments, but is also a pathogen of plants, animals, and humans. Infections are rare in healthy individuals, but the organism is an opportunistic pathogen that can be devastating to immunocompromised people. Burn, wound, urinary tract, skin, eye, ear, and respiratory infections all occur. *Pseudomonas* also causes "swimmer's ear," and is a frequent cause of rash problems in hot tubs and whirlpools. It can also cause pneumonia. *Pseudomonas* is very resistant to antibiotics and drug combinations must be used in some cases.

▌ STAPHYLOCOCCUS

Wound infections are frequently caused by staphylococcal infections. *Staphylococcus aureus,* a Gram-positive cocci, is a major human pathogen. In addition to wound infections, it can cause impetigo, a skin infection; toxic shock syndrome, a serious acute infection sometimes caused by high-absorbency tampons; septicemia, a blood infection; and endocarditis, an inflammation of the lining of the heart and heart valves. It is the common organism found in "boils," a painful lump caused by infection through a sweat gland or hair follicle. These infections can be very serious, as many staph organisms have become drug resistant.

Staphylococcus is the most common bacterial food poisoning and is caused when food containing the enterotoxin is ingested. This type of food poisoning is spread by food handlers who have the organism on their hands. Improperly refrigerated chicken salad, cottage cheese, cream-filled bakery products, custard, ham, hollandaise sauce, ice cream, and processed meats are foods that are often implicated. The food is normal in odor, appearance, and taste, but 4 to 6 hours and 86°F allows enough production of toxin to produce this food poisoning. Symptoms appear abruptly 2 to 6 hours after ingestion of the food and consist of severe cramping, abdominal pain, nausea, vomiting, and diarrhea. Recovery is in 6 to 8 hours.

▌ BACTEROIDES INFECTIONS

Bacteroides species account for about 10 percent of wound infections in North America. *B. fragilis*, the common pathogen from this group, is an opportunistic pathogen and is the most common cause of Gram-negative infections in North America. It can also cause pulmonary and soft tissue infections. Treatment is with antibiotics other than penicillin to which this organism is usually resistant.

▌ LYME DISEASE

Lyme disease has received much publicity in recent years and is caused by the spirochete *Borrelia burgdorferi*. Although it is Gram-negative, the presence of this organism is usually demonstrated with either the Wright or Giemsa stains. It is spread by a tick bite that causes a characteristic skin lesion, a red bump with a "bull's eye." Fatigue, headache,

stiffness, muscle pain, and swollen lymph glands are common symptoms. Weeks to months after the skin lesion, 10 to 15 percent of people develop neurological symptoms, and 6 to 10 percent develop cardiac symptoms. Treatment is with antibiotics.

The tick reproduces on deer and feeds on mice to become infected. There is no person-to-person transmission, but transmission through the placenta has been documented. In North America, Lyme disease occurs only in the Atlantic coastal states from Maine to Georgia; the upper midwestern states, concentrated in Minnesota and Wisconsin; and California and Oregon. The tick is also present in areas of British Columbia.

▌ INSECT-BORNE DISEASES

Like Lyme disease, plague (*Yersinia pestis*), tularemia (*Francisella tularensis*), endemic (*Rickettsia typhi*) and epidemic typhus (*Rickettsia prowazekii*), scrub typhus (*Rickettsia tsutsugamushi*), spotted fevers (*Rickettsia rickettsia*), rickettsial pox (*Rickettsia akari*), and Q fever (*Coxiella burnetii*) are all spread when an infected vector (an insect) bites a human. *Yersinia pestis* is a Gram-negative bacillus and *Francisella tularensis* is a Gram negative coccobacillus. All of the other organisms are rickettsia and their shape varies from coccus to bacillus, causing them to be called coccobacilli. Their cell wall, which resembles a bacterial cell wall, stains poorly with the Gram stain, but is Gram-negative. These organisms are more frequently identified with other stains.

While the diseases caused by each of these organisms has slightly differing symptoms and complications, headache, chills, fever, muscle pain, and rash are common to

Plague Still a Concern

Plague, caused by Yersinia pestis, *is an infection of rodents and small mammals and is transmitted to humans by the bite of infected fleas. It has two major clinical forms, bubonic and pneumonic. In bubonic plague, painful swellings known as bubos appear in the infected lymph nodes. Without treatment, the patient can progress to a fatal bacterial infection. In pneumonic plague, people develop necrotic, hemorrhagic pneumonia, and survival is rare without specific therapy.*

The plague was the cause of the most virulent epidemic in human history, the Black Death of the Middle Ages. Pandemics continued until the end of the 19th and early 20th centuries in spite of all quarantine efforts and treatments. After the causative agent was discovered in 1894, treatment efforts improved. However, effective treatment still depends on accurate and timely diagnosis and treatment.

Plague continues to infect people today. It is enzootic (present in animals in certain locations) in the western United States, including Arizona, California, Colorado, Utah, New Mexico, Oregon, and Wyoming. Animals and infected fleas have been detected from Mexico to the eastern half of the state of Washington. Delay in diagnosing and treating plague increases the potential for pulmonary involvement and the spread from person to person. Physicians should consider plague in any person with fever and swollen lymph glands who has a history of recent travel or residence in areas where plague is enzootic.

them all. Likewise, the insect vector is different for each organism, but includes ticks, mites, fleas, lice, and chiggers. Animal reservoirs include squirrels, rats, mice, rabbits, sheep, cattle, goats, and other animals. The areas in which these diseases occur are governed by the presence of the vector and reservoir animal.

■ TREATMENT OF BACTERIAL INFECTIONS

Antibiotic therapy is the usual treatment for most bacterial infections. When it is indicated, determining antibiotic sensitivity is just as important as identifying pathogenic bacteria. An effective therapeutic agent must be determined, as well as the concentration level at which it will be effective against the bacteria. As antibiotic usage has increased substantially, more and more bacteria are becoming resistant to antibiotics, thus increasing the importance of the sensitivity test.

The practice of giving antibiotics to animals in order to reduce disease, speed meat production, and improve meat quality has played a major role in this developing resistance. The meat we eat contains residual antibiotics unless it has been obtained from a special antibiotic-free source.

In addition to treatment with antibiotics, specific immunotherapy extracts, and hands-on allergy treatment, the following substances will aid recovery from bacterial infections.

- *Vitamin A:* Aids repair of mucous membranes.
- *B complex vitamins:* The intestinal mucosa, which produces B complex, may be damaged by bacterial infections. B complex supplements serve as replacements until normal bacterial flora can resume vitamin B production.
- *Vitamin C:* Stimulates the immune system.
- *Co-enzyme Q$_{10}$:* Increases immune defense.
- *Essential fatty acids:* Aid repair of mucous membranes and deter colonization of harmful organisms.
- *Organic germanium:* Provides an oxygen medium that will deter the growth of anaerobic organisms (bacteria which live in the absence of oxygen).
- *Lactobacillus acidophilus:* Replaces the helpful bacteria "killed" in the bowel by antibiotic therapy.
- *Thymus extract:* A glandular preparation that supports the thymus gland, which plays a major role in fighting infection.
- *Echinacea:* An herb that strengthens the immune system.
- *Goldenseal:* An herb that strengthens the immune system. However, it should not be used during pregnancy.
- *Colloidal silver:* A broad-spectrum antimicrobial that is nontoxic and appears to have no interactions with other drugs.

Viruses

For those with poor immune system function, a viral infection can tip the scale toward hypersensitivity, chronic fatigue syndrome, or an autoimmune disease spiral.

These tiny, opportunistic invaders have ravaged humans, plants, and animals for centuries. Viruses were unknown by sight prior to the invention of the electron microscope in 1931. However, victims of viruses were well aware of the effects of disease they caused, even though the viruses themselves could not be seen. The face of Ramses V provided evidence that he had been a victim of the smallpox virus 3,000 years ago. Spanish conquistadors provided contaminated blankets to the South American Aztecs and Incas. The blankets had been taken from homes in Europe whose inhabitants had died from smallpox, and the unsuspecting natives died by the thousands.

The first antiviral treatment was given in 1798 in England, when Edward Jenner inoculated a patient with cowpox exudate in an attempt to prevent the dreaded smallpox. Jenner took this drastic measure after observing that farmhands who contracted the milder cowpox did not contract smallpox.

Scientists in the late 19th century were able to observe bacteria under their microscopes, but viruses were small enough to pass through porcelain filters that would trap the smallest known bacteria. They can be as small as 16/1000 the size of a pinhead, yet their potential for devastation cannot be correlated to their miniscule size.

■■ TYPES OF VIRUSES

Viruses are a very heterogeneous group of organisms. They vary in size one-hundredfold from the smallest virus, hepatitis B, to the largest, the herpes virus. They also vary in morphology, complexity, host type, and their effect on the host. However, viruses share certain characteristics.

- They all contain a genome (genetic material) of either RNA (ribonucleic acid, containing the sugar ribose as a structural element) or DNA (deoxyribonucleic acid, containing the sugar deoxyribose as a structural element).
- The RNA and DNA are covered with a protective protein shell that may be enclosed in an envelope containing protein and lipid.
- They grow and multiply only in living cells.
- Their genomes separate from their protective shells as the first step in their multiplication cycles.

The principal content of all viruses is protein, which serves as a particle building block. They also contain glycoproteins in their envelope that appear as spikes or projections. Some viruses look like soccer balls with triangular faces while others resemble space vehicles, with angular appendages. The influenza virus, for example, looks very like a Roman mace, complete with spikes extending in all directions; the AIDS virus is spherical.

Some viruses contain hemagglutinins that clump the red blood cells of animals. They often contain enzymes that have various functions, including facilitating the release of viruses from the cells in which they were formed. The envelopes contain a mixture of lipids (fats) that resemble the membranes of the cells in which they multiplied.

Viruses are classified according to:
- morphology (form and structure)

Transmission of Viruses

Viruses enter our bodies through the mucous membranes, respiratory tract, skin, oral-fecal route, and bloodstream via insect and animal bites. They live in our nerves and blood, and they invade every organ. We transmit them on our fingers and with our breath and saliva. They can also be carried by insects and in animal saliva.

- physical and chemical nature of viral components
- gene sequences—DNA and RNA content
- strategies used for gene expression and replication

The following is the most common classification of viruses. Not all viruses for each family are listed.

DNA viruses include the following virus families.

- *Poxviridae:* variola (smallpox) and related diseases
- *Herpesviridae:* herpes, cytomegalovirus (CMV), *Varicella zoster,* and Epstein-Barr virus (EBV)
- *Adenoviridae:* Adenovirus
- *Papovaviridae:* warts (flat, plantar, papilloma, common)
- *Hepadnaviridae:* hepatitis
- *Parvoviridae:* parvovirus

RNA viruses are a larger group, which includes the following virus families.

- *Picornaviridae:* enteroviruses (polio), *Coxsackie,* ECHO (enteric cytopathogenic human orphan)
- *Togaviridae:* encephalitis, rubella

- *Flaviviridae:* yellow and dengue fever
- *Coronaviridae:* coronavirus
- *Reoviridae:* rotavirus
- *Rhabdoviridae:* rabies
- *Filoviridae:* Ebola virus
- *Paramyxoviridae:* parainfluenza, measles, respiratory syncytial virus, mumps
- *Orthomyxoviridae:* influenza
- *Retroviridae:* leukemia, lymphoma, HIV (human immunodeficiency virus)
- *Bunyaviridae:* encephalitis, hemorrhagic fever, hantavirus
- *Miscellaneous:* do not fit any other group

When the specific shape of the virus meshes with its counterpart on a cell, like a lock and key mechanism, the cell accepts the virus, unaware that it is welcoming its own death. The cell membrane envelops the virus, which proceeds to exploit and alter the cellular machinery to its own advantage in order to replicate.

Some viruses gain access to the cell by synthesizing an enzyme that dissolves a portion of the cell membrane. After entry, the viral shells or coats are dissolved, leaving the viral RNA or DNA free to suppress the RNA or DNA of the host cell. The virus then proceeds to control the cell function with its own nucleic acid pattern. It reprograms the cell to use its own raw materials and machinery to make new virus particles, called virons. Some viruses can assemble these parts like a jigsaw puzzle, while others produce enzymes to aid in viron assembly. Thousands of virons are manufactured in each cell of the host. Viral replication occurs at different speeds and in different sequences.

These replicated viruses are then shed from the host cell in two ways—one is a "budding" mechanism through the cell membrane, while the other causes the death of the cell by rupturing its membrane and leaking out the virons and cell contents. A "clever" virus uses its host in a long-term symbiotic or cooperative relationship. If the virus is poorly adapted to its host and destroys it, it also destroys itself and all of its clones.

Viruses mutate into many shapes that are both species and type specific. A particular virus can attach itself to only one type of cell—bacterium, plant, animal, or human—and it must attach to a specific receptor site on a specific cell. For example, the hepatitis virus finds its way to the liver; the AIDS virus meshes with a T-cell; the polio virus seeks out an exact subset of nerve cells in the spinal column; and the rabies virus makes its way to particular cells in the brain. Mutations have allowed viruses to adapt to pre-existing receptor sites for hormones and other substances vital to the cell's function.

Viruses do not grow equally in all cells. A particular virus can usually grow in only very few types of cells. This is called permissiveness. If viruses infect nonpermissive cells or cells that are not fully permissive, they cannot multiply. Cellular permissiveness can be changed, which changes infectivity. Infection with one virus may allow other unrelated viruses to multiply. Interferon is a protein released by cells infected with viruses. It keeps uninfected cells from becoming infected.

The diversity of viruses is evident in acute diseases such as the common cold or poliomyelitis, where rapid cell death occurs. Another form is the latent virus, which can lie undetected and dormant for long periods between flare-ups. Each successive viral burst weakens the host's immune defenses. Yet another type of virus causes a slow viral infection, which builds up over a long period of time and causes a form of progressive dementia. Some viruses mutate rapidly by changing their surface antigens. By the time the immune system produces an antibody to one form, the virus has already changed the antigen beyond recognition.

■■ EFFECTS OF VIRAL INFECTION

Any living cell is susceptible to a viral invasion. Viruses can have many different effects on cells, including a cytopathic effect, in which infected cells are killed. Areas of dead cells called plaque are formed, and viruses are released from the dead cells.

Some viruses can live in cells over a long period of time without replicating, and do not produce classic viral syndromes. Research done in 1989 by Michael Oldstone and his colleagues at Scripps Clinic and Research Foundation in La Jolla, California, has demonstrated that these insidious viruses alter a specialized cell function, such as the production or secretion of a hormone. The affected cell is not in danger of rupture or death, but the overall function and health of the host organism is greatly affected. The invaded cells do not show any abnormality or inflammation when seen under a microscope. This mode of viral activity is suspected to be a factor in such diseases as neuropsychiatric disorders, diabetes, growth retardation, hypothyroidism, and some autoimmune diseases.

Viruses can trigger acute infections that are self-limiting, such as upper respiratory infections or gastrointestinal symptoms of vomiting and diarrhea. They can also cause progressive infections of the central nervous system that persist for years. Maternal infections can result in congenital malformation of their offspring.

The many and varied symptoms of viral infection are caused by cell alteration and the resulting effects on the immune system. Viruses can inhibit host protein synthesis, change gene expression (their genetic makeup), and form new antigens on the cell surface that modifies the outer cell membrane. They can also cause host cells to fuse, forming a giant syncytia, a mass of protoplasm bounded by one membrane and containing hundreds of nuclei.

Some viruses lie dormant in nerve centers or ganglia, where no drug or antibody can reach them. This occurs with such viruses as *Herpes simplex*, which causes chronic recurring genital or mouth sores. Epstein-Barr virus hides in B-cells, the same cells that produce antibodies to viruses. The hepatitis B virus continues to multiply slowly in the liver and surfaces 20 to 30 years later to cause extensive liver damage. A less lethal virus, the papilloma virus, causes warts on the skin and mucous membranes. Recently, however, a strain of this virus has been linked to some forms of cervical cancer. Still another strain known as a retrovirus (such as HIV) can produce an enzyme that converts the cell's RNA to DNA. It then lies dormant, hidden away from the functions of the immune system, to wait for an opportune time to resurface and cause disease.

Latent viruses may be reactivated when

the balance between host and virus is upset. Some factors in upsetting this balance are prolonged stress; hormonal or immunological shifts; overgrowth of other pathogens; nutritional deficiency; age; drug, alcohol, or tobacco misuse; fatigue; genetic and hereditary factors; changes in diet; sudden temperature changes (either extreme cold or the sun's ultraviolet rays); deterioration of the environment; and excesses of anything, including exercise.

Research conducted worldwide shows that many forms of cancer are linked to a variety of viruses. Viruses have been tied to liver cancer, Burkitt's lymphoma, leukemia, and cervical cancer. It is believed that viruses further damage the DNA of some cells that are already stressed, and weaken a host's immune system that is already compromised.

Oldstone and his colleagues found in recent research that only a small number of viruses are needed to cripple immune function to a state of immune suppression. Researchers believe it is possible that this form of immune suppression may be present in cytomegalovirus, hepatitis B, and HIV, since these diseases all include the infected lymphocyte phenomenon.

▮ MUTATION AND INTERACTION OF VIRUSES

Viral genomes are subject to change by mutation. Some mutations are spontaneous and occur during viral multiplication. They can cause change in plaque size, host cell specificity, drug resistance, enzyme production, noncoding regions of viral genomes, and temperature growth ranges.

Cells can be infected by more than one virus. If they are closely related, the viruses interact. They may undergo recombination in which a new genome is formed. This is the mechanism by which the influenza virus mutates, causing the necessity for the influenza vaccine to be changed yearly.

Interference can also result, with one virus diminishing the reproduction of the other. In complementation, genomes interact indirectly to allow both mutants to multiply. Some virus particles are defective and cannot multiply on their own, but must multiply in cells simultaneously infected with helper viruses.

▮ DIAGNOSIS OF VIRAL INFECTIONS

Viral infections may be diagnosed by several methods:

- *Cell culture:* Viruses are cultured in living cells.
- *Tissue pathology:* Tissue is stained to demonstrate giant cells and inclusion-bearing cells.
- *Electron microscopy:* Negative staining with metal salts allows visualization of viruses that cannot be grown in cell culture.
- *Antigen detection:* Precipitation tests allow electron microscope identification of extracellular antigens.
- *Immunofluorescence:* Cells are examined by direct or indirect immunofluorescence. In this method, antibodies that attach to the cells are tagged with a substance that fluoresces in the presence of light, allowing rapid, specific identification.
- *Antibody titers:* Comparison of antibodies

in samples taken early in the illness and a convalescent sample.

COMMON VIRAL INFECTIONS

There are numerous viral infections. The following are the more common viral infections encountered by most people.

COMMON COLDS

The rhinovirus and other similar viruses cause the common cold. Over 200 different viruses can cause a cold. A successful vaccine to protect against colds has never been developed because of the number of viruses involved and the rapidity with which they mutate.

The cold is the most common upper respiratory infection in the world. It causes a mild syndrome in all age groups, especially older children and adults. The incubation period is two to three days and acute symptoms last three to seven days. Symptoms include swelling of the membrane lining the upper respiratory tract and mucus formation that results in congestion, stuffiness, nose blowing, postnasal drip, "scratchy" throat, and cough. Colds can occur any time of the year, with epidemic peaks in early fall or spring. The virus causing the cold can live for three hours outside the body, on the skin and on hard surfaces.

RESPIRATORY SYNCYTIAL VIRUS

Respiratory syncytial virus (RSV) is the single most important cause of respiratory infections in young children worldwide. Nearly every child will have an RSV infection during the first few years of life. It occurs annually, between late fall and early spring, and most commonly manifests as a pneumoni-

> ## Better Diagnoses
> *Some of the better adapted forms of viruses were probably classed together simply as "flu" in past decades. With today's sophisticated diagnostic methods, the viruses are now seen to have specific characteristics that can be recognized.*

tis or bronchiolitis in children less than six months old, although older children may also have the infection.

Transmission appears to be by large droplets, and this virus is very contagious. The incubation period is one to four days and begins with a nasal discharge, with the severity of the illness progressing to a peak in one to three days. Fever is variable, and the acute illness can last for 10 to 14 days. The virus is spread to the upper respiratory tract by contact with infective secretions. The child can shed the live virus in their discharges and secretions for three to seven days, during which time they are contagious. The shedding period may be longer in infants. The virus can survive on the skin for 15 minutes and for hours in droplets and on surfaces in the environment.

Immunity to RSV is weak and short-lived, allowing repeated infections, and one percent of children with RSV may need to be hospitalized. The virus can be very severe in immunocompromised children and adults, and in premature infants.

Death can result from RSV when it is not suspected or diagnosed, and procedures that would be helpful for other conditions are

RSV and Asthma

The connection of RSV with asthma has been the subject of continuing controversy. A Swedish study at the Borås Central Hospital in Borås, Sweden, examined a group of children hospitalized with RSV bronchiolitis (inflammation of the bronchioles) in infancy and a group of children who had not been infected with RSV. The frequency of both asthma and allergic sensitization was significantly higher in the RSV group at a follow-up study done when the children were seven and a half years old.

performed. It is frequently a nosocomial infection, and its spread in hospitals is a serious problem. Careful handwashing between contact with patients is of utmost importance, as is control of personnel and visitors with any respiratory illness.

▌ INFLUENZA (FLU)

Influenza symptoms can range from minor two- to three-day upper respiratory problems to a severe, fatal syndrome. The influenza virus mutates rapidly, creating new strains each year to which we must adapt. Epidemics of virulent new strains also appear from time to time, causing worldwide fatalities.

There are three serotypes (strains) of influenza, A, B, and C. A is the most extensively studied and mutates most often, with major shifts every 8 to 10 years. It has three subtypes, and new subtypes occur at irregular intervals. This strain causes the serious epidemics and is the reason that influenza

vaccines must be reformulated yearly. Influenza B can also cause severe illness, while influenza C occurs infrequently and causes milder disease.

Influenza is spread by airborne droplets in enclosed spaces, and with direct contact with the mucus of an infected person. The incubation period is one to two days. Symptomatic care is important once the flu begins, with its symptoms of nasal discharge, sore throat, and hoarseness. Cough, headache, and profound fatigue are common. Accompanying fever can last from one to five days. Respiratory symptoms and malaise will last another 7 to 14 days. An influenza virus can survive for up to three days on a nonporous surface, but lives on the skin for only 10 minutes.

▌ CROUP

Croup in children is caused by several species of the parainfluenza viruses. It affects children from six months to three years of age and can be the cause of serious illnesses. These viruses can be demonstrated in the respiratory tract for as long as six days before the onset of symptoms. The acute illness lasts for 4 to 21 days. Inhalation of large drops transfer the infection.

Symptoms include a cough that sounds like a seal's bark, difficulty breathing because of swelling beneath the vocal cords, fever, and a runny nose.

Croup is responsible for 15 to 20 percent of all nonbacterial respiratory diseases requiring hospitalization in infancy and childhood. Outbreaks occur most commonly in the fall, but can occur in any season. There is no specific therapy except for supportive measures.

■ ROTAVIRUS

The major cause of diarrhea in infants and small children is the rotaviruses. These viruses cause at least 30 to 50 percent of the diarrheas severe enough to require hospitalization. Peak infections in North America occur in the winter months, and the virus is excreted in the feces for about 8 days after the onset of symptoms. The most common means of transmission is the oral-fecal route.

There are three groups of rotavirus—A, B, and C—with A the most common in infants and children, and B in older children and adults. These viruses have been found worldwide and account for 40 to 60 percent of cases of acute gastroenteritis. The incubation period is one to three days, followed by an abrupt onset of vomiting. Watery, brown, copious, frequent stools will follow vomiting. Severe dehydration is a major complication, and death can result in malnourished infants.

■ ADENOVIRUS INFECTIONS

There are 41 serotypes (strains) of adenoviruses, which cause respiratory illness, conjunctivitis, pneumonia, croup, laryngitis, gastroenteritis, and cystitis. Symptoms include fever, rhinitis, pharyngitis, and cough. However, an adenovirus can produce infection without disease; the virus has been found in tonsils and adenoids removed from healthy children. Prolonged shedding of the virus from the pharynx and intestinal tract occurs after the initial infection. Infections occur most frequently during the late winter or early spring.

These viruses are spread by inhalation of droplet nuclei or by oral route. Direct spread

> ## A "Wheel" Virus
>
> *The name is from Latin "rota" for wheel because of the shape of the virus. Many people think the name is "roto," because it cleans out the body like a roto-rooter!*

by hands or contaminated towels and eye medications may also occur. Viremia (viral infection of the blood) can occur and spread the virus to the kidney, bladder, liver, lymphoid tissue, and occasionally the central nervous system.

■ CYTOMEGALOVIRUS

At least 80 percent of adults have antibodies to cytomegalovirus (CMV), and there is a very high rate of acquisition during the first five years of life. It has the most serious effects on newborns, and some infants are infected in utero. Ten to fifteen percent of mothers excrete CMV from their cervix during delivery. One-half to one-third of infants born to mothers excreting the virus will acquire the disease.

The symptoms of CMV vary with age, antibody status, and the immune response of the person. CMV has been implicated in learning disabilities. Like its close cousin Epstein-Barr virus (EBV), it can amplify an already existing problem and cause a variety of neurological symptoms. Specific antibody titers indicate the presence of cytomegalovirus. When the host's immune system overcomes the virus, the immunity prevents further outbreaks. However, excessive antibodies or viral debris can remain, causing a chronic stimulation of the immune system.

▌HANTAVIRUS

Much publicity was generated in 1993 when an unexplained pulmonary illness occurred in the "Four Corners" area of the United States. This region is shared by Arizona, New Mexico, Colorado, and Utah. About half of the previously healthy young adults who suddenly developed acute respiratory symptoms died. The culprit was the hantavirus, which is transmitted by rodents, and its principal carrier is the deer mouse.

The disease appeared in the Four Corners area because the heavy rains in the spring of 1993 produced a plentiful supply of foods that the rodents eat. Hantavirus pulmonary syndrome (HPS) has been identified in over half of the states in the U.S. and in Canada's western provinces. Hantaviruses are found worldwide and each variety appears to infect specific rodents. The most common mode of transmission is by the inhalation of dust or dried particles that carry dried saliva or waste products of an infected rodent. No arthropod vector has been established for hantaviruses, and there appears to be no person-to-person transmission.

Any activity that puts people in contact with rodent droppings, urine, or nesting materials can place them at risk for infection. Activities where people may touch rodents or their droppings, such as opening cabins and sheds or cleaning outbuildings that have been closed during the winter, puts them at risk. When the weather turns cold, some houses become shelters for rodents. The chance of being exposed to hantavirus is greatest when people live, work, or play in closed spaces where rodents have been actively living.

▌RUBELLA (GERMAN MEASLES)

German measles, or the "three-day measles" is caused by a member of the togavirus family. The incidence of rubella has dramatically decreased with the development of a vaccine in 1969. The "R" in the MMR vaccine stands for rubella. While the disease that rubella causes is relatively benign in children and adults, it is the most serious cause of birth defects when women contract German measles during the first four months of pregnancy.

The incubation period for German measles is 14 to 21 days. The illness is usually very mild with low-grade fever, upper respiratory symptoms, and swollen lymph glands. The rash lasts for one to three days, appearing on the neck, neck, and trunk. There may also be lesions on the soft palate. It occurs most often during the winter and spring months. Only 30 to 60 percent of infected people will develop a clinically apparent disease.

▌RUBEOLA

Rubeola, commonly called the five-day measles or "hard measles," was recognized as a disease as early as the seventh century. It is one of the M's in the MMR vaccine, and is caused by a virus in the paramyxovirus family. It has an incubation period of 7 to 18 days, and begins 9 to 11 days after exposure.

Cough, nasal drainage, conjunctivitis (inflammation of the mucous membrane lining the eyelids), and fever, accompanied by gray-white spots surrounded by redness on mucous membranes, signal the onset of this disease. These spots are the most apparent on the throat mucosa and are called Koplik's spots. The rash begins on the head and trunk within a day of the appearance of the spots, and spreads to the arms and legs. It persists for three to five days before fading, with the fever and systemic symptoms diminishing as the rash progresses to the extremities. Measles can be very severe in immuno-compromised or malnourished patients. Treatment is based on supportive measures and observation for complications.

▌ MUMPS

Mumps are caused by a paramyxovirus. Hippocrates first described mumps in the fifth century. The average incubation period is 16 to 18 days, and symptoms of mumps include fever, swelling, and tenderness of the salivary glands, especially the parotid glands. Swelling may be on one or both sides and will last for 7 to 10 days. Mumps are highly infectious, but immunity to reinfection is permanent after the primary infection.

Mumps can be accompanied by infrequent complications, including meningitis, encephalitis, pancreatitis, and neuritis. Other complications include orchitis (swelling and pain in both testicles). Orchitis occurs in 10 to 20 percent of males and infertility may result. Oophoritis, an unusual benign inflammation of the ovaries, can occur in women. A vaccine is available and is part of the MMR.

▌ HERPES

Herpes has been known since biblical times. *Herpes simplex I* causes the familiar fever blisters (oral cold sores), and *Herpes simplex II* causes genital lesions. *Herpes simplex II* is the most common cause of genital ulcers in North America.

Fever blisters are contagious. Kissing and oral sex can spread the infection and children can develop fever blisters by being kissed by an infected adult or being in close contact. The small blisters on the lips can affect the mouth, nostrils, eyelids, and even fingers. They will burst after a few days to several weeks, dry, crust over, and disappear. Fever, neck ache, enlargement of neck lymph nodes, and fatigue may accompany the first fever blisters. However, the first infection may also go unnoticed.

Because the virus is dormant in nerve cells, *Herpes simplex I* will be a lifelong problem, and 40 percent of people will have recurrences, often during times of stress. *Herpes simplex I* has also been implicated in ulcerations of the cornea, damage to nerves in the eyes, and swelling of the brain (encephalitis).

Herpes simplex II is sexually transmitted, highly resistant, and contagious. Infants can be infected as they pass through the birth canal, which can be devastating and can cause corneal blindness, sepsis (acute infection), brain damage, and death. Unless the first herpes outbreak is during pregnancy, it does not cause problems prior to delivery. If the mother's herpes is active at the time of delivery, the baby must be delivered by Cesarean section.

Herpes simplex II first appears as a systemic illness with fever, swollen glands, severe genital pain, and or discomfort when urinating. There will be tingling and burning or itching of the skin before the rash breaks out. The small red pimplelike bumps turn into blisters and heal in 7 to 14 days. Women may develop blisters on their buttocks, external genitals, cervix, and around the rectum. Men may develop blisters on the glans, foreskin, shaft of the penis, and around the rectum.

People can contact herpes without having noticeable symptoms, and because the virus is latent, they can have their first outbreak 20 years after infection. The virus remains in the nerves for a lifetime. Most people have recurrent attacks triggered by stress, anxiety, menstruation, sexual activity, food allergy, drugs, and minor infections.

■ CHICKEN POX

Another herpes virus, *Herpes zoster* (formerly called *Varicella zoster*), causes chicken pox. Nearly all people contract chicken pox before they are 10 years old. Chicken pox usually appears as a generalized blister-type rash on the back of the head and ears, and spreads to the face, neck, trunk, and extremities. There is a low-grade fever early in the disease, and the lesions, which are itchy, become pus-filled, then crust over. Chicken pox is contagious from the day before the rash appears until it crusts over five days later. Some children develop secondary bacterial infections of the rash, and complications can include pneumonia and encephalitis. Chicken pox lesions can rarely become infected with the "flesh-eating" bacteria, a species of *Streptococcus.*

After the initial infection, the virus can lie dormant in nerve cells. If the host is overly stressed for any reason, the virus can re-emerge in the form of painful "shingles" that follow the nerve paths. Pain warns of the eruption, which occurs days later. Postherpetic neuralgia (severe pain after resolution of the shingles), is common in older people.

During early days of exploration, sailors carried this rather mild infection to people of the New World. Since they had never encountered the disease and had no immunity, many of the affected natives experienced severe symptoms and died within days.

■ ROSEOLA

Human herpes virus VI, also called roseola, begins with a sudden onset of fever for three to five days. A rash forms on the abdomen after the fever subsides and spreads to the rest of the body. The incubation period is 10 days, and it usually occurs in children under four years of age. There have been febrile (fever) seizures in a few cases. As many as 90 percent of people in North America and Japan demonstrate antibodies to roseola, which is not a recurring infection.

■ EPSTEIN-BARR VIRUS

In the initial stages of another herpes virus, Epstein-Barr virus (EBV), antibodies are almost undetectable. As the immune system recovers from the early invasion, the antibodies can be detected. Symptoms of this infection include debilitating fatigue; sore throat; headaches; muscle and joint pains; swollen lymph tissue, spleen, and liver; and elevated liver enzyme levels.

EBV infections are widespread, with antibodies found in 90 to 95 percent of adults in North America. Most early infections are asymptomatic. It is the causative agent of "heterophile positive" (a special lab test) infectious mononucleosis that is most frequently seen in young adults. Symptoms of mononucleosis include fever, swollen lymph glands, sore throat, fatigue, and malaise that may last from days to several weeks. It is not very contagious and is spread by repeated contact. Treatment is largely supportive. Because rupture of the swollen spleen can occur, contact sports and heavy lifting are restricted. The virus remains in the body for life, and most people do not have recurrences. However, in people with cancer and chronic fatigue immunodeficiency syndrome, recurrences are seen.

▋ COXSACKIE

The coxsackie virus strains belong to the family of enteroviruses (intestinal). The symptoms are similar to EBV and appear to affect muscle function. When first identified, coxsackie strains were thought to be polio. Enteroviruses are spread by the oral-fecal routes and cause meningitis, myocarditis, hepatitis, respiratory disease, and febrile conditions accompanied by rash. The many different serotypes of coxsackie make it possible to have recurring infections with this virus. However, infection with a given serotype confers immunity for that particular serotype.

▋ HEPATITIS

Although hepatitis is not as common as the other viral infections discussed, its seriousness when it does occur merits its inclusion here. Hepatitis is an inflammation of the liver. It may be acute and eventually heal, or it may be chronic and continuous. Several types of viruses cause hepatitis, including types A, B, C, D, E, F, and G. All types can cause acute infection, with types B, C, and D resulting in chronic infection. Symptoms of hepatitis include fever, nausea, vomiting, loss of appetite, rashes, joint pain, and ex-

treme fatigue with rapid weight loss. The urine will be dark, the stools light, and jaundice will occur.

Type A is called infectious hepatitis and is spread though oral-fecal contact and contact with infected items. It is contagious two to three weeks before jaundice symptoms appear and for one week afterward.

Hepatitis B is called serum hepatitis and is the most lethal. It is spread through infected blood products and needles, as well as sexual contact. Six to ten percent of infected adults become carriers, and over 300 million people are carriers worldwide. There are 200,000 new cases annually in North American and 6,000 die from it each year. Ten percent of cases progress to the chronic state. High-risk groups for hepatitis B include healthcare professionals, inmates and staff of institutions, dialysis patients, household contacts and sexual partners of carriers, international travelers, intravenous drug abusers, sexually active adults with more than one sexual partner, and sexually active bisexual and homosexual men. Hepatitis B is not very contagious except among those with high-risk behavior, which includes anal sex and the use of IV drugs. Some hepatitis B cases develop liver cancer.

Hepatitis C can be contracted through sexual contact, intravenous drug abuse, broken skin, or mucous membranes. In 40 percent of cases, no risk factor is identified. Hepatitis C causes 90 to 95 percent of all hepatitis contracted from blood transfusion. All blood is screened for both hepatitis B and C, but because it takes six months for hepatitis C to develop, it is impossible to identify all infected blood. Acute hepatitis causes a mild illness, but 80 percent of cases become chronic and lead to liver disease. Chronic hepatitis C affects 3.9 million North Americans.

Hepatitis D is called a "defective" virus because it causes infection only in the presence of hepatitis B, but can cause both acute and chronic hepatitis. Hepatitis E and F are transmitted through oral-fecal contact. Hepatitis E is rarely seen in North America, but both water- and food-borne transmission have been documented. Although recovery from hepatitis F confers specific immunity, its importance in human infection is not yet established. Hepatitis G is transmitted by blood and is the cause of some post-transfusion hepatitis. It is found in 2 percent of blood donors in North America.

■ HUMAN IMMUNODEFICIENCY VIRUS (HIV)

One of the most dreaded viruses is human immunodeficiency virus. As its name suggests, it creates a rapidly mutating form that debilitates the immune system and often leads to death. HIV mutates by changing the structure of its surface protein markers (antigens). It attaches itself to the T-cells of the immune system and changes the host RNA to DNA (the master molecule of life). More than 20,000 North Americans have succumbed to this tiny invader, and it occurs throughout the world. HIV is contagious only through intimate contact or by exposure to contaminated body fluids. It can be passed to babies if their mothers are HIV positive, and infection of babies through breast milk has been documented. At this time, prevention is the best weapon against HIV.

HIV usually presents as the sudden onset of fever, sweats, fatigue, muscle pain, joint pain, headaches, sore throat, diarrhea, generalized swelling of the lymph glands, and skin rashes. It may also have a gradual onset, with unexplained fatigue, weight loss, fever, diarrhea, and generalized swelling of the lymph nodes. It can directly infect the brain and cause dementia. People can also develop recurrent, unusual, and severe infections and lymphomas. Some HIV-positive people may not develop symptoms for years.

■ PAPILLOMA VIRUS (WARTS)

Warts are caused by the papilloma virus and range from the common skin wart to plantar and genital warts. Skin warts occur mainly in children and young adults and are believed to be spread through contact and minor abrasions. Genital warts are transmitted sexually.

Most human papilloma viruses, including those that cause common, plantar, and flat warts, are completely benign and are not associated with development of carcinomas. However, some species, especially those that cause warts on the cervix, vagina, and vulva, can convert to a malignant form. Therapy for warts is usually directed toward removal of the lesion rather than treatment of the papilloma virus infection. Topical application of caustic agents, cryosurgery, and laser surgery are used.

■■ TREATMENT OF VIRAL INFECTIONS

In treating viral infections, the goal is to stop viral replication as quickly as possible in order to prevent the spread of infection to other host cells. Many viral diseases result from a series of growth cycles. Unfortunately, symptoms do not occur until after a number of viruses have entered host cells and altered cell function and machinery enough to start rapid replication.

Inoculations for some viruses are considered to be very effective. The incidence of these diseases decreased at the time that vaccines for measles, rubella, mumps, and polio were introduced. Vaccines have also essentially eradicated smallpox; the last case was reported in 1978. When people are at high risk, hepatitis B or influenza vaccines may be administered.

However, some physicians fear that the viral antigens and debris from vaccines may adversely affect the immune systems of hypersensitive people. Some healthcare practitioners question the effectiveness and safety of vaccines. For example, polio declined in Europe at the same time that it declined in North America, and there was no polio vaccination in Europe. Serious side effects result from vaccinations in some people, including contracting polio.

Donor immunoglobulin is used to prevent extreme symptoms in some viral infections. Human serum containing specific antibodies is the preferred source of this artificially acquired immunity. This method provides only temporary protection, however. With the advent and increase of AIDS, human blood products are frequently no longer available. Manufacturers of human blood products feel they cannot guarantee the absence of the AIDS virus in their products and are reluctant to market them.

While drug therapy is limited for treat-

> ## Antibiotics Ineffective Against Viruses
>
> *Viruses do not respond to the antibiotics that eradicate bacteria. Treatment with drugs is extremely difficult, considering the evasion tactics that the viruses employ. It is virtually impossible to kill a virus hidden in lymphocytes or nerve cells without also destroying the host cells.*

ing viral infections, a drug named acyclovir (Zovirax) is being used to control some forms of herpes virus with effective results. Some people with chronic fatigue syndrome have also improved after a course of acyclovir. Amantadine and Rimantadine have been successfully used both as preventive agents and to treat influenza A infections. These are very selective drugs, which appear to interfere with the viral nucleic acid injection of the host cell.

Doctors Robert Cathcart and Linus Pauling have used large dosages of vitamin C to control a number of viruses. Vitamin C is known to have active antiviral properties, as well as being an important nutrient for immune system repair. Dr. Cathcart recommends that patients take up to 150 grams every 24 hours over several days to effect a remission in severe viral infections. During infection, our body uses up to four times more vitamin C than normal. The indicator introduced by Dr. Cathcart for optimal intake is known as the bowel tolerance level, the point just short of the amount that produces a liquid type of stool. (See Vitamin C: A Key Nutrient in chapter 20.)

A nontoxic material, Monolaurin, is effective against a number of viruses. Its action is twofold: it disintegrates the virus envelope or shell, and it also stimulates the host immune response. Monolaurin can also prevent viral attachment to the cell. This therapy is most effective if started early in a viral infection, before the viral injection of host cells. In this case, many infections can be aborted. If given later, Monolaurin it will not abort the infection, but can lessen the severity of the disease.

Another effective nontoxic viral treatment is lysine (an amino acid). It, too, should be started as early as possible when a viral infection begins. Viruses change the host cell's metabolism to demand more arginine (also an amino acid) in order to replicate within the cell. Arginine is found in nuts, beans, and chocolate. It is wise to reduce or eliminate these foods during a viral infection. Lysine is effective because it has a similar chemical structure to arginine and is taken into an infected cell in its place. The virus uses lysine for food but cannot use it for replication.

Several homeopathic remedies are available that also aid in the relief of symptoms from viral infections. Glycyron is available in oral preparations. This material detoxifies the host from the harmful effects of the virus. Engystol, another homeopathic preparation, can be taken both orally and by injection. This material stimulates immune system function and detoxification pathways, but has no direct effect on the virus. Oscillococcinum is effective for influenza infec-

tions and has been proven in double-blind trials. Health food stores carry these homeopathic remedies.

Parasites

Parasitology is the science dealing with organisms that take up residence, either temporarily or permanently, on or within other living organisms for the purpose of obtaining food. The term parasite applies to the organism that obtains food, shelter, and other benefits from the association. The harboring organism is called the host.

Parasites are classified in several different ways:

- *Ectoparasite:* Lives outside the host on skin or hair, causing infestation.
- *Endoparasite:* Lives within the body of the host, causing an infection.
- *Facultative:* Lives independently or as a parasite.
- *Obligate:* A permanent resident, totally dependent on the host.
- *Incidental:* An organism established in a host in which it does not ordinarily live.
- *Temporary:* A free-living organism that seeks a host intermittently to obtain nourishment.
- *Permanent:* Remains in or on the host from early life until maturity.
- *Pathogenic:* Causes injury to the host by mechanical, traumatic, or toxic activities.

The relationship between a parasite and a host may be symbiotic, constituting a permanent association between two organisms that cannot exist independently. It may be mutual, where both organisms benefit, or it may be commensal, where one partner benefits and the other is unaffected. However, many organisms that were previously thought to be commensal are not; the host is damaged. The host may suffer functional or organic disorders when the parasite is pathogenic. Hosts are classified as follows:

- *Definitive host:* Harbors the adult or sexual stage of the parasite.
- *Intermediate host:* Harbors the larval or asexual stage and may be a primary or secondary intermediate host.
- *Incidental host:* An infected host not necessary for parasite survival or development.
- *Reservoir host:* Another animal harboring the same parasite. It ensures continuation of the parasite and is a source of human infection.

Knowing parasite life cycles is important; these cycles tell us how we become infected, as well as helping to identify the stages in which preventive measures can be applied. Parasite life cycles can be simple or complex. A more complicated life cycle decreases the organism's chances of survival, so these organisms compensate with increased reproduction and multiplication.

Medical parasites include protozoa (one-celled animals); helminths (worms); and arthropods (insects, arachnids, and crustaceans—including flies, ticks, mites, spiders, and scorpions). Parasitic diseases caused by these organisms have no geographical boundaries or class distinction. Parasites have been carried all over the world by travelers and immigrants. For example, the slave trade introduced hookworm and schistosomiasis to this continent. The fish tapeworm was carried to the United States by immigrants from the Baltic region. With today's extensive travel, parasites are regu-

Prevalence of Parasites

Parasitic disease is believed to be a thing of the past in the more industrialized parts of the world, but this is untrue. Parasites are the most misunderstood of the organisms. Many people in North America unknowingly harbor parasites and far more people have been exposed to them. Parasitic diseases are among the major causes of human misery and death in the world today. They represent enormous obstacles to the development of countries that are economically poor and have inadequate sanitation and unsafe water.

larly transported all over the world, making diagnosis more complicated.

Although parasites are distributed worldwide, they abound in the moisture and humidity of the tropics. Short summers in the temperate zones prevent the growth of species that require higher temperatures in their larval stage, since low temperatures arrest the development of larvae and eggs. Moisture is essential for parasites with free-living stages.

In some parts of the world, people cannot walk barefooted because of the risk of getting hookworms in their feet. Many insects, such as mosquitoes, black flies, and tsetse flies, carry developmental forms of parasites that are spread when these insects bite humans. Streams and rivers can be polluted with several types of parasites, including flukes, and infection can result from any contact with the water, whether it is used for drinking, wading, and bathing. In Africa, the rate of parasite transmission is so high that control measures have had little effect.

Economic and social conditions affect the prevalence of parasites. Low standards of living, lack of information, and inadequate personal and community sanitation play a large role in the spread of parasites. The use of human feces for fertilizing agricultural crops in some developing countries constitutes a major factor in the spread of parasitic infections. Produce imported into North America from these countries can infect the people who eat it.

The spread of parasites depends on the source of the infection, the mode of transmission, and the presence of a suitable host. Humans may be the only host, the main host (together with animals), or an incidental host, with animals as the principal host. Transmission can take place through direct contact, indirect contact, contaminated food or water, soil, vertebrate and invertebrate vectors (a living carrier such as an insect that transports the parasite to the host), and in rare cases, from mother to offspring.

Pathological effects due to parasites depends on the number of parasites, their tissue specificity, and their mechanisms of tissue damage. Damage to the host is caused by:

- sheer numbers of the parasites as they multiply
- mechanical damage by obstructing vessels
- destruction of host cells by parasite invasion
- inflammatory or allergic reaction to the parasite or its metabolic products, causing symptoms that affect many systems of the body

- competition for nutrients, depleting the host body

Several factors affect resistance to parasites. Some people have innate or natural resistance; genetic factors may give resistance to parasitic infections. Remaining parasite-free as we age may represent an acquired or a natural resistance. People in a state of nutritional deficiency may experience an increase in the severity of a parasitic infection, while good nutrition can decrease the severity of an infection.

▐▌ PREVENTION OF PARASITIC INFECTION

Sources of parasitic infection are many and varied. Contaminated water, food, dirt, and dust are primary sources of infection. Wild animals as well as household pets are often infected with parasites, and can transmit these parasites to humans. However, there are measures we can take to limit our risk of becoming infected with a parasite.

▐ FOOD AND WATER

Observing the following guidelines can aid in preventing parasitic infections:

- Drink only safe water. It should be either filtered or treated with a stabilized oxygen product such as Aerobic 07. If you add 6 drops per gallon, it acts as a germicide. Ten to 15 drops per glass of water acts both as germicide and oxygenator. If there is any doubt concerning the water, boil it for 20 minutes.
- Wash all fruits and vegetables. Use $1/2$ teaspoon of Clorox bleach (this brand only) to 1 gallon of water, and soak food 15 to 30 minutes. Clorox-sensitive people may substitute hydrogen peroxide, NeoLife Green,

Nature Clean Veggie Wash, soap and water, or ozonated water. Rinse thoroughly in a fresh bath of plain water, then store or cook. Whenever possible, peel fruits and vegetables.

- Rinse meat, fish, and poultry thoroughly in cold water before cooking. Be sure to cook it well. Improperly cooked or raw meat, fish, and poultry may transmit tapeworms and other parasites. Meats and poultry (except ground meat) may be thawed in a Clorox bath, then placed in clear water for 10 minutes. Meats may also be frozen to kill larvae. Fish require 0°F (–18°C) for 48 hours and beef and pork require 24 hours at 6°F (–20°C).
- Minimize your sugar intake; parasites thrive on high-sugar diets.
- Control insects such as flies, cockroaches, mosquitoes, and ticks that can carry parasitic diseases.

▌ PERSONAL

Simple, practical hygiene practices can prevent your getting parasites.

- Wash your hands before each meal, and *always* wash your hands with soap and water after using the toilet, having sexual intercourse, changing a diaper, or handling pets.
- Keep fingernails short and scrub under them with a nailbrush.
- Use sterilized lens cleaning preparations or safe water (never water from the tap) to clean and sterilize contact lenses.
- Keep your immune system strong, and your intestines healthy. (See Candidiasis in chapter 17, and see chapter 23, Detoxification, for general information.)
- Be aware of sexual risk factors: oral sex, anal sex, and multiple sex partners.

▌ PETS

To minimize the possibility of your pets passing parasites to you, use the following precautions.

- Never allow children to eat dirt, or to play in sand or dirt where cats and dogs relieve themselves.
- Change cat litter daily and wear gloves when you do so. Pregnant women and immunocompromised people should have someone else do this chore.
- Keep your pets wormed, and brush and clean them outdoors.
- Make certain that all food preparation and eating areas are totally off limits to pets.

▌ TRAVEL

Exercise care when traveling out of the country. The following precautions can help you to avoid parasites.

- Wipe or protect toilet seats with toilet paper before sitting; squatting is better. But be sure to wipe off the seat to prevent leaving toilet seats dirty for the next person!
- Drink only bottled water from reliable sources, carry a portable water filter, or carry a bottle of stabilized oxygen such as Aerobic 07 or Dioxychlor to treat the water.
- Avoid ice cubes in drinks, as they are usually made from tap water. Do not brush your teeth with tap water.
- Eat only cooked or peeled fruits and vegetables and do not eat from salad bars.
- Avoid regional foods that are not well cooked and may have been fertilized with human feces, and dishes containing pickled, raw, dried, or smoked fish, crabs, and crayfish. All meat should be thoroughly cooked.
- Stay covered up in the tropics; wear long

sleeves and long pants to avoid insect bites. Do not walk barefoot. Sleep under netting.

▌▌ SYMPTOMS OF PARASITIC INFECTION

In some people, a parasite infection is chronic with few or no symptoms. These people are carriers and represent the normal state of infection, in which there is an equilibrium between host and parasite, or infection without disease. In others, the infection is acute.

Parasitic infections can cause the following symptoms, and people who have these symptoms should be tested for parasites.

Gastrointestinal symptoms include:
- diarrhea, colitis, dysentery, and chronic bowel symptoms
- bloating, excessive gas
- abnormal stool formation and appearance: frothy, floating, blood-tinged, mucus laden, or crumbling
- alternating diarrhea and constipation
- nutrient malabsorption and metabolism disruption
- increased food intolerance

Symptoms of other systems include:
- chronic or unexplained fatigue
- stimulation of detoxification enzymes (the mixed-function oxidase system and cytochrome P-450, a complex system of enzymes that processes chemicals)
- eosinophilia (an increase in specific white blood cells)
- immune suppression
- allergic responses to many substances
- joint pain
- night sweats

- fever
- asthma

You do not have to be experiencing bowel symptoms for a parasite infection to be a problem. Anyone who has camped extensively or who has traveled outside of North America should be tested for parasites. University or preschool students should be tested if they suddenly develop symptoms, since they are often in contact with many people from other areas of the world. Others at high risk for infection include prisoners and patients in institutions and long-term medical facilities.

It is advisable to have a parasite test twice a year if you travel frequently, eat out regularly, or have pets.

In sensitive people, there are three main areas in which symptoms manifest. Even when infection has been long term, many of these effects are reversible with treatment.
- chronic gastrointestinal distress, including irritable bowel, malabsorption, nonspecific symptoms, and severe food allergies
- fatigue resembling Epstein-Barr virus (EBV). Intestinal symptoms are not the major presenting symptoms.
- allergic and inflammatory symptoms linked with chronic immune dysfunction. These include allergy symptoms that have nothing to do with the intestinal tract, such as aching joints and muscles and chronic asthma.

▌▌ COMMON PARASITIC ORGANISMS

There are hundreds of parasitic organisms that can affect humans. However, for purposes of this discussion we will consider only the more common medical parasites.

▌ PROTOZOA

The most common parasitic infections that result in symptoms are those caused by protozoa, or one-celled microscopic animals. Although most are free-living, some are parasitic. They have anaerobic metabolisms, allowing them to live without oxygen in the lumen (interior space) of the intestines. Their presence contributes to immune dysfunction.

These pathogenic protozoa secrete:
- proteolytic enzymes that decompose protein
- hemolysins that rupture red blood cells
- cytolysins that destroy cell membranes
- toxic and antigenic substances

Intestinal parasites obtain their nutrition through liquids absorbed from the intestine of the host. Some ingest solids, and many utilize both solids and liquids. Several species ingest red blood cells and bacteria.

All protozoa have a trophozoite form (a vegetative form) and a cyst form (an inactive state). The cysts are able to resist more environmental insults and are the infective stage. Cysts enter our bodies through:
- wells, springs, and other water supplies contaminated by feces
- vegetables and fruits contaminated with feces
- food contaminated by houseflies and cockroaches
- food contaminated by infected food handlers
- direct transmission by cyst carriers
- carelessness in personal hygiene

Methods of locomotion and reproduction divide protozoa into four major classes: rhizopods (amebas), flagellates, ciliates, and Sporozoa.

▌ *Rhizopods*

Amebas are rhizopods, the most primitive protozoa. They move by forcing liquid endoplasm into projections called pseudopodia (false feet). These move the organism forward and engulf food sources in its path. Amebas multiply by simply binary fission (dividing in half).

Amebas are a common human parasite, and the following species have been established as parasites in humans: *Entamoeba histolytica, Entamoeba coli, Entamoeba gingivalis, Entamoeba hartmanii, Dientamoeba fragilis, Endolimax nana, Iodamoeba butschlii, and Blastocystis hominis.* All of them live in the intestine, except *Entamoeba gingivalis,* which is found in the mouth.

Entamoeba histolytica. A tissue-invading ameba, and the second most common protozoan infection in North America, *Entamoeba histolytica* is the cause of amebiasis, amebic dysentery, and amebic hepatitis. The wall and the lumen of the colon are the area of the body inhabited by *E. histolytica.* It is considered anaerobic, but it can consume oxygen. Its distribution is worldwide, but *E. histolytica* infections are most prevalent in the tropics.

The mature cysts are very hardy and are resistant to the acid of the stomach, but disintegrate in the alkaline medium of the small intestine. Infected people shed large numbers of infective cysts every seven days.

Entamoeba histolytica uses its cell-destroying enzymes to leach nourishment from host tissues. After tissue invasion, this ameba no longer depends on the bowel nutrients, instead ingesting red blood cells, tissue fragments, bacteria, and intestinal contents.

In the large intestine, *Entamoeba histolytica* causes lesions that become ulcerous, forming nodules of inflamed tissue. The degree of damage depends on the resistance of the host, the virulence of the ameba, and the conditions in the intestinal tract.

Entamoeba histolytica infections can be impossible to distinguish from ulcerative colitis. Appropriate tests for amebiasis should be performed on anyone with ulcerative colitis because steroids, a common treatment for ulcerative colitis, can cause death if the patient has amebiasis.

If the *Entamoeba histolytica* organisms migrate from the intestine, every organ can be affected. Some people develop systemic amebiasis, or amebic infection. The liver can then be invaded and diagnosis becomes difficult. Lung amebiasis accompanied by fever and chills may develop. Brain abscess, although rare, can also occur. Infected people can suffer from ulcerative vaginitis, cervicitis, and lesions on the penis. Secondary bacterial infections frequently follow the amebic invasion.

Entamoeba coli. This ameba has a life cycle similar to that of *Entamoeba histolytica*, and is often mistaken for it. While *Entamoeba coli* is not considered a pathogen, it can cause difficulties to those with immune system problems. It occurs with a 10 to 30 percent frequency in America and is even more prevalent in Europe. This ameba is transmitted by ingesting the cysts in food, in drink, on the fingers, and on other objects.

When *Entamoeba coli* is found in the stool, this indicates ingestion of fecal contaminants. It lives in the intestine in the same area as does *E. histolytica*, and feeds on enteric bacteria and possibly red blood cells.

Entamoeba gingivalis. An inhabitant of the mouth, this ameba is found in the tartar and gingival pockets. While *Entamoeba gingivalis* is considered a nonpathogen, it is found in 10 percent of people with healthy mouths and in 95 percent of those with diseased teeth and gums. The presence of this ameba suggests the need for better oral hygiene. Transmission takes place through droplet spray from the mouth and through contaminated drinking glasses or dishes.

Entamoeba hartmanii. Because *Entamoeba hartmanii* resembles *E. histolytica* except for size, it was at one time thought to be a "small race" of *E. histolytica*. This ameba does not digest red blood cells and is identified by the size of its cysts. Ingesting contaminated food or water transmits it. *E. hartmanii* can cause diarrhea in otherwise healthy people.

Dientamoeba fragilis. A small amoebaflagellate, *Dientamoeba fragilis* has been identified worldwide and has a 4 percent incidence of infection. *D. fragilis* lives in the human intestine, causing moderate, persistent diarrhea, gastrointestinal symptoms, some low-grade fever, and vomiting.

Endolimax nana. Formerly classified as a commensal organism, this ameba is now believed to be the fifth most common pathogen, living in the lumen of the intestine. It feeds on bacteria and has a 10 to 20 percent prevalence rate. Methods of infection include ingesting viable cysts in polluted water or contaminated food, from contaminated objects, or through poor personal hygiene.

Iodamoeba butschlii. Another ameba that was formerly believed to be only commensal, *Iodamoeba butschlii* has a prevalence rate of 8 percent. It is distributed worldwide, with a higher incidence in tropical regions. *I. butschlii* lives in the lumen of the large intestine and feeds on intestinal bacteria. Contaminated food, drink, and soiled objects transmit it.

Blastocystis hominis. There has been much controversy over the classification of *Blastocystis hominis,* and at one time it was thought to be a fungus. It is now classified as a protozoan, and by most authorities as an ameba. *B. hominis* is frequently mistaken for the cyst form of other protozoa because of its spherical central mass, thick outer protoplasm, and thin cell membrane.

Blastocystis hominis is also now recognized as a pathogen that causes diarrhea in humans, and has been reported in epidemics of gastrointestinal disease in subtropical areas. Symptoms accompanying infection by this ameba include diarrhea, pain, cramps, nausea, fever, vomiting, headaches, gas, chills, and malaise. It is transmitted by the same methods as other ameba. It is frequently found in the bowel with *Candida albicans,* and is an obstacle to the cure of Candida.

I *Flagellates*

A second class of protozoa, the flagellates are one-celled animals that have developed special organs to enable them to withstand the peristaltic (contraction) action of the intestine. They also have flagella, whiplike structures that aid in propulsion. Flagellates have both a trophozoite and cyst form but, unlike the ameba, the trophozoite is also infective in some species. Flagellates infect both humans and other animals; however, it is difficult to determine whether the species are the same.

Giardia lamblia. The most widespread protozoan intestinal parasite in North America is the flagellate *Giardia lamblia.* It lives in the duodenum and jejunum (parts of the small intestine), and possibly in the bile ducts and gallbladder. This parasite causes increased permeability of the gut and allows larger food particles to pass through the gastrointestinal mucosa into circulating blood. The immune system does not recognize these particles as food, and so allergic responses develop. These allergies resist treatment until the *Giardia* infection is treated. Giardiasis is a problem in 30 to 40 percent of allergy patients.

Giardia has both trophozoite and cyst forms. The trophozoite form has four pairs of flagella and a concave sucking disk that attaches to the intestine. By attaching itself to the intestine, *Giardia* is able to maintain its position in spite of peristaltic action. It obtains food from the intestinal contents and from the intestinal wall through the sucking disk.

Giardia proliferates in an alkaline environment. Hypochlorhydria and achlorhydria (low or no acid in the stomach) and a carbohydrate-rich diet enhance multiplication. Multiplication occurs by mitotic (complex) division during the cyst stage. The

Beaver Fever

Some authorities believe that over half of our the North American water supply is contaminated by Giardia lamblia. *Campers should be particularly careful, since even chlorine treatment does not always kill these parasites. There have been reported cases of giardiasis in campers who obtained their water from ice runoff.*

Wild animals are thought to be capable of infecting humans and to be one of the causes of water contamination in the wild. Beavers are natural reservoirs and are leading contributors to water contamination, which has resulted in an alternate name for giardiasis, "beaver fever." Household pets can also be reservoirs for the parasite.

cysts, which make up the infective stage, are very resistant and may remain viable for months outside the host.

Giardia is transmitted by food and water contaminated by sewage, food handlers, flies, and from hand to mouth in cases of poor hygiene. It is prevalent in mountain regions, and people can become infected from swimming in contaminated water. Infection is more common in children than in adults; outbreaks are frequently reported in daycare centers and nurseries. The incidence of giardiasis is highest in areas with poor sanitation and among populations unable to obtain clean water or maintain adequate hygiene.

Some people may become infected with-

out having symptoms. Others may suffer diarrhea, total malabsorption, steatorrhea (excess stool fat), or irritable bowel syndrome. Giardiasis also promotes small intestine bacterial overgrowth. While bowel symptoms are common in giardiasis, it is possible to have a serious Giardia infection and experience no intestinal symptoms at all. Chronic infection with *Giardia lamblia* resembles an Epstein-Barr virus infection because of the persistent, chronic fatigue. Anyone suffering from fatigue should be checked for Giardia.

The following factors increase the risk of giardiasis:
• hypochlorhydria or achlorhydria
• IgA deficiency
• candidiasis
• anal sexual habits or multiple partners
• type A blood

Trichomonas vaginalis. This protozoan flagellate inhabits the vagina of the female, and the urethra, epididymis, and the prostate of the male. It causes a persistent vaginitis in females and is accompanied by a burning, frothy, creamy discharge. Women develop vaginal and cervical inflammation accompanied by itching and burning. *Trichomonas* causes urethritis, and prostatitis in males. However, the infection rate in husbands of infected wives is surprisingly low.

There are several modes of transmission, sexual intercourse being probably the major mode. However, *Trichomonas* infections occur in young virgins, suggesting that contaminated toilet articles and toilet seats can transmit the infection. Infections in babies are probably acquired when passing through an infected birth canal.

Diagnosis is based on symptomology and demonstration of the organism on microscopic examination. Cultures are sometimes positive even when microscopic examinations are negative. Restoration of vaginal pH will suppress trichomonas. Attention to personal hygiene is extremely important, as is the detection and treatment of all infected males.

Ciliates

These protozoa are distinguished by threadlike cilia that cover their bodies and are appendages of locomotion. Ciliates reproduce by binary fission (dividing in half).

Balantidium coli. The only pathogenic parasite of the *Ciliate* class, *Balantidium coli* is the largest of the intestinal protozoa. Its trophozoites live in the lumen, mucosa, and submucosa of the upper region of the large intestine, and in the terminal portion of the small intestine. Its threadlike cilia allow rapid propulsion. This parasite also has a boring action, allowing it to invade the mucosa and submucosa of the intestine with the aid of a cell destroying enzyme. There it divides rapidly and forms "nests" containing many organisms.

There is a high incidence of *Balantidium coli* in hogs, which, together with their contaminated feces, are an important source of human infection. It is transmitted when people ingest cysts in contaminated food and water. Infection causes liquid stools containing blood and pus, sometimes alternating with constipation. Although a *Balantidium coli* infection can be present without symptoms, in someone who is debilitated it can be fatal. Sanitary control is probably the best means of prevention.

Sporozoa

The species of this fourth class of Protozoa have no method of locomotion, and have both sexual and asexual reproduction.

Cryptosporidea. The third most common protozoan intestinal pathogen, *Cryptosporidea parvum* parasites infect the stomach and small bowel, causing enterocolitis (intestinal inflammation), nausea, low-grade fever, intestinal cramps, and diarrhea in humans. These organisms have also been found in the respiratory system, gallbladder, liver, and pancreas, in addition to the gastrointestinal tract. Symptoms come and go, but will subside in less than 30 days in a healthy person. Immunocompromised people may not be able to clear these parasites, and the infection can become prolonged and contribute to their death.

Cryptosporidea have been documented as causing disease in people who practice anal sex and in immunocompromised individuals, such as AIDS patients. It has also been found in preschoolers attending daycare. An oral-fecal route of transmission is suspected, from contaminated fingers, food, and water, and there is no known treatment.

In 1993, the water supply in Milwaukee, Wisconsin was contaminated with *Cryptosporidea*. Over 400,000 people developed an infection and over 100 people died. It is thought that the *Cryptosporidea* came from untreated water from Lake Michigan that entered a water-treatment plant and were inadequately removed by the coagulation and filtration process. The source of the *Cryptosporidea* in Lake Michigan remains speculative.

Effective water treatment and personal

hygiene are the most importance preventive measures for *Cryptosporidea*. Careful handling of animal excreta and hand washing by those in contact with animals that have diarrhea, particularly calves, may also be important.

Pneumocystis carinii. This organism is a lung parasite and has both a trophozoite and cyst form, which spreads the infection when it is inhaled. Its multiplication in the lungs causes secretion of fluid and cells, resulting in death by respiratory failure. Its mode of transmission in humans is unknown, as is the period of communicability. Symptoms typically appear in 1 to 20 months after the onset of immunosuppression.

Symptoms include dry cough, fatigue, fever, weight loss, night sweats, and cyanosis (blue skin due to deficient oxygenation of the blood). It causes a pneumonia that is often fatal in premature infants, as well as in malnourished, chronically ill and immunocompromised adults. Two chemotherapeutic agents are available, but the prognosis is still poor. This is a common infection in patients with AIDS or people who are immunocompromised. It affects 60 percent of people with HIV disease.

Plasmodium. Malarial parasites of humans are species of the genus *Plasmodium* and include *Plasmodium malariae, P. vivax, P. falciparum,* and *P. ovale*. These organisms have a very complicated life cycle that involves two hosts, a vertebrate and a mosquito. The asexual life cycle takes place in the vertebrate host, and the sexual cycle takes place in the mosquito.

After an incubation period of 9 to 30 days, an infected individual begins to exhibit symptoms of malaria, including headache, lassitude, vague pains in the bones and joints, chilly sensations, and fever. They then begin regular episodes of chills and fever, and the spleen can become enlarged. The person is quite well in between these episodes, which occur at regular intervals. Without treatment, all species of malaria can result in self-cure except *Plasmodium falciparum*, which can be fatal and has become resistant to a number of drugs. However, some people may suffer recurrent episodes for the rest of their lives.

Although it is more common in the tropics, there have been malaria outbreaks in North America. Many outbreaks are among migrant workers and war veterans. However, two cases were reported in New Jersey in 1991 among people who had not traveled outside the state. The potential exists for the disease to become established in North America. Competent mosquito vectors are present, and there are areas with substandard sanitary control. Travelers returning from other countries, people entering North America for the first time, and the high numbers of immigrants from Mexico all increase the possibility of malaria. However, mosquito control is the most important method of prevention.

▮ WORMS

There are many species of worms, which are called "helminths," from the Greek word meaning worm. Most are free-living, but some are parasites of humans. Parasitic worms usually have some type of structure that helps them to attach, penetrate, or abrade the tissues of the host. The majority also have secretory glands near the mouth that are lytic (capable of disintegrating tissue), allowing the worm to digest the host's tissue for food or to migrate through the tissue to the site where it matures.

In the majority of species, eggs or larvae hatched from eggs pass out of the definitive host's body into an external environment where they wait for another host. Some species require several intermediate hosts. Many eggs and larvae perish from desiccation (drying), overgrowth by bacteria and fungi, inability to find an intermediate or definitive host, or death of the intermediate host. However, under favorable conditions, helminths can develop into epidemic proportions.

Malnutrition plays a major role in helminthic infections, both for the host and the parasite. It interferes with antibody production and can decrease inflammatory reactions, thus lowering host resistance. Diet alterations, including fasting, and deficiency of nutrients can cause the spontaneous loss of worms from the host.

Worms are classified into several phyla, according to structure.
- *Annelida*—segmented worms (leeches)
- *Nemathelminthes*—roundworms
  —*Nematoda*
- *Platyhelminthes*—flatworms
  —*Cestoda*— tapeworms
  —*Trematoda*—flukes

❚ Leeches

The leeches in *Annelida* are ectoparasites (living outside the host) and occur mainly in the Far East. Leeches of medical importance are both aquatic and terrestrial and have muscular, oval bodies with hard jaws and

Tapeworm Diet Pills

People have been fighting the "battle of the bulge" for years. In the United States, early in the 20ᵗʰ century, tapeworm segments were sold as a diet aid. The theory behind this action was that the tapeworm segment, containing viable eggs, would give the person a tapeworm. People with a tapeworm experience irritability, gastric discomfort, nausea, diarrhea, and weight loss. After the appropriate amount of weight had been lost, the person would be treated to rid him or her of the tapeworm. Needless to say, this venture was soon abandoned, but not before some people suffered severe physical and psychological problems.

suckers at both ends. Larger aquatic leeches may suck the blood of swimmers, and the smaller leeches, taken into the body in drinking water, infest the upper respiratory or digestive passages. They may even invade the vagina, urethra, and eyes of swimmers.

Terrestrial leeches live in damp forests in the Far East and attach themselves to travelers. They will crawl inside clothing and boots. Their bites bleed easily and are slow to heal because of the anticoagulant substance injected by the leech.

❚ Roundworms

The nematodes are roundworms that range in size from the *Ascaris,* which can be as long as 13 to 14 inches and *Dracunculus medinensis,* which can be 3 feet long, to *Trichinella spiralis,* a microscopic worm that infects mus-

Common Helminth Infections of Human Beings

Nemathelminthes Roundworms

	COMMON NAME OF PARASITE OR DISEASE	SITE IN HOST	PORTAL OF ENTRY	SOURCE OF INFECTION, INTERMEDIATE HOST OR VECTOR	MOST COMMON CLINICAL SIGNS OR SYMPTOMS
Ancylostoma braziliense	Creeping eruption, cutaneouslarva migrans (hookworm larva)	Intradermal	Skin	Dog and cat hookworm larvae in soil	Spreading skin lesions, itching
Ancylostoma duodenale	Old world hookworm	Small intestine, attached	Skin, usually feet	Infective filariform larvae in soil	Anemia, growth retardation, G.I. symptoms
Ascaris lumbricoides	Large roundworm	Small intestine	Mouth	Eggs from soil or vegetables	Vague abdominal distress, failure to thrive
Enterobius vermicularis	Pinworm, seatworm	Large intestine, appendix	Mouth	Eggs in environment; autoinfection	Anal itching, irritability
Necator americanus	New World or tropical hookworm	Small intestine, attached	Skin, usually feet	Infective filariform larvae in soil	Anemia, growth retardation, G.I. symptoms
Strongyloides stercoralis	China diarrhea (now called Vietnam diarrhea)	In wall of small intestine	Skin	Larvae in soil, sometimes direct fecal contamination, autoinfection	Abdominal discomfort, diarrhea
Toxocara canis *Toxocara cati*	Visceral larva migrans	Liver, lung, brain, eye	Mouth	Eggs from soil	Inflammation of the lungs, eosinophilia
Trichinella spiralis	Trichinosis	Adult: small intestine wall. Encysted larva: striated muscle	Mouth	Encysted larvae	Edema around eyes, muscle pains, eosinophilia
Trichuris trichiura	Whipworm, threadworm	Cecum, large intestine, ileum	Mouth	Eggs from soil vegetables	Abdominal discomfort, anemia, bloody stools
Wuchereria bancrofti	Filariasis	Lymph system	Skin	Mosquitoes	Inflammation of lymph nodes, fever

	COMMON NAME OF PARASITE OR DISEASE	SITE IN HOST	PORTAL OF ENTRY	SOURCE OF INFECTION, INTERMEDIATE HOST OR VECTOR	MOST COMMON CLINICAL SIGNS OR SYMPTOMS
Platyhelminthes Tapeworms					
Diphyllobothrium latum	Fish or broad tapeworm	Small intestine	Mouth	Infectious form in fresh-water fish	Digestive disturbances, anemia
Dipylidium caninum	Dog tapeworm	Small intestine	Mouth	Flea and louse	Usually none
Echinococcus granulosus	Hydatid cyst	Liver, lungs, brain, bones	Mouth	Eggs from dog feces in soil	Pressure symptoms in various organs
Hymenolepis diminuta	Rat tapeworm	Small intestine	Mouth	Cysts from insects	Usually none
Hymenolepis nana	Dwarf tapeworm	Adults and cysts in small intestine	Mouth	Eggs from feces in soil Autoinfection	Abdominal discomfort, failure to thrive
Taenia saginata	Beef tapeworm	Small intestine	Mouth	Cysts in beef	Usually none
Taenia solium	Pork tapeworm	Small intestine	Mouth	Cysts in pork	Usually none
Taenia solium (cysts)	Cysticercosis Verminous epilepsy	Muscles, brain, eye	Mouth	Eggs from feces, regurgitation of eggs	Intracranial pressure, epilepsy
Platyhelminthes Flukes					
Clonorchis sinensis	Human liver fluke	Bile ducts	Mouth	Fresh-water fish	Indigestion, diarrhea, enlargement of the liver
Fasciola hepatica	Sheep liver fluke	Liver	Mouth	Encysted infectious form on watercress or in water	Enlarged, tender liver, eosinophilia with fever
Fasciolopsis buski	Intestinal fluke	Small intestine	Mouth	Water nuts and vegetables	Diarrhea, edema, abdominal pain
Paragonimus westermani	Lung fluke	Lungs	Mouth	Fresh-water crustaceans (crabs)	Coughing up blood, cough, abdominal pain, fever
Schistosoma haematobium	Schistosomiasis "Bilharzia"	Veins of urinary bladder	Skin	Infectious form in fresh water, from snail	Urinary disturbances, blood in the urine
Schistosoma japonicum	Schistosomiasis "Bilharzia"	Veins of small intestine	Skin	Infectious form in fresh water, from snail	Dysentery, fibrosis of the liver
Schistosoma mansoni	Schistosomiasis "Bilharzia"	Veins of large intestine	Skin	Infectious form in fresh water, from snail	Chronic dysentery, fibrosis of liver

cles, and *Strongyloides stercoralis,* which is less than 1/8 inch in length. The parasitic species of nematodes live in plants, mollusks, annelids, arthropods, and vertebrates. More than 80,000 species are parasites of vertebrates and can live in the intestine, blood, and tissue.

I *Flatworms*

Platyhelminthes, the flatworms, consist of two classes, Cestoda, which includes the tapeworms, and Trematoda, which includes the flukes. The adult tapeworms live in the intestine of vertebrates, and their larvae inhabit the tissues of vertebrates and invertebrates. The life cycle of the tapeworms is complicated, and depends on several intermediate hosts. Humans are occasional hosts for the tapeworms of other animals.

Tapeworms vary in size, from the beef tapeworm reaching up to 36 feet long, to the dwarf tapeworm, which is about 1 1/2 inches long.

The majority of the trematodes (flukes), are endoparasites (living within the host), and are primarily a problem in the Far East. However, an increase in travel and in the number of immigrants from these areas has increased the number of parasitic infections caused by flukes in this country. Flukes infect the intestine, liver, blood, and lungs of human beings.

While there are other parasitic worms in these phyla, the helminth chart includes the major and most common roundworms and flatworms seen in North America. However, with the international travel that is now common, more species of parasites are being discovered in North Americans. Parasites that once were uncommon can become es-

tablished if adequate hosts exist to promote their life cycles. Suspecting and detecting the presence of parasites is extremely important for the health of an individual.

▮▮ DIAGNOSIS OF PARASITES

Recent improvement in diagnostic techniques has shown that gastrointestinal and systemic parasites are more significant in immune system suppression than previously recognized. Parasites are diagnosed after demonstration of ova and parasites in a fresh stool specimen. This method, however, poses many problems. Stool examination, even with purged specimens, is frequently negative even when a person has an active parasitic infection. Parasites typically grow in the intestinal mucosa. Unless the parasite breaks off from the mucosa into the stool on the day the specimen is obtained, it will not be visible on examination. Sometimes the specimen is too old when it reaches the laboratory, and there may be excess material to deal with, calling for complicated concentration techniques.

New diagnostic techniques involve examining smears taken from the rectal mucosa. This specimen is then stained with immunofluorescent stains for examination with specialized microscopy. It is a highly sensitive and specific test. However, insufficient swabbing for the smears can miss parasites. The best results are obtained by using both a purged stool examination and a rectal smear.

Blood tests can be used to demonstrate eosinophilia, a general indicator of parasites. Antibodies to many parasites can be demonstrated in blood serum. Malarial and filarial infections can be identified by examining blood and blood smears. Abnormal levels of liver enzymes, vitamins, and minerals may be indicative of parasitic infection. Urine, sputum, and radiological tests may demonstrate some parasitic infections. Tissue scrapings, biopsies, cultures, and aspirations of fluids from body cavities can also be used to diagnose parasites.

■■ TREATMENT OF PARASITES

The type of parasite determines the treatment method. There have been significant advances in parasitic infection treatment, and in some cases toxic drugs are not necessary to eradicate the parasites.

Because some parasitic infections can be transmitted throughout a family, all family members must be treated. Even symptom-free members should be treated to prevent reinfections, since person-to-person contact is the most important factor in the spread of parasites.

■ PROTOZOAN TREATMENTS

One of the best current treatments for protozoan intestinal parasites is twofold, involving the use of ParaMicrocidin and Par-Qing. These substances are distributed by Allergy Research Group and are available at health food stores. (For more information on ParaMicrocidin, see chapter 17.)

Par-Qing is a nontoxic, noncarcinogenic, generally well-tolerated herbal product. Its major ingredient is *Artemesia annua*, which is presently being studied as an antimalarial agent. This variety of *Artemesia* has become available only recently in North America; other species of *Artemesia* are not effective. Par-Qing also contains anise seed, cinna-

mon, marjoram, and valerian. No alcohol should be consumed during treatment with this herbal product, and it should not be used by pregnant or lactating women.

You may experience some die-off symptoms (the Herxheimer reaction) when you begin treatment as the body reabsorbs protein from dead parasitic cells. These proteins are toxic to the body, and will cause symptoms such as fever, chills, sweating, diarrhea or constipation, headaches, irritation, muscle aches, memory loss, poor concentration, hormonal imbalances, or depression. Die-off may also include a worsening of symptoms already present; these symptoms will subside as treatment progresses.

Begin all treatment gradually—increase the dosage slowly in increments. Never begin any parasitic medication program at full strength. This helps minimize die-off levels and lessens the shock to the body, since our bodies respond poorly to sudden or large changes. If a particular dosage causes die-off symptoms, remain at that level of treatment until you can take the medication without experiencing symptoms, then increase your dosage. Hypersensitive people should be checked for material compatibility before starting the use of either ParaMicrocidin or Par-Qing because they are derived from plant material.

Begin with one capsule of ParaMicrocidin per day, taken with meals. Gradually increase the dosage to two capsules three times daily as die-off permits. Add Par-Qing when you have had no die-off symptoms with ParaMicrocidin for two weeks. Start Par-Qing with one capsule taken with meals and gradually increase the dosage, as die-off permits, to three capsules three times daily.

Children's doses are dependent upon body weight; your physician will determine the dose for each child. For everyone, however, treatment will vary depending on the following factors:
• progress of the individual
• severity of the infection
• duration of the infection
• organism(s) causing the infection
Because there is a very high relapse rate in parasitic infections, treatment must be continued long enough to ensure that the infection is gone. Repeat parasite tests must be performed at your physician's discretion to confirm that treatment is complete. If any of the repeat tests are positive, treatment will be continued or changed as determined by your physician.

Multiple organism infections and infections with more virulent organisms are more difficult to treat. Treatment requires consistency, and stringent personal hygiene is essential in order to prevent reinfection.

Vitamin C, taken at bowel tolerance levels, can relieve symptoms caused by toxins and released during die-off. Coenzyme Q_{10} (30 mg) taken three times a day, and organic germanium (150 mg), from one to three times daily, aid in restoring immune function. It is also important to take an acidophilus supplement both during and after treatment. This encourages "good" bacteria growth on the intestinal mucosa to prevent reinfection of fungi or parasites. Consuming fluids and exercising are important during treatment, to flush out toxins.

A treatment regimen combining ParaMicrocidin and Par-Qing has a failure rate of less than 10 percent for protozoan intestinal parasites. Drugs should be considered for those who do not respond to this treatment. Such drugs include Yodoxin, Humatin, Vermox, Flagyl, Aralen, Atabrine, Furoxone, and others. Their toxicity varies, and repeated trials of the less toxic drugs is preferable to directly beginning the more toxic substances.

Paratox 22 is an herbal remedy to treat protozoa. It contains grapefruit seed extract, garlic, slippery elm, and cranberry concentrate. This combination penetrates the intestinal mucosa where protozoa and fungi are growing. It is taken in four cycles to ensure that all the organisms have been eliminated.

▌ WORM TREATMENT

Niclocide and Biltricide are used for tapeworm, and Vermox, Antiminth, or Zentel are used to treat hookworm and ascariasis. Herbs can be effective against worms also. A combination of wormwood, black walnut hull tincture, and ground cloves will help eliminate many parasitic worms.

Paratox 11 is an herbal remedy that is effective against worms. It contains black walnut, senna blend, pink root, slippery elm, and garlic. This preparation is taken in four cycles to be certain that all parasites are gone.

CHAPTER 17

Fungi, Yeast, and Mold

FUNGI MAKE UP A portion of the plant world that does not contain chlorophyll and therefore cannot synthesize food from water and carbon dioxide. Many of these fungi are familiar to us: mushrooms, toadstools, puffballs, and various yeasts and molds. There are over 100,000 fungi, which fall into the classes listed below:

- *Lichens:* Grow in gray-green patches on rock
- *Phycomycetes:* Water molds
- *Basidiomycetes:* Mushrooms, toadstools, puffballs
- *Ascomycetes:* Yeasts used in industrial processes and manufacturing
- *Fungi imperfecti:* Pathogenic yeasts (*Candida* species) and molds

These fungi, yeasts, and molds have pronounced differences in structure and physiologic properties. Fewer than 300 species are directly implicated in human or animal disease. Less than a dozen cause 90 percent of all fungal infections (called mycosis).

The class of fungi containing the organisms that cause disease in humans is called *Fungi imperfecti.* These fungi are divided into two general classes: yeasts, which are typically oval or round, and molds, which are composed of tubular structures, called hyphae. Yeasts usually reproduce by budding, while the hyphae of mold grow by branching and longitudinal extension. However, not all fungi can be classified as a yeast or a mold. Some of them are round in shape, but do not bud. Some can grow either yeastlike in a host at body temperature, or as a mold at room temperature. These organisms are called dimorphic, and the nutrients available, carbon dioxide levels, and the age of the colony regulate their structure.

In this chapter we will discuss infections caused by different classes of fungi. Those organisms that are commonly referred to as yeasts and molds will be discussed under those headings, and the others will be presented under fungi.

Fungi

The word fungi comes from the Greek word meaning mushroom, and the study of fungi

303

is called mycology. Of course, not all fungi are mushrooms, and the taxonomy (classification) of fungi undergoes constant revision. All fungi reproduce by spore formation. Asexual spores are formed by mitosis (splitting apart), and sexual spores are formed by a few species as a result of mating. Classification of fungi depends primarily on the type of spore formation that follows sexual reproduction. All fungi for which a sexual reproductive cycle has not been discovered are lumped under the class *Fungi imperfecti*.

Fungi live in nature and accidentally cause infection, which is not advantageous for the fungus. Transmission usually does not occur from person to person. A fungal infection that involves the actual growth of fungus on or in a human or animal depends on host defenses, the route of exposure, the port of entry into the body, the size of the inoculum, and the virulence of the organism. Mycotic infections may be superficial infections of the skin; cutaneous infections of the mucosa, skin, and nails; subcutaneous infections that involve subcutaneous tissues, lymphatic vessels, and surrounding tissues; and deep-seated systemic infections. Diagnosis of fungal infections is made by microscopic examination of specimens, laboratory culture, and serology (blood tests that measure antibodies produced by the body to fungal antigens).

■■ COMMON FUNGAL INFECTIONS

■ DERMATOPHYTOSIS

Dermatophytosis is a fungal infection of the skin, hair, or nails. These infections are caused by any of a group of keratinophilic fungi called dermatophytes. These fungi secrete keratinases, which are proteolytic enzymes that digest keratin, the structural protein of hair, nails, and epidermis, the outer layer of skin. The species are similar in morphological, physiological, and biochemical composition. They cause a variety of specific clinical conditions, and a single species may produce several types of skin diseases. However, several species may also be the causative agent of the same disease.

Dermatophytoses are the most prevalent fungal infections in the world and can spread from person to person. The incidence varies considerably, but is higher in the tropics. The attack rate is higher in institutions and crowded living conditions. Their biology is unique and they are predominantly saprophytes, living on dead tissue.

The dermatophyte organisms causing infections include 22 species of *Trichophyton*, 18 species of *Microsporum*, and 2 species of *Epidermophyton*. Each of the diseases caused by these organisms has been given a clinical name. The most common infections are listed in the following chart.

Symptoms of dermatophytosis of the scalp and hair include dull, gray, circular patches of alopecia (loss of hair), scaling, itching, and acute inflammatory infection of the hair and follicle. Dermatophytosis of the beard, arms, legs, torso, feet, and hands may present as round, scaly lesions embellished with redness and vesicles (blisters). The thickness and duration of the lesion and the extent of the inflammatory response are determined by the nature of the fungus-host interaction.

Jock itch causes dry, expanding lesions

Forms of Dermatophytosis

CLINICAL NAME	SITE OF LESIONS	ORGANISMS FREQUENTLY ISOLATED
Tinea capitis – infection of the scalp	Scalp	*Trichophyton tonsurans, Microsporum audouinii*
Tinea capitis, nonepidemic	Scalp	*Microsporum canis, Trichophyton verrucosum*
Tinea capitis, epidemic	Scalp	*Trichophyton tonsurans, Microsporum audouinii*
Tinea favosa – severe, chronic ringworm	Scalp, torso	*Trichophyton schoenleinii, Trichophyton violaceum*
Tinea barbae – infection of the beard	Beard	*Trichophyton rubrum, Trichophyton verrucosum*
Tinea corporis – infection of parts of the body not covered with hair, ringworm	Arms, legs, torso	*Trichophyton rubrum, Microsporum canis, Trichophyton mentagrophytes*
Tinea cruris – infection of the groin and perineum – jock itch	Genitocrural folds	*Trichophyton rubrum, Trichophyton mentagrophytes, Epidermophyton floccosum*
Tinea pedis and manus – infection of the feet and hands, athlete's foot	Feet, hands	*Trichophyton rubrum, Trichophyton mentagrophytes*
Tinea unguium – infection of the fingernails and toenails	Nails	*Trichophyton rubrum, Trichophyton mentagrophytes, Epidermophyton floccosum*
Tinea imbricata – infection scattered over the body	Torso	*Trichophyton concentricum*

in the groin, and athlete's foot has chronic involvement of the toe webs. Athlete's foot may also cause vesicles, ulcers, or cover the foot like a moccasin, as well as causing thickening of the sole.

Onychomycosis, a fungal infection of the fingernail or toenail, causes white, patchy, or pitted lesions on the surface of the nail. If the hyphae of the fungus is under the nail, digestion, discoloration, and deformation of the nail occurs.

Diagnosis of dermatophytosis is made by direct examination of hairs under a microscope or by dissolving skin and nail clippings in 20 percent potassium hydroxide and looking for hyphae under a microscope. Hair, skin, or nail specimens can be cultured at room temperature on Sabouraud's agar (a special culture for fungi) containing antibiotics. The fungi are identified on the basis of colony appearance, growth rate, surface texture, pigmentation, and morphology of reproductive structures.

Treatment is usually with daily applications of a topical antifungal ointment. Some oral medications that are helpful for a particular organism are used. Griseofulvin deposits in the skin and inhibits fungal growth. Oral ketoconazole (Nizoral) is effective in some people, and Lamasil is used in other cases. Nail infections may require a year or longer to heal.

■ HISTOPLASMOSIS

Histoplasmosis is a common pulmonary mycosis of humans and animals caused by *Histoplasma capsulatum*, a dimorphic fungus. It occurs worldwide and develops after inhalation of the fungi. Ninety percent of infections are not apparent and are detected by residual lung calcifications, delayed hypersensitivity, or both. This disease is endemic in the Ohio-Mississippi Valley, in Missouri, Tennessee, Kentucky, Indiana, and southern Illinois. This area has a large population of starlings, and the excrement from the birds is an excellent growth medium. In South America, chicken coops and bat caves are a reservoir for this organism.

It is estimated that 40 million people are exposed to *Histoplasma capsulatum*, with 500,000 new infections each year. Of these cases, 55,000 to 200,000 will be symptomatic, 1,500 to 4,000 will require hospital-ization, and 25 to 100 deaths will occur. Histoplasmosis manifests as acute and chronic pulmonary episodes and is seen most often in adult men. If large areas of the lung are affected, cavitary histoplasmosis may occur, which results in holes in the lungs. Its symptoms are indistinguishable from chronic cavitary tuberculosis. Chronic episodes may be accompanied by low-grade fever and productive cough, as well as progressive weakness and fatigue. In the past, mistaken diagnosis caused some histoplasmosis patients to be hospitalized in TB sanitariums.

The disseminated form (which spreads throughout the body) form ranges from benign to progressive, and damage can occur in any part of the body. The tissues of the spleen, liver, lymph nodes, and bone marrow are the next most common sites. In this progressive form, the pulmonary symptoms are insignificant, and the patient may have an enlarged spleen and liver, weight loss, anemia, and increased leukocytes. These severe cases are often rapidly fatal.

Diagnosis of histoplasmosis is by microscopic examination of sputum, tissue material from biopsy, spinal fluid, and blood. Culture of an early-morning sputum specimen or bronchial wash can be diagnostic, as can several blood test techniques. Skin tests are positive within two weeks of infection. A negative test rules out histoplasmosis in an immunocompetent person, but not in a person who cannot mount an allergic response.

Most cases of histoplasmosis are not detected and need no treatment. Rest allows the body to heal. For the most progressive cases, Amphotericin B is used, and other drugs are available for less severe cases. Prevention involves exercising care in endemic areas around bird droppings.

CRYPTOCOCCOSIS

Cryptococcosis is caused by a yeastlike fungi, *Cryptococcus neoformans*. This fungus is encapsulated and reproduces by budding. It occurs worldwide and frequently grows in pigeon droppings, although the birds are seldom infected. In the soil it is killed or inhibited by bacteria, sow bugs, amebas, and mites.

Most infections begin in the lungs and may then spread to the brain, urinary tract, skin, or bones. Although many cases may be asymptomatic, symptoms of a respiratory infection include coughing and chest pain with occasional scant sputum. With a central nervous system infection, the symptoms will be headache, nausea, dizziness, irritability, clumsiness, and drowsiness. Immediate treatment is necessary to prevent life-threatening complications. The number of cases of cryptococcosis was very low until the advent of AIDS, which allows many opportunistic infections to affect patients. In addition to being seen in AIDS patients, cryptococcosis occurs in diabetics, patients with kidney transplants, and people on corticosteroid therapy.

Culture, tissue sections, and blood tests diagnose this disease. The best treatment is with combination therapy with Amphotericin B and flucytosine. The mortality rate is 25 to 30 percent, and the relapse rate is 20 to 25 percent.

COCCIDIOIDOMYCOSIS

Coccidioides immitus is a dimorphic fungus that normally lives in the soil in a highly restricted geographic area confined to southwestern U.S., northern Mexico, and areas of Central and South America. This fungus causes coccidioidomycosis, which until 1930 was thought to be a disseminated and severe disease. However, a more common form causes a mild, respiratory ailment also called valley fever or San Joaquin Valley fever. This disease is infectious, but not contagious, and resembles tuberculosis.

Primary coccidioidomycosis follows inhalation of arthroconidia (spores). The incubation period is 10 to 16 days and the disease resolves in three weeks to three months. In most people it is asymptomatic, but when the disease manifests, symptoms include fever, chest pain, cough, or weight loss. X-ray exam shows discrete nodules in lower lobes. Twenty percent of people have allergic reactions and erythema nodosum (reddened nodules) on the shins, legs, and occasionally other areas. They may also have fever, muscle and joint pain, and malaise.

Disseminated coccidioidomycosis is a complication of the primary form. It is a chronic and progressive pulmonary disease and may be fulminant (severe) or chronic, with periods of remission and exacerbation. Lesions may also occur in the meninges (covering of the spinal cord and brain), skin, or bone.

Diagnosis is by skin test that will become positive within two weeks of onset of symptoms, and through blood tests. A positive skin test is not diagnostically significant unless there are accompanying symptoms. A negative test excludes coccidioidomycosis except in anergic individuals (those who are unable to mount an allergic response). Laboratory diagnosis includes spherules in sputum, culture, chest X-ray, and tissue appearance. Blood tests eliminate the infectious hazards of working with cultures.

Treatment for primary coccidioidomycosis is usually symptomatic. Amphotericin B, miconazole, and ketoconazole are used for disseminated cases. Prevention is important and involves wearing protection, particularly a mask, when working with soil in endemic areas.

Yeast (Candida albicans)

Yeasts are a class of fungus that is round or oval in form and reproduces by budding. Although there are many different yeasts, our discussion is limited to the strain of body yeast belonging to the genus *Candida* that can cause health problems for humans.

There are many strains of *Candida* in our environment, but the two that most commonly affect humans are *C. albicans* and *C. tropicalis*. In our discussion, Candida will refer to *C. albicans*, and the disease that its overgrowth causes is referred to as candidiasis. Overgrowth from *C. tropicalis* is not common.

Candida albicans is a very complex organism. It releases over 80 known toxins that adversely affect our body. If left untreated, a chronic Candida infection and overgrowth can severely debilitate us, leaving us susceptible to more serious diseases. Two chemicals produced by Candida are acetaldehyde and ethanol. Acetaldehyde disrupts cell membrane function and alters protein synthesis. (Acetaldehyde is also a breakdown product of alcohol and is thought to cause the "fuzzy brain" symptoms of a hangover.)

Since our metabolism cannot convert these materials into useful compounds, it must detoxify them. When the circulating load of these materials is too great, poor memory, lightheadedness, fatigue, inability to concentrate, and depression can result.

Candida normally has a rounded, yeast-like shape. However, it can mutate and develop branching threads called mycelia, which penetrate the mucous membrane of the intestinal tract. This mycelial form is more difficult to eradicate. Candida has the ability to change its cell membrane structure in order to escape the effect of single drug therapy. Dr. David Soll of the department of biology at the University of Iowa has demonstrated at least five rapid mutations of the Candida cell membrane. This mechanism is known as "switching."

▮ CAUSES OF CANDIDIASIS

Although candidiasis is typically seen as a minor infection of mucous membranes, skin, and nails, Candida overgrowth is not a new problem. The overuse and prolonged use of antibiotics kills the "good" bacteria, allowing Candida to proliferate and become a chronic intestinal infection. Also, many meats contain high levels of antibiotics, which is an unexpected and in some cases constant source of antibiotics. The optimum growth media provided in the moist and dark areas in the gut and vaginal tract make us excellent hosts for Candida overgrowth. Low stomach acid also fosters Candida growth.

Birth control pills, cortisone and other steroids, and nonsteroidal anti-inflammatory drugs cause hormone imbalances in our body, encouraging Candida to grow more abundantly. The chemicals produced by the yeast attack our immune system, and if it weakens, the Candida will spread and involve more tissues: membranes swell; organisms multiply; and nasal, throat, sinus, ear, bronchial, bladder, vaginal, and other infections develop. Antibiotics are then usually prescribed, promoting further yeast growth. Health problems will continue until this cycle is interrupted by appropriate treatment.

Candida also seriously interferes with the digestion and absorption of nutrients from the intestinal tract; as a result, prolonged, untreated infection can lead to overt nutrient deficiency. Other conditions that may upset the normal symbiotic relationships of microflora in our body are debility due to other infection, diseases, or aging; drug or alcohol abuse; suppression of the immune system to avoid organ transplant rejection; and use of chemotherapeutic agents in cancer treatment.

The most common place for Candida growth is the gastrointestinal tract (the entire digestive tube from the mouth to the anus). Its only food source is sugar. A diet with excess refined or simple carbohydrates such as candies, sweets, cookies, and junk food contributes greatly to Candida overgrowth. The average North American eats over 100 pounds of sugar annually.

▪▪ SYMPTOMS OF CANDIDIASIS

Men, women, and children can have candidiasis. Men may have prostatitis (inflammation of the prostate gland). Because women have more complex hormone sys-

> ## Opportunistic Yeast
>
> Candida albicans *is a body yeast that lives in small amounts in all of us. Normally its presence is limited to the skin, the vagina, and the mucous membranes of our gastrointestinal and upper respiratory tracts. Candida growth is kept in balance by beneficial or "good" bacteria and our immune system. However, Candida is an opportunistic organism and if our immune system becomes depressed, inefficient, or overwhelmed, the tenuous balance is upset and the good bacteria are destroyed. Candida then multiplies and an overgrowth (chronic infection) results.*

tems, candidiasis occurs in them more frequently, and with more severe effects. Candida overgrowth is suspect in women's infertility problems. It attacks children who have received large quantities of antibiotics or who consume excessive sugar and junk food. Babies can be infected with Candida as they pass through the birth canal if their mother has a yeast vaginitis.

Candida is known as the great masquerader—any symptom is possible, and any organ can be targeted. Many people with severe yeast problems have never described all of their symptoms to their doctors for fear of being labeled neurotic or a hypochondriac.

Candida symptoms can fall into several categories.

• *Emotional and mental problems:* Severe depression, confusion, extreme irritability, anxiety, memory lapses and short-term memory loss, inability to concentrate, difficulty in reasoning, drowsiness, insomnia, lethargy, and loss of self-confidence can all point to Candida overgrowth.

• *Hormonal:* Disrupted hormone production in the thyroid, adrenal glands, ovaries, pituitary gland, or testes causes the entire endocrine system to function poorly. *Candida albicans* also interferes with the receptor sites for hormones, further contributing to the problem.

• *Hypersensitivity reactions to Candida or its byproducts:* Asthma, headaches, bronchitis, hay fever, earaches, hives, skin rashes, and severe chemical and food sensitivities result from these reactions.

• *Intestinal and genitourinary tracts:* Yeast vaginitis; menstrual complaints; bowel problems, such as bloating, constipation, diarrhea, and gas; and inflammations of the prostate, esophagus, stomach lining, colon, and bladder can signal the presence of Candida.

• *Nose and throat:* Severe sinus headaches may be caused by colonies of Candida growing in nasal passages. The increased sinus congestion and pressure can cause loss of equilibrium and may be confused with a middle-ear infection. A white, "furry" tongue is also a symptom of Candida overgrowth.

• *Skin:* Unrelenting skin itching and deep ear itching are aggravating symptoms of *Candida albicans.* The itching occurs deep beneath the surface of the skin with no visible rash. Scratching or rubbing does not relieve the itching. It may be caused by a hypersensitivity reaction either to antibodies produced by our body or to metabolic toxins produced by the yeast.

• *Worsening of existing symptoms:* Weakness, fatigue, fleeting muscle and joint pains, dizziness, difficulty in swallowing, easily detected body and breath odor, and acne and other distinctive skin rashes can all be indicators of Candida. Sugar cravings and hypoglycemic symptoms are common.

■ DIAGNOSIS OF CANDIDIASIS

A history of exposure to oral contraceptives, steroids, anesthesia, and multiple doses of antibiotics together with these chronic symptoms point to a Candida problem. Positive allergy tests for yeast, mold, and fungus may also indicate candidiasis.

Several diagnostic blood tests for Candida are now available at specialized laboratories. It is possible to detect high levels of Candida antibodies from three classes of immunoglobulins: IgA, found in mucous membranes in the mouth, vagina, and intestinal tract; and IgG and IgM from the blood. Some laboratories perform blood titers of these specific immunoglobulins against Candida organisms to aid in diagnosis. Testing for Candida Specific Immune Complexes is also useful for diagnosis, as well as for monitoring the effectiveness of treatment. The immune complexes contain Candida antibodies, Candida antigens, and fragments of complement (immune) enzymes. These complexes are present in direct proportion to the Candida antigen load, and drop quickly when the Candida load is reduced.

Culture surveys for *Candida albicans* can be done using smears from the nose, throat, rectal area, genital area, and vagina. Anyone with a positive culture and accompanying symptoms should be treated. In some cases, evidence of the infection cannot be ascertained unless repeated cultures are run. Women with chronic vaginal yeast infections do not always show growth of yeast from a vaginal culture. Finally, response to treatment confirms the diagnosis of Candida overgrowth.

▌▌ TREATMENT OF CANDIDIASIS

Treatment is intended to reduce the organism's colonization to a tolerable level. It is essential to change the environment of Candida. This can be accomplished in four ways:
- Deny it food (sugar).
- Provide an acid medium.
- Increase its natural enemy, "good" bacteria.
- Introduce antifungal agents that the body can tolerate.

A combination of treatment modalities is necessary to prevent "switching," the cell membrane mutation mentioned earlier.

Treatment should be cumulative; do not stop taking one material when the next is added. It is important to proceed slowly with treatment and target all areas in and on the body simultaneously. Since most Candida infections are long-standing and well established, treatment must be persistent and continued for as long as necessary to prevent symptoms from returning. Unfortunately, there is no quick fix. Treatment duration will vary—some people may require treatment for only a few months, but most will have to be treated for a year or more.

Treatment must be long term, consis-

> ### Yeast Unaffected by Blood
>
> *In one 1983 study, done by Steven Witken and others at Cornell University Medical College in New York, the blood of women with chronic vaginal yeast infections was added to a culture of yeast. It did not kill the yeast. The blood of women without yeast infections was added to another culture of yeast, and it killed the yeast. When the two bloods were added together, they did not kill the yeast, demonstrating that something blocked the destruction of yeast in women with chronic vaginal yeast infections.*

tent, and continual because the Candida organism is a very resistant, natural symbiotic inhabitant of the gut. When it is not in balance with the normal flora, the Candida organism is encouraged to bury itself deeper into the tissues by developing the mycelial form.

However, if the Candida organisms are killed off too rapidly, our body is flooded with overwhelming amounts of toxins from ruptured yeast cells. The body immediately reacts with an inflammatory immune response that can cause unbearable symptoms, known as "die-off" or Herxheimer reaction. You may feel slightly dizzy, lightheaded, or depressed; experience tightness in your chest; or have muscle aches, diarrhea, or an upset stomach. Some people have nightmares and night sweats.

These die-off symptoms can also be an exaggerated form of the symptoms you experienced prior to treatment. As each yeast cell dies, the cell ruptures and its toxic contents are released. An accumulation of these toxins produces the symptoms, which will pass within a few days. Although you may feel a little discouraged by temporarily not feeling well, die-off symptoms are a sign that the treatment is working.

Treatment is complete when there is no relapse after treatment is withdrawn. The immune system must recover sufficiently to keep the Candida under control, since Candida overgrowth will return with a vengeance if therapy is stopped too soon. When therapy is complete, substances and dosages should be reduced slowly, one at a time, under the supervision of a healthcare professional. Watch for a subtle return of symptoms; if they reappear, resume full treatment. When all therapy is discontinued, your diet should continue to remain low sugar or sugar-free.

When one family member has candidiasis, other members are often infected. It is wise to have the whole family checked for infection and treated if necessary. Otherwise, the one who is being treated will be constantly re-exposed, making the treatment less effective. Candida can be passed back and forth between sexual partners.

If Candida overgrowth is not treated, it will continue to spread and break down our body's ability to fight off other serious infections and diseases. Merely destroying the Candida organism does not immediately undo its damage to our immune and endocrine systems. It takes about one to three years or longer for our body to rebuild its immunocompetence against *Candida albicans* infections. Each of us is unique; therefore, treatment programs must be tailored to each person's specific needs. Faithfully following a treatment program will speed the rate at which candidiasis is controlled. For this type of treatment, you need a long-term commitment to being fully involved in your recovery. This requires a process of education about our body functions and a willingness to share the responsibility for a return to wellness.

We are in control of our health, and symptoms from Candida are a signal that something in our lifestyle needs to be altered. Exercise, diet improvements, nutritional supplements, and active Candida treatment are necessary to keep Candida under control. Once this has been achieved, our healthier bodies—together with altered lifestyles—will keep the organism suppressed.

For more information about *Candida albicans* and candidiasis, please see Recommended Books. The more informed you are, the better you will understand your problem and how to fight it.

■ BASICS OF CANDIDA TREATMENT
The following instructions are basic principles you should follow when treating Candida, regardless of the treatment materials you use.

• Begin each treatment substance separately and gradually increase your intake at weekly intervals as die-off permits. Build up to top dosage as rapidly as possible so the treatment time will not be prolonged and die-off will not be constant. The speed of therapy varies with the severity of the symptoms and the length of time the infection has been present.

- Treat any other suspected illness (including allergies) and infections to lower the total load on the immune system.
- Avoid antibiotics, steroids, and nonsteroidal anti-inflammatory drugs unless absolutely necessary.
- Avoid birth control pills and hormones, particularly progesterone (also known as Provera). Women will have difficulty recovering from candidiasis if they continue to take birth control pills, as progesterone and the higher than normal levels of estrogen cause Candida to proliferate.
- Avoid environmental molds at home and at work. Continued exposure to molds inhibits recovery from candidiasis.
- Avoid chemicals in the environment as much as possible in order to lower the total load of the immune system.
- Take supplements of additional vitamins and minerals, glandulars, and enzymes that will enhance proper functioning of the digestive, immune, and endocrine systems. (See chapter 20, Nutrition and Allergies.)
- Take detoxification baths or dry saunas to rid the body of toxins produced by the Candida organism. (See chapter 22, Detoxification.)
- A brisk five-minute walk or other tolerated exercise several times daily will help the body rid itself of excess toxins.
- Have your stool checked for parasites.
- Proper bowel function (at least two soft stools daily) is very important. Increase vitamin C intake to help accomplish this. (See Vitamin C: A Key Nutrient, in chapter 20.)

■ HYGIENE FOR CANDIDA TREATMENT

In addition to other treatments, exercise stringent hygiene practices.

- Brush your teeth and gums, including your tongue, three times daily.
- Use Orithrush mouthwash and gargle (see Nonprescription Therapy below).
- Refrain from oral sex and have protected sex to prevent reinfection until you have completed treatment.
- Cleanse all affected skin areas with soap and water before applying any of the treatment materials.
- Wash your hands with soap and water after using the toilet, and after sex.
- Also wash your hands with soap and water after touching infected areas on skin, scalp, ears, or nose.
- Wear only cotton underwear and stockings.
- Avoid polyester or nylon clothing, as these fabrics cannot "breathe" and help to create a moist environment for Candida.

■ NONPRESCRIPTION THERAPY

Several nonprescription materials derived from plant sources are effective treatments for candidiasis. All of these materials are available at health food stores. However, many people with candidiasis require a prescription medication in addition. It is best to begin treatment with the materials from the health food store and then consult your physician regarding the need for a prescription medication.

▌*Lactobacillus*

Lactobacillus acidophilus is the name of the "friendly" bacteria normally present in the lower bowel. It naturally deters overgrowth of Candida and other undesirable organisms by competing for nutrients, altering the gastrointestinal tract pH, and by occupying "attachment" sites. As the Candida colonies are destroyed by antifungal agents, other strains of yeast will flourish if "good" bacteria are not recolonized in the intestinal tract. Use of this material is mandatory. Unhealthy flora can lead to ammonia and histamine release, irritating the mucosal lining of the intestinal tract, and causing inflammatory reactions and toxic accumulations.

Use high-quality preparations, containing at least 10 billion viable *Lactobacilli* per 1/4 tsp. Acidophilus preparations are made by culturing beneficial bacteria on milk, soy, carrots, or other plant materials, giving food-sensitive persons a choice of culture media. Acidophilus should be refrigerated at all times to maintain its potency.

Acidophilus therapy starts with 1/4 tsp. acidophilus and gradually increases to 1/2 tsp. three times daily. An initial die-off period may temporarily increase intestinal gas. Acidophilus can also be sprinkled on food (it tastes like powdered cream), put on your tongue and swallowed with water, added to beverages, or put into capsules. (A well-packed "oo"-size capsule holds 1/4 tsp.) It is very effective for treating your mouth, throat, and esophagus if it is put under your tongue and left there to dissolve slowly. Acidophilus is also helpful in soothing viral sore throats. It is best to take acidophilus immediately before meals, as the food will provide a good medium for continued growth of these helpful bacteria.

Acidophilus or plain yogurt can also be diluted and used as a vaginal douche, as suggested by your healthcare professional. Yogurt is not effective orally as a treatment for Candida because it does not contain adequate amounts of live *Lactobacillus acidophilus* organisms. Used as a vaginal treatment, however, yogurt can be very soothing because it alters the pH of the vaginal tract, discouraging Candida growth.

Lactobacilli strains also have beneficial effects on vitamin and nutrient synthesis. They aid in lowering blood cholesterol and blood fats; they have antiviral properties; and they produce enzymes that improve digestion and absorption. After Candida problems are under control, Lactobacillus use should be continued at a lower level as a regular dietary practice.

▌*Caprylic Acid*

There are several preparations of caprylic acid, a contact fungicide, available in health food stores. Some of these products are enterically coated tablets that release the caprylic acid slowly throughout the large and small intestines. Swallow these tablets intact to protect the coating. Other caprylic acid products are packaged in capsules designed to release in the stomach and upper intestine. Next to the esophagus, the stomach is the most common site of Candida infection, and occurs in people with low stomach acid. A combination of enteric coated tablets and capsules is very effective in treating candidiasis because of the distribution of these fatty acid complexes from the stomach throughout the intestinal tract.

The required total dosage for caprylic acid varies from person to person. Begin with one tablet per day and gradually work up to the dosage suggested by your healthcare professional. The usual dosage ranges from six to nine tablets per day, taken in divided doses. The usual dosage for caprylic acid capsules is one capsule three times per day. If taken in conjunction with enteric coated tablets, the dosage of the tablets is reduced. When Nystatin or other prescription medications are added, caprylic acid can be reduced, but not eliminated. Unless you experience gastrointestinal distress when doing so, take caprylic acid on an empty stomach, once hour before or two hours after a meal, for better absorption.

Caution: Do not use caprylic acid if you are pregnant, as its effects during pregnancy have not yet been determined.

Be certain to read labels as some caprylic acid products contain additional materials that may be allergenic for some people. Caprylic acid is usually derived from coconut and can be a problem for people sensitive to coconut.

I *Grapefruit Seed Extract*

A broad-spectrum, antimicrobial agent extracted from grapefruit seed is effective against Candida, as well as against parasites. One such product, ParaMicrocidin, is available from Allergy Research in three strengths, 75 mg, 125 mg, and 250 mg, as well as in liquid form (see Recommended Sources and Organizations). The most effective dosage is two to three capsules three times daily of any dosage, depending on the severity of infection.

Most liquid grapefruit seed extract has a very bitter taste that some people are unable to tolerate. It should be used only in diluted form, 2 to 6 drops stirred into 8 ounces of water or juice, two to three times a day with meals. The maximum intake is usually 36 drops per day, depending on the product you purchase.

I *Essential Fatty Acids*

As Candida colonies grow in the small intestine, they interfere with and obliterate the absorptive surface of the bowel. This interference particularly affects the absorption of essential fatty acids (EFAs), which are necessary for normal growth and skin quality. Because our bodies cannot synthesize EFAs, we must consume them in our diets.

Essential fatty acids aid in rebuilding the immune system. They also strengthen cell membranes to prevent the invasion of organisms into cells. One of the EFAs, oleic acid, helps to prevent conversion of the Candida organism from its yeast form to its invasive, mycelial fungus form. Fish oils, flax oil, evening primrose oil, black currant oil, borage oil, and cold-pressed sunflower or safflower oils are the best sources of EFAs. These nutrients can be used on alternating days for people on rotation diets. Take 1 to 5 Tbsp. of a vegetable oil daily. The dose for evening primrose oil is one to two capsules three times daily.

I *Mathake and Taheebo Tea (Pau D'Arco or La Pacho)*

These teas are made from the inner bark of two different species of tropical trees, and clinical studies have demonstrated their natural antifungal properties. They are best used with other therapeutic agents. While these teas may induce die-off symptoms, they will pass in a few days.

The teas can be steeped or ground and put into capsules; they can also be used as a soothing douche. If applied topically, they can deter the growth of athlete's foot and skin rashes. As with other anti-Candida preparations, some people may not be able to tolerate these teas. Drink 2 to 3 cups daily, as die-off symptoms will allow.

❙ *Garlic*

Many people shy away from eating garlic because of its odor, but garlic has excellent antifungal properties. Odorless capsules are available that still retain the antifungal ingredient, allicin. In addition to inhibiting Candida growth, garlic also inhibits the conversion of the yeast form to its mycelial form.

A food or chemically sensitive person should exercise care in selecting a garlic supplement, choosing only chemical- and yeast-free products. Garlic is more effective if taken on an empty stomach, as it is enhanced by acid. For dosage, follow the directions on your product.

❙ *Organic Germanium*

Organic germanium is an organically bound trace mineral that stimulates energy production. The immune system is composed of high-energy tissue and requires extra oxygen and nutrients during inflammatory and infectious processes, and during periods of stress. Germanium affects the immune system by stimulating gamma interferon, and macrophage and natural killer-cell func-

tions. It also provides an oxygen-rich medium that acts as a deterrent to the growth of yeast colonies, which thrive in anaerobic (oxygen-free) conditions. Take 1 to 5 capsules of 150 mg of organic germanium daily during Candida treatment. A maintenance dose is two 150 mg tablets daily.

❙ *Coenzyme Q_{10}*

Coenzyme Q_{10} is produced naturally in the body. When used as a supplement, this enzyme stimulates greater energy production in each cell and restores the integrity of all cell membranes, enhancing overall functioning of the immune system. This coenzyme also activates the body's macrophages (specialized killer white blood cells of the immune system). Take up to 30 mg three times daily.

❙ *Fructo-Oligo-Saccharides (FOS)*

Fructo-oligo-saccharides are polymers of simple sugars that occur naturally in some foods (including asparagus, bananas, barley, garlic, Jerusalem artichokes, onion, tomato, and wheat), but are technically a soluble fiber. They do not behave like simple sugars in the body and can be used as a sweetener because they are half as sweet as sugar (sucrose). Humans do not have an enzyme to break down FOS and cannot use it. They absorb very little of it and therefore receive only a very small, if any, caloric value.

FOS is of benefit in Candida treatment because it selectively promotes the growth of friendly bacteria in the intestines. These bacteria are able to utilize FOS, and proliferate, making the gut healthier. They also help to maintain a slightly acidic environment, which is less hospitable to unfriendly bacteria and Candida. At high doses, intestinal gas may develop from the increasing intestinal flora. Take ¹/₂ to ₁ level tsp. two to three times daily.

▌*Orithrush*

Orithrush (or other specially buffered forms of sorbic acid) is designed to inhibit the proliferation of *Candida albicans*. It can be used on several areas of the body. When diluted, Orithrush can be effective as a mouthwash or vaginal douche; it can also be used full-strength on infected areas on toes, fingers, the external ear, and skin. When first using the liquid, treat only a small infected area in order to test for allergenicity.

▌*Thyme Oil*

Thyme oil (available in health food or herbal shops) is naturally aromatic and has a natural antifungal action on the skin. Thyme oil is very concentrated and should be kept out of reach of children. *Caution:* Do not use thyme oil internally.

For external use on Candida lesions on the scalp, skin, toes, and fingers, dilute it with oil (₁ part thyme to ₃ to ₄ parts oil). Alternate it with Nystatin cream (see below) or other tolerated skin lubricants, because thyme oil can be somewhat drying to the skin. A phenol-sensitive person may not tolerate thyme oil.

▌*Goldenseal Douche*

For persistent vaginal itching, the following vaginal douche recipe may be soothing and helpful. Sensitive women should be certain that they can tolerate all of the ingredients. *Caution:* Do not use goldenseal if you are pregnant.

Mix ₁ ounce goldenseal tincture (available at herb shops) with ₁ cup witch hazel. Use 2 Tbsp. of the mixture in 2 cups boiled water. Add ¹/₂ tsp. salt, ¹/₂ tsp. acidophilus, and ₁ Tbsp. yogurt. Let stand for 10 minutes. Use as a slow douche, keeping bag at hip level. Use daily for 10 consecutive days, and then only as needed or after intercourse.

▌*Tea Tree Oil*

Available at health food or herbal shops, tea tree oil is an undiluted plant oil that has antifungal properties. *Caution:* Do not use tea tree oil internally.

Rub it into rashes on the skin, either diluted or full-strength. Try it on one small rash area to see if it is tolerated and effective. Its odor is objectionable to some people.

▌*Myrrh*

Myrrh is an herb that has antifungal properties. It is effective for some people with candidiasis. The dried form is taken orally, mixed with water. It is also frequently used as a mouthwash. However, many sensitive people do not tolerate herbs.

Prescription Medications

The following treatments for Candida overgrowth are available only by prescription. Your physician will prescribe the medication that will be the most effective for you.

▌*Formula SF722*

Formerly called Mycocidin, Formula SF722 contains another fatty acid (undecylenic acid), which has antifungal activity. It occurs naturally in body perspiration. This product, derived from the castor bean, is contained in an olive oil base. As SF722 is gradually released in the digestive tract, it inhibits yeast growth. It is an excellent alternative for those who cannot tolerate caprylic acid preparations, and does not interfere with normal bacterial intestinal flora. There is no drug-nutrient interaction with this material, and it can be used in combination with prescription medications.

Formula SF722 must be ordered directly from the manufacturer, Thorne Research. (See Recommended Sources and Organizations.) A prescription form signed by a physician is required to purchase this material. Suggested dosage begins with 1 perle daily and gradually increases, as die-off permits, to 9 to 12 perles daily (3 perles three times a day).

Nystatin

An antifungal drug that kills yeasts and yeastlike fungi on contact, Nystatin is thought to bind with the yeast cell membrane. This causes changes in cell wall permeability, allows leakage of fluids into the yeast, and causes the cell to burst, releasing the intracellular components. Nystatin is a yellow, bitter-tasting powder, and has been demonstrated to be safe through more than 30 years of medical application. Nystatin is well tolerated by all age groups, even on prolonged administration.

Although Nystatin comes in several forms, produced by several companies, use only the chemically pure Nystatin powder that contains no additives. It is usually not available at pharmacies unless it has been specially ordered when your physician prescribes it. The Nystatin powder most pharmacies keep in stock contains talc, and is intended for topical use on a localized area, such as a skin rash. It is not for internal use.

Nystatin is a contact fungicidal agent, killing the yeast when it touches it. It is poorly absorbed and significant blood levels are difficult to attain. Only minor absorption takes place from the gastrointestinal tract, and from sublingual usage if the powder is held under the tongue. For this reason, you must use more than one treatment method—at least one for localized intestinal treatment and one for systemic treatment, depending on the severity and location of the candida infection.

Before starting Nystatin treatment, take a warm-water enema to cleanse the lower bowel so the Nystatin can have closer contact with the mucous membranes (see Nystatin Enema, below).

How to Take Nystatin. The most effective way to take Nystatin is to stir the powder in 1/2 to 1 ounce of water. Hold the Nystatin solution under your tongue for three to five minutes before swallowing. Do not allow the solution to sit after mixing it, as it will become more bitter. Nystatin is also more effective when it is taken on an empty stomach, because its action is enhanced by acid. Avoid food and drink for one to two hours after a dose to receive maximum benefit. Take 1 to 2 grams of ascorbic acid (vitamin C) with your Nystatin to increase the amount of acid in your stomach.

Those who experience nausea may have to take Nystatin with meals. If you cannot tolerate the taste of Nystatin, you can put it into capsules, available at drug or health food stores, but you will not receive the esophageal coating obtained when swallowing the powder. (The lower part of the esophagus is a common site of Candida growth.) Nystatin tables are also available, but they may contain cornstarch and dye, to which some people are sensitive. Some people do not tolerate Nystatin.

The prescribed amounts for starting

doses of Nystatin will vary from person to person, depending on the length and severity of the infection and on the severity of die-off symptoms. Always divide your daily dose into three to four doses. The length of time you will have to take oral Nystatin will depend on the severity of your case, your consistency and response to treatment.

Begin your Nystatin therapy slowly to determine whether or not you are going to have die-off symptoms. Begin with 1/4 tsp. per day, and gradually work up as your die-off allows to 3 tsp. per day, taken in divided doses. In more severe cases, you may need to take a fourth dose at bedtime—consult your physician. If your daily schedule makes taking Nystatin four times a day difficult, increase the amount of the other three doses instead.

Children's doses are half that of the adult dose, or 1/2 tsp. three to four times a day. Older teenagers usually require adult dosages.

It is important to refrigerate Nystatin to preserve its potency. If you are going on a long trip, carry it in an ice chest or an insulated soft-side bag, available at sporting goods stores. Nystatin is stable enough to last through only a short trip without refrigeration, but do not leave the medication in a hot car. Carry a small amount with you and leave the remainder at home in the refrigerator.

Nystatin Nose Drops. If there is a possibility that you have Candida in your sinus cavities, your physician may prescribe Nystatin nose drops. They are used as follows: First, place three drops of the solution into each nostril while holding your head back. Then swing your head forward rapidly and hold it down between your legs for two min-

utes to force the solution into your sinuses. Finally, sit up and let it trickle down your throat.

Nystatin nose drops are usually taken at least twice a day, and may increase your symptoms for several days due to yeast die-off in your nasal passages. Continue treatment; your symptoms will improve in a short time. Use Nystatin nose drops until you are certain that all the yeast cells in your nasal passages are dead.

Nystatin Vaginal Treatment. If you have yeast vaginitis, your physician may prescribe Nystatin for vaginal treatment along with other supplemental treatment. For yeast vaginitis, use one or more of the methods listed below. Itching, burning, or excessive discharge may increase temporarily due to die-off, but these symptoms will subside. Use Nystatin vaginal treatment every night for two weeks. If severe symptoms have subsided, you may alternate its use with Ori-thrush douche or acidophilus suppositories. You may need to repeat this course of treatment several times over several months.

- Mix 1 tsp. Nystatin powder in 3 to 5 ml water. Draw the solution into a 5-ml syringe (with needle removed) and insert carefully into the vagina. Squeeze the plunger gently to release the solution. Retain as long as possible. This procedure is more easily done at night.
- Pack a "oo"-sized gelatin capsule with Nystatin powder. Prick both ends of the capsule with a needle and moisten the capsule with water. Insert vaginally (it is usually more convenient to do this procedure at night).
- Use commercially prepared Nystatin sup-

positories, available from some pharmacies. These suppositories are usually compounded in a cocoa butter base. However, some people do not tolerate cocoa butter.

- Use a Nystatin douche occasionally, as needed to control symptoms. Use 1 Tbsp. Nystatin per pint of warm water for a slow douche, to provide longer contact with the mucous membranes.

Nystatin Enema. If you have large numbers of Candida organisms in your intestine, your physician may prescribe a Nystatin retention enema. Do not use this enema on yourself or your children unless a physician familiar with your health status has prescribed it. This method is adapted from *The Yeast Syndrome*, by John Trowbridge, MD, and Morton Walker.

- First take a warm-water cleansing enema before using a Nystatin preparation. (See enema instructions in Relief for an Allergic Reaction in chapter 21, Solving Everyday Problems.
- Mix 1/4 tsp. sea salt and 1/4 tsp. Nystatin in 1 cup (8 ounces) of warm, tolerated water.
- After making sure the mixture is at body temperature, put it into a rectal syringe or enema bag. Lubricate the nozzle with vitamin E or nonpetroleum jelly.
- Lie on your back with your knees bent, insert the nozzle, and squeeze the entire contents into your rectum.
- Remove the nozzle and roll onto your left side for about five minutes to allow the solution to travel to the left side of your colon.
- Roll over onto your back again (for five minutes), propping up your buttocks to allow the solution to travel up the left side of your colon.

- Roll over onto your right side for five minutes to allow the solution to travel across your transverse colon.
- Get up and walk around, which will allow the solution to travel down the right side of your colon.
- Retain the solution as long as it is comfortable before evacuating.

Nystatin Topical Treatment. Rashes caused by Candida and other yeasts can be treated with Nystatin cream, available by prescription. You can also make your own topical treatment by mixing Nystatin powder with liquid vitamin E.

I *Nizoral*

Nizoral is the brand name for a synthetic, broad-spectrum antifungal agent known as ketoconazole. In some cases of deep-seated infection, Nizoral is more effective than Nystatin in eliminating Candida. It is also useful in killing strains of yeast that may be resistant to Nystatin, since Nizoral has a more systemic effect. Dr. John Trowbridge in *The Yeast Syndrome* has described its action as "punching holes in the yeast cell wall and letting it slowly bleed to death."

Nystatin remains in the bowel, but Nizoral enters the tissues. Nizoral can cause some side effects, but most patients tolerate it well. A liver screen blood test to check liver enzyme levels should be performed before beginning treatment, and these levels must be checked monthly as long as Nizoral is taken.

The usual dosage of Nizoral is one 200 mg tablet daily for approximately six months. However, in some difficult cases, longer treatment and/or two tablets daily may be required. Nizoral should be taken on an empty stomach since it is absorbed better under acid conditions. To ensure adequate acid, take Nizoral with 1 or 2 grams of ascorbic acid (vitamin C). While you may experience die-off symptoms with Nizoral, they generally are less severe and of shorter duration than those caused by Nystatin. Some men experience lowered sex drive when they take Nizoral, which is usually restored to normal when they stop taking the drug.

▌ *Diflucan*

Diflucan, or fluconazole, has a systemic effect on the body similar to that of Nizoral. Its action is more rapid than that of Nystatin or Nizoral. Diflucan specifically inhibits fungal cytochrome P-450, an enzyme essential to fungal cell survival. It is very efficient for treating Candida overgrowth. As with Nizoral, a liver screen blood test to check liver enzyme levels should be performed before beginning treatment.

Diflucan should not be used during pregnancy unless its benefits outweigh the risk to the fetus. It is secreted in human milk and its use is not recommended for nursing mothers. The safety profile for infants has not been established for infants less than six months old but can be safely used in children over that age.

Diflucan is taken in 50-mg, 100-mg, or 200-mg tablets once daily. Diflucan tablets contain a dye that some people cannot tolerate. Those who demonstrate sensitivity to other azole drugs, such as itraconazole, terazole or miconazole, should not use this drug.

▌ *Sporanox*

Sporanox is the trade name for the antifungal agent itraconazole. It inhibits a step in the cytochrome P-450–dependent synthesis of ergosterol, a vital component in the cell wall of fungi. It is effective against several fungal, mold, and yeast infections, including Candida. It is less toxic than Nizoral, and unless there are pre-existing liver function abnormalities, regular liver screening is not necessary.

No studies have been done with Sporanox during pregnancy. It is excreted in human milk and should not be used by nursing mothers. Efficacy and safety for children has not yet been established.

Sporanox is administered in capsules of 200 mg once daily, and it is better absorbed when taken with food. Some people experience die-off during the first few days of treatment.

Nizoral, Diflucan, and Sporanox should not be taken with Hismanal, or Claritin. The combination can cause fatal heart arrhythmias.

▌ IMMUNOTHERAPY

Seek out immunotherapy for allergies—specific to yeast and mold—to help build the immune system's resistance to yeast infection and reduce cross-reactivity symptoms between molds and Candida. Testing and treatment with Candida and T.O.E. (Trichophyton, Oidiomycetes, and Epidermophyton—a mixture of common skin fungi) extracts relieves many of the hypersensitivity symptoms associated with Candida overgrowth. These extracts will also stimulate immune response. Clinical trials have shown that people respond better when treated with both of these antigens, rather than only one or the other.

Testing for T.O.E./Candida should be

Restoring Balance with Diet

An inadequate diet is a major factor in enabling candidiasis to flourish. Nourishment must rebuild your body, rather than encouraging Candida overgrowth. Your diet must restore cells and metabolic systems that are not functioning properly. You cannot eliminate Candida totally from the mouth, vagina, and intestines, but you must reduce it to a minimal level and rebalance the interactions between the yeast and your body.

carried out after you have begun treatment with antifungal medications—your health must be stable enough so that testing will not cause an overload. An effective neutralizing dose can then be determined.

■ HANDS-ON ALLERGY TREATMENTS

Hands-on allergy treatment for Candida and T.O.E. is also helpful. It will relieve the allergic response to *Candida albicans,* and will also stimulate the immune system to fight these organisms. Sensitivity to mold should also be treated to ensure recovery.

■ HOMEOPATHIC REMEDIES

Some health food stores carry complex homeopathic Candida remedies that are helpful for some people. Classical homeopathic remedies, such as *Lycopodium, Medorrhinum, Pulsatilla,* and *Thuja,* are useful in treating Candida overgrowth.

■■ CANDIDIASIS AND DIET

Diet is very important in candidiasis treatment—medications and acidophilus are not enough. You must eliminate or severely limit foods that promote Candida growth to reduce your overgrowth. Everyone is unique, and your dietary requirements may differ in many ways from the requirements of others with candidiasis. Some people will experience symptoms unless they adhere closely to their diets, while others can "cheat" a little without severe symptoms returning. Keep in mind that the less you cheat, the faster you will get well!

If diet is not improved, progress will be negligible. Your diet should contain proteins, vegetables, some complex carbohydrates, and unsaturated fats and oils. You may need to increase the volume of food intake in order to keep the caloric intake high enough to prevent weight loss. Cutting down on carbohydrates causes many people to lose weight.

■ SUGAR AND CARBOHYDRATES

Eating refined sugars weakens our immune system and promotes yeast growth. Honey (which sometimes contains yeast), molasses, maple syrup, date sugar, turbinado sugar, cane sugar, beet sugar, corn sugars (including dextrose, high fructose corn syrup, and glucose), corn syrup, fructose (found in fruit), lactose (found in milk products), and other refined carbohydrates/sugars are known promoters of yeast growth. Reducing or eliminating these in your diet will help minimize yeast growth.

A low-carbohydrate diet is extremely important in the management of Candida. Many people with candidiasis may have hyperinsulinemia, a metabolic disorder in which too much insulin is released in response to food intake, particularly carbohydrates. If you have a very severe case of Candida or hyperinsulinemia, consume no more than 60 to 80 grams of any carbohydrates per day. The yeast feeds only on sugars and simple carbohydrates, such as are found in white bread, soda, candy, and ice cream.

Some people report strong cravings for carbohydrates during early stages of candidiasis treatment. This "appetite" can be compared to the yeast organisms crying, "feed me, feed me!"—but if you think of this as the yeasts' craving and not yours, it will be easier not to succumb to their insistent pressure. Your "sweet tooth" will lessen within a few weeks on your improved diet. A diet this restrictive will be very difficult for those who are accustomed to high-carbohydrate diets. Each day, work toward reducing refined carbohydrates and congratulate yourself as you accomplish more and more.

Sugar is highly addictive. One of our patients became addicted to morphine as a result of an attempt to control the pain she experienced after a very serious automobile accident. She confessed to us that it was easier for her to wean herself from morphine than it was for her to quit eating sugar.

▌ MOLD AND YEAST

Foods that contain yeasts, molds, or fungi can also cause problems and should be restricted. The cell walls of Candida and baker's and brewer's yeast contain a common carbohydrate. Because of this, our bodies cannot distinguish between these different yeast species, and will produce the same reaction to each. When eaten in foods or even breathed in high concentrations, yeasts will trigger symptoms. (See Yeast in chapter 9, Food Allergies, for additional sources of yeast.)

Molds build up on foods while drying, smoking, curing, and fermenting. Foods to avoid include:
- pickled, smoked, or dried meats, fish, and poultry
- bacon, sausage, ham, hot dogs, and luncheon meats
- all cheeses, including Swiss, cottage, and cream cheese (moldy cheeses such as Roquefort contain the largest amounts of mold)
- buttermilk, sour cream, sweetened yogurt or yogurt with fruit, and sour milk products
- dried and candied fruits (frequently made from fruit that has molded)
- all fungi, including all types of mushrooms, morels, and truffles

Be sure that your condiments are fresh. Dry spices, seasonings, and some teas, including herb teas, may mold during the drying process. In damp climates, spices and teas may mold as they sit in the cupboard.

▌ ALLOWED FOODS

You will feel less deprived if you concentrate on foods you can eat rather than on the avoidance lists. The following foods are safe to eat:
- any meat as long as it is fresh, including chicken, duck, pheasant, quail, turkey, beef, veal, venison, goat, lamb, pork, rabbit, frog's legs, fish, and seafood of all kinds
- eggs
- complex carbohydrates, such as fresh vegetables, limited fruits and whole grains
- milk (may be restricted initially) and yogurt
- unprocessed, toasted nuts and seeds
- oils

A good rule of thumb for remembering what

you may eat is the letters MEVY (meat, eggs, vegetables, and yogurt). If possible, buy organic foods to avoid ingesting antibiotics and other substances.

Be sure the yogurt you buy contains *Lactobacillus acidophilus*, which aids in recolonizing the gut. However, remember that yogurt is a milk product and still a source of lactose, so you should limit the amount you eat. Its acidophilus content is also too low for sufficient treatment levels.

Begin eating MEVY, then gradually add fruits in limited amounts. After your immune system has had time to repair—toward the end of your treatment—you may slowly reintroduce a few yeast-containing foods.

You may eat vegetables of all kinds, except mushrooms. Eat fresh vegetables as much as possible. Canned, bottled, boxed, and other packaged foods usually contain refined sugar products. Frozen vegetables are sometimes processed with yeast. Mold grows on all vegetables; wash them well before cooking or eating them. Vegetables that grow beneath the soil, such as potatoes, carrots, beets, onions, turnips, and sweet potatoes, should be washed, peeled, and cooked. Do not eat them raw. A potato may be baked with the skin on, but do not eat the skin.

You may eat fresh fruits and juices on a limited basis. However, some people have to restrict their fresh fruit intake during the first few months of treatment. An increase in symptoms indicates you have consumed too many sugars and refined carbohydrates. Even when you can eat fruits without provoking symptoms, do not overdo them. Bottled, canned, and frozen fruits or juices frequently contain yeast. Also, the fruit used to make juices is frequently moldy. Melons, particularly cantaloupe, often accumulate mold in the rinds as they grow. They can be eaten if they are washed thoroughly and then peeled carefully. Do not cut the fruit in sections while the rind is still intact because the cutting knife will draw mold from the rind across the flesh. Bananas, pears, and apples can be reintroduced first because their sugar content is lower. Avoid raisins and dates, as they have a high fructose concentration.

You may eat limited amounts of whole grains as long as doing so does not worsen your candidiasis symptoms. Some people also have to restrict their intake of gluten-containing grains. Gluten is found in wheat, oats, rye, spelt, kamut, and barley, but not in corn, teff, rice, and millet. To avoid yeast, make breads with baking powder or baking soda. Waffles make a good substitute for bread. There are several types of yeast-free crackers, snacks, rice cakes, and oatcakes available at health food stores, and they make good bread substitutes.

Milk may have to be restricted during the first part of treatment since it contains lactose, which is a simple sugar.

Nuts and seeds need to be roasted to destroy any molds that may be present. Bake them at 325°F for 10 to 15 minutes until they are a golden color.

▌ DIET TIPS

Increase natural fiber in your diet (raw vegetables, fruits, and whole grains, as tolerated, on a rotated basis). Apple pectin and psyllium seed are also good sources of fiber. When intestinal bacteria work on fiber, they release fatty acids that inhibit yeast growth. Fiber also decreases bowel transit time, decreases toxin absorption from the gut, and stimulates secretion of digestive enzymes.

If you eat packaged foods of any kind, read the labels carefully. Remember that anything labeled "enriched" usually contains yeast. Manufacturers of such foods have removed nutrients during processing and then have attempted to add them back. "Fortified" foods have substances added to make them "better," and may be made from yeast products. Fresh is always best. When reading labels, you often cannot be certain of the contents in a product without checking with the food manufacturer.

Be sure to drink at least six to eight 8-ounce glasses of tolerated water daily. This will help to flush out the accumulated toxins from die-off. Also chew your food well; small, softened amounts of food can be more easily digested.

The less you eat of the avoidance foods, the faster you will get well. Dr. Trowbridge says in *The Yeast Syndrome* that "we provide a luxurious home for yeast colonies and provide 'yeast feasts' for their growth with our poor-quality diets." Individual differences may allow some people to eat small to moderate amounts of the avoidance foods without experiencing symptoms. Each person will have to determine tolerance levels, first by total omission of a food from the diet, and later by readmission trials.

Your diet is something you control completely, and it is not necessary to feel victim-ized by Candida. You may want to make your dietary changes gradually so it will not be a shock, but you must change your dietary lifestyle to starve out the yeast. If you continue to eat simple carbohydrates while taking antifungal agents, you will be on a constant seesaw, feeding the yeast one minute and attempting to eradicate it the next. This action causes the yeast to be drawn more deeply into affected tissues, and it is then much more difficult to eliminate. Continuing sugar intake also makes your treatment more prolonged and expensive as you buy medications to kill the yeast, then eat sugar to feed it.

You may design your own Candida diet or, as indicated by your healthcare professional, you may follow a diet from one of the books listed in Recommended Books. Of all the therapies available to combat Candida, appropriate diet most effectively rebalances your body and will lead you back to good health.

Molds

In addition to symptoms caused by an allergic reaction to mold, it can cause clinical symptoms from an infection by mold organisms. Many people with chronic sinus problems have mold colonizing their nasal passages and sinuses. The possibility of mold growing in the lungs should be examined in those with asthma and bronchitis-type symptoms.

Mycotoxins are poisons produced by molds when they grow on particular food substances. Only certain species of mold produce these poisons, and only under particular environmental conditions and on particular foods, such as rye, peanuts or wheat. These toxins can cause mild to severe symptoms in animals and humans. Symptoms include destruction of blood vessel and liver tissues, overgrowth of fibrous tissue, convulsions, hematomas, vertigo, rashes, swelling of the heart, destruction of brain cells, hemorrhage, and even death.

▮▮ COMMON MOLD INFECTIONS

Many clinical conditions are attributable to mold, although at times distinguishing whether an organism should be called a mold or a fungus is difficult. The two common molds discussed below cause numerous symptoms.

▮ ASPERGILLUS INFECTIONS

A wide spectrum of diseases is caused by the *Aspergillus* mold species. These molds occur worldwide and can adapt to a wide range of environmental conditions. *Aspergillus* grows on almost anything including all types of organic debris: decaying vegetation, soil, manure, spilled food, wet paint, cracked dialysis bags, opened medications, refrigerator walls, "sanitizing" fluids used in dressings, and many other substances. There are over 600 different species, but the most common include *Aspergillus fumigatus, A. flavus, A. niger, A. terreus, A. ustus,* and *A. versicolor.*

Aspergillus can cause the mold allergy symptoms that were discussed in chapter 13, Inhalant Allergies. It also causes aspergilloma, in which the fungi colonize pulmonary cavities, paranasal sinuses, and ear canals. It can also cause localized infections of the eyes, and skin lesions. If conidia (spores) are present in the operating room, they can enter the site of cardiac surgery, or the eye during cataract surgery.

Invasive aspergillosis is usually localized in the lung, but can be generalized and involve a number of other organs. It causes cough, sputum production, and a chest X-ray that resembles cavitary tuberculosis. It occurs in people with serious health problems, but causes a milder disease in middle-aged people with some health problems. Aspergillosis is the lung disease developed by explorers of the Egyptian pyramids. If untreated, aspergillosis can be fatal.

Diagnosis for aspergillosis is by microscopic examination of sputum or by culture. *Aspergillus* grows readily on most routine media. Blood testing techniques are also used for identification.

Corticosteroids and antifungal therapy are prescribed for aspergillosis. The treatment varies with the severity of the disease. At times, surgical intervention may be necessary to remove the diseased tissue, both externally and internally.

▮ MUCORMYCOSIS

Mucormycosis refers to several diseases caused by *Mucorales,* a group of molds that include *Rhizopus* and *Mucor.* These molds grow on decaying matter, with *Rhizopus* frequently seen as mold on bread. While these molds are widespread, disease caused by them is limited. They gain entry to the body through the respiratory tract or through abraded skin.

In order to cause disease, they must overcome the natural immunity of the host. Symptoms caused by these molds are the same, regardless of which species of mold may be causing the infection.

These molds can cause six separate clinical manifestations:

- *Rhinocerebral:* This condition is found in patients with diabetes mellitus, in the presence of metabolic acidosis, in patients with leukemia, in cases of long-time neutropenia (low neutrophils, a type of white blood cell), and in cases of long-time broad-spectrum antibiotic use. Headache, fever, and facial pain are symptoms. There will be eye infection and thrombosis of the retinal artery, resulting in loss of vision. Complications of mucormycosis of the eyes and nose can include cerebral abscess. An X-ray of the sinus cavity or a CAT scan will show destruction of bone.
- *Pulmonary:* This type of mucormycosis occurs in seriously immunocompromised individuals, in people receiving chemotherapy, and in people on long-term antibiotics. Fever and shortness of breath are the only symptoms. Chest X-ray usually shows involvement of one lung, but the disease can spread to the other lung. The infection is worse in people with low white blood count than in those with leukemia. This form of mucormycosis is frequently seen as a nosocomial pneumonia, contracted while in a hospital or institution. It frequently is fatal.
- *Cutaneous:* Sporadic cases of cutaneous mucormycosis are normally seen. However, in the U.S. in the 1970s there was an epidemic caused by contaminated bandages. Cellulitis formed under the bandages, with the adhesive acting to inoculate the skin. Failure to recognize and treat mucormycosis allows it to go into the body more deeply and affect other tissues and organs. Using sterile bandages helps prevent the condition. Recently, mucormycosis has been reported in burn wounds.
- *Gastrointestinal:* This type of mucormycosis is seen in cases of malnutrition. The mold enters the body with food, and the stomach, ileum, and colon are the sites commonly affected. This condition is acute and fatal, the diagnosis usually being made after death. Pain, abdominal distention, nausea, and vomiting are its only symptoms.
- *Central nervous system:* This rare condition occurs in debilitated people. Infection in the nose and sinuses goes into the brain. The mold can also get into the brain through open head trauma or be implanted with surgery. In these cases it is usually fatal.
- *Other:* At times the heart, bones, kidneys, and bladder can be affected by mucormycosis, and the condition can be fatal.

The primary characteristics of these molds are vascular invasion and tissue necrosis (death). A black nasal drainage should not be dismissed as blood, and black necrotic lesions of the nasal mucosa or hard palate may reflect the presence of mucormycosis.

Diagnosis is by examination of biopsy tissue. Treatment of the underlying condition is extremely important, as is surgical debridement of the affected area. Amphotericin B is the usual treatment, as the "conazole" drugs have not been found to be effective. Oxygen therapy has helped a small number of people, used in conjunction with medications. Early diagnosis and treatment and clearing of the predisposing illnesses are imperative for recovery from mucormycosis.

▮ TREATMENT OF MOLD INFECTIONS

Mold infections are difficult to treat with natural remedies and usually have to be treated with drugs. Even with drug therapy, many times molds are refractory to treatment and must be treated with drug combinations. It is very important to correct the underlying disease processes that are making the person either immunocompromised or more susceptible to the infection.

All steroid drugs and long-term antibiotic use should be stopped, and body acidosis corrected. In acidosis, the body tissues are extremely acidic, providing a medium conducive to mold growth. Many times diet can help reverse the acidosis. Limiting food intake to those foods that produce alkaline residue in the body will help reverse the acidosis. These foods include avocados, corn, dates, fresh coconut, honey, maple syrup, molasses, raisins, soy products, and most fresh fruits and vegetables. Low-level alkaline-forming foods such as almonds, blackstrap molasses, Brazil nuts, buckwheat, chestnuts, lima beans, millet, and soured dairy products are almost neutral in their effect.

At times surgical intervention to debride necrotic tissue is necessary with a mold infection. With extremely invasive mold infections, reconstructive surgery may be required to correct extensive tissue removal.

The use of nutrients to strengthen the immune system can be helpful in preventing, as well as controlling, mold infections. See chapter 20 for nutrients that strengthen the immune system.

CHAPTER 18

The Role of Infections in Allergies

WE MAY SUFFER FROM unwanted symptoms caused by bacteria, viruses, parasites, fungi, yeasts, or molds. They can grow in our bodies and cause infection. These organisms can be the primary cause of an attack on the immune system that can exacerbate sensitivities. They may also play a secondary role as a result of lowered immunity caused by other factors, such as chronic stress from allergic reactions.

Microorganisms can affect us in many ways other than the infections themselves. Toxins produced by the organisms—and our sensitivities to them—add to the effects of illness. Because the bodies of the organisms contain protein, carbohydrates (polysaccharides), and lipids, they can be allergenic to us. Metabolic waste products of the organisms can also cause problems. Much of the inflammation of any disease caused by an organism is the result of an allergic response to the organism. IgE antibodies may contribute to certain types of gastrointestinal reactions, and the allergic component of infectious diseases.

Cell fragments of the organisms, as well as inactive organisms, can trigger an allergic or hypersensitivity response. When these organisms die as a result of treatment, the metabolic products released when the cell walls of the organism rupture cause further symptoms. Immunotherapy is very helpful in relieving this type of allergic and hypersensitivity symptoms, as is hands-on allergy treatment for the specific organism.

Latent infections that surface during continued treatment of environmentally ill people are most often not single, primary causes of the symptoms, but rather the result of lowered immunity and resistance to these opportunistic organisms. An allergy or sensitivity response to the latent organism contributes to the person's symptoms and is often difficult to determine.

Bacteria and Allergies

Bacterial infections can cause problems aside from the disease they initiate. Some people have an "allergy of infection," in which they become allergic to the bacteria it-

Infectious Symptoms

Microorganisms may also cause symptoms even when there is no infection. Their presence in the environment can trigger allergic symptoms. For example, molds in both the indoor and outdoor environment can trigger symptoms associated with viral or fungal infections in a sensitive person.

self or the bacterial metabolic products of the organism.

Dr. D. Bernard Amos states in *Zinsser Microbiology* that an allergic response to bacteria, in addition to the infection itself, should be suspected when symptoms are unusually severe or prolonged, or when they occur in an allergic person.

Another allergic phenomenon that may occur in response to bacterial infection is the Jarisch-Herxheimer reaction seen in syphilis. Chills, fever, headache, muscle pain, and rapid heartbeat may develop 2 to 24 hours after treatment is begun, apparently due to immune response to antigens released as the syphilis spirochetes are killed.

Because bacterial infections contribute significantly to total immune system load, it is crucial to treat and eliminate all sources of infection. These infections, whether acute or chronic, can make allergies worse. Common chronic hidden infections include vaginosis, pelvic inflammatory disease, and dental problems. Both root canals and cavitations can be hidden sources of dental infection. (See Dental Care for Allergic People in chapter 22, Finding Safe Healthcare.)

Even after an infection has subsided, people can continue to have an allergic response to the cellular debris from the bacteria and from excess circulating antibodies. Symptoms will be low grade, but over a period of time will contribute significantly to the total immune system load.

Normal intestinal bacteria can provoke an immune response. Some intestinal bacteria contain protein that resembles human protein, and this tricks the immune system, causing the body to attack itself. Fragments of dead bacteria from the intestine may leak into the intestinal wall or the bloodstream because of increased intestinal permeability. Bacterial debris circulating through the body is deposited in joints, provoking an attack on these tissues by the immune system as it tries to remove foreign material.

Clinical experience has shown that extracts or hands-on allergy treatment for any bacteria to which a person tests positive will help relieve both acute and chronic, low-grade symptoms caused by those bacteria. Among the organisms we have encountered that can be treated with extracts or hands-on allergy treatment are:
• *Chlamydia trachomatis*
• *Enterococcus*
• *Escherichia coli*
• *Gardnerella vaginalis*
• *Haemophilus influenzae*
• *Mycoplasma pneumoniae*
• *Pseudomonas aruginosa*
• *Salmonella*
• *Staphylococcus aureus*
• *Streptococcus*
This type of testing and treatment is particularly effective for people who have recurrent

strep throat. Skin conditions caused by staph infections are also extremely responsive.

Viruses and Allergies

Many of the symptoms of a viral illness are an allergic reaction to the protein of the viral body, and treating for this sensitivity stops the allergic response of the body. During an acute illness, if the exact virus or the viral family causing the infection can be determined, an extract or hands-on treatment can significantly lower, if not eliminate, most of the symptoms of the illness. This type of treatment is particularly effective for the influenza virus, and will dramatically shorten the duration of the illness.

Testing for viruses can be done by several methods, and several types of extracts are available. Neutralizing dosages can be determined by provocative neutralization testing (see chapter 8, Testing and Treatment). Homeopathic dilutions for viral extracts are also very helpful.

Because viruses and viral proteins are antigens, our bodies produce antibodies against viral surface components. We may require several antibody molecules to neutralize one viral body. These antibodies interfere with replication of the virus, and protect us against disease. However, the antibodies may stay in the body for years, and can cause us problems even after the infection has resolved.

In chronic infections, latent viruses can remain dormant in the body for years. However, their protein continues to be allergenic to their host. After an acute infection, viral debris can remain attached to the cells and will continue to trigger an allergic response.

Viral Crazies

A viral infection can sometimes trigger cerebral symptoms. One of our patients has what she describes as the "viral crazies." Viral infections, regardless of the infecting virus, cause her to have cerebral symptoms. Each time she has a virus she feels that if the world has not already come to an end, it will do so immediately. She feels that she cannot cope, and that if she ever had any skills and ability in life, they are gone. These mental symptoms are caused by an allergic response to the viral body, and always pass as soon as she begins to recover from the infection.

Testing for the causative virus, whether from a latent or an acute infection, and treating with an extract or hands-on allergy treatment for the virus can dramatically improve the health of the person. Fatigue, headaches, and muscle pain will gradually improve or disappear.

In certain patients, the damage caused by the respiratory syncytial virus (RSV) may be caused by the formation of virus-antibody (IgG) complexes and the accompanying inflammatory response. Evidence suggests that there is also an immediate hypersensitivity reaction to virus-IgE interactions, and "nonimmunologic" triggers of inflammation may also play a role. These mechanisms may also play a role in other respiratory infections. Patients can be helped with an RSV extract or hands-on treatment.

Extracts made from influenza vaccine

material can control fever blisters from *Herpes simplex* types I and II, as well as symptoms of infectious mononucleosis and *Herpes zoster* (shingles). Some people use the extracts only when experiencing acute symptoms, while others with chronic symptoms use them daily. *Herpes simplex extracts* and *Herpes zoster extracts,* as well as hands-on allergy treatment for these organisms, will also help eliminate both acute and chronic symptoms.

Several of our patients have responded with violent reactions when tested for SV40 (Simian virus 40), a contaminant of the polio vaccine between 1954 and 1963. The intensity of their reaction may indicate that they have a latent infection of SV40, as opposed to remaining antibodies. One person with a particularly incapacitating reaction had polio as a child and was given the polio vaccine after being dismissed from the hospital.

Many people who had polio in the past are now developing post-polio syndrome, in which many of their polio symptoms are recurring. Muscle pain, stiffness, weakness, difficulty swallowing, and fatigue are common. The allergic component of this syndrome responds well to a polio extract or hands-on treatment for polio. Other people who did not have polio, but who lived with a polio victim, also respond to this treatment, finding that their muscle aches, pains, and malaise clear.

Viral extracts or hands-on allergy treatment for the following viruses have been successful for our patients:
- Hepatitis A, B, C
- *Herpes simplex* I and II
- Human parvovirus
- Influenza
- RSV
- Polio
- SV40

Parasites and Allergies

As with viral and bacterial infections, our body responds with allergic reactions to parasitic infections. This response is twofold: reaction to the parasite itself and reaction to the parasite's metabolic products. Parasites stimulate the production of antibodies (IgE, IgG, and IgM) by the B-cells. The histamine and other mediators released when these antibodies attach to basophils or tissue mast cells contribute to the pathogenicity of the parasites. Parasitic infections cause marked elevation of serum IgE, and high levels of parasite-specific antibodies are useful in diagnosis for some cases.

Intestinal parasites do not provoke an allergic response as long as the barrier formed by the intestinal lining is intact, so that parasites cannot attach to the wall of the bowel. The attachment of the parasite and the excessive permeability this causes triggers a cascade of reactions. There will be excess absorption of antigens and parasitic fragments from the intestine, overstimulating the immune response, leading to allergy and autoimmune reactions.

Eosinophilic pneumonia, a pneumonia in which white blood cell infiltrates are present in the lungs, can be caused by an allergic bronchopulmonary response to such parasites as *Ascaris, Ancylostoma* species, *Toxocara* species, and *Strongyloides stercoralis.* With an echinococcal (or tapeworm) infection, a sudden release of foreign protein in the body of the host may cause anaphylactic shock. This can happen when hydatid fluid (from the larval cyst of a tapeworm) is released by the cyst's rupture in a body cavity.

Treating parasites may temporarily worsen die-off symptoms. As the parasites die, the host is exposed to greater levels of parasitic antigens, which exacerbate symptoms. Exposure to parasitic antigens also increases when egg deposition begins in egg-producing parasites. Severe systemic symptoms may result as a result of increased allergic response to the higher levels of parasitic antigens.

People who have had parasitic infections in the past may suffer from malaise and vague symptoms for which no cause can be determined. Many times, these symptoms are a result of the antigenic response to parasites that may continue long after the parasitic infection has subsided. Remaining cellular debris and toxins of the parasites causes this response. As long as the debris or toxins are in the body, they continue to be allergenic. Allergy extracts or hands-on treatment for the specific organism will help relieve these symptoms and reduce the total immune system load of the infected person.

In our clinical experience, treatment extracts or hands-on allergy treatment have been helpful for the symptoms of both current and past infections of the following parasites:

- *Endolimax nana*
- *Entamoeba hartmanii*
- *Entamoeba histolytica*
- *Giardia lamblia*
- *Enterobius vermicularis*

- *Iodamoeba butschlii*
- *Blastocystis hominis*
- *Taenia saginata and Taenia solium*

Fungi and Allergies

Pathogenic fungi have a rigid cell wall and are potent antigens. Humans and animals do not have the enzymes to degrade the cell wall polysaccharides of the fungi. As a result, they are excreted slowly and contribute to the disease-causing aspects of a fungal infection.

Pathogenic fungi usually do not produce toxins. However, the fungi and their spores are often highly allergenic to people. These organisms release enzymes and other chemicals in an effort to convert the substance on which they are growing into nutrients for their use. Many of these substances elicit an allergic response in people.

Fungal allergies are largely respiratory allergies because the respiratory tract is constantly exposed to spores. Many of these spores contain potent allergens that can cause a strong hypersensitivity reaction. This response does not require growth or viability of the fungus, although the inflammation produced may allow the spores to colonize in the respiratory tract. Spore concentration varies with the season, time of day, geographic location, and weather conditions. The outdoor average spore concentration is 10^5 spores per cubic meter of air, and indoor spore concentration may exceed 10^9 spores per cubic meter of air.

The host and nature of the fungus exposure determine response to the fungus. This includes the immune response of the host, and the size, antigenicity, and amount of fungus exposure. People may have rhinitis (inflammation of the nose accompanied by discharge), bronchial asthma, alveolitis (sometimes called farmer's lung), or generalized pneumonitis. In farmer's lung, there is an allergic response to inhaled fungi from moldy hay, characterized by coughing, difficulty breathing, nausea, chills, fever, and rapid heartbeat.

People may also have a dermatophytid (skin eruption) or "id" reaction to fungus. This is caused by an allergic response to fungal antigens. A dermatophyte (skin fungus) infection in one area can elicit an allergic reaction elsewhere caused by circulation of allergenic products from a primary site of infection. Diagnosis is based on negative microscopic and cultural examination of the site and finding dermatophytosis (skin fungus) elsewhere on the body.

Allergy extracts for the specific fungi involved are helpful in controlling and eliminating the allergic response to the infection. Hands-on allergy treatments are also very effective.

Yeast and Allergies

Besides the direct invasion of body tissues accompanying an overt infection, some people experience hypersensitivity reactions to either surface antigens on the Candida organism or to the metabolic byproducts and toxins released by it. Hypersensitivity reactions can occur throughout the body. These immune responses increase the body burden for the hypersensitive person and can worsen already existing reactions to foods, chemicals, molds, and other inhalants.

Allergic symptoms or aggravation of pre-existing allergy following antibiotic use should suggest yeast overgrowth. Hypersensitivity reactions to Candida overgrowth or to byproducts of the organisms include abdominal pain, asthma, bronchitis, hay fever, headaches, earaches, hives, skin rashes, and severe chemical and food sensitivities.

Candida has the ability to "hide" from the immune system. It is able to shut down the response of the immune system to it as a pathogen. An allergy extract of Candida and TOE or a hands-on treatment will stimulate the immune system to fight the overgrowth of the organism and bring it under control.

Mold and Allergies

Molds can be significant in many clinical disorders caused by an allergic response to the mold. When they are inhaled, mold spores can be an important cause of nasal symptoms. Respiratory complaints, such as hypersensitivity pneumonitis, an inflammation of the lungs, can result from contact with airborne spores or mycelial fragments of several molds, including *Penicillium*, *Cladosporium*, *Aureobasidium*, *Alternaria*, *Aspergillus*, *Rhizopus*, and *Mucor*. Allergic bronchopulmonary mycoses due to *Aspergillus*, and more rarely by *Penicillium*, *Curvularia*, or *Helminthosporium* species, can cause eosinophilic pneumonia.

Urticaria or hives (raised, itchy skin patches), secretory otitis (fluid behind the eardrum), gastrointestinal distress, and other complaints can all be caused by mold sensitivity. Dermatitis (inflammation of the skin) can be caused by the inhalation of allergenic mold material, as well as by absorption from skin colonization. Dermatitis can also result from invasion of other tissues by mold.

In addition, a mold allergy can cause cerebral symptoms that can be quite severe, the most common of which is depression. Anger, confusion, irritability, anxiety, hostility, fear, inability to concentrate, and hyperactivity can also be triggered by mold exposure. Mold allergy is always a consideration when symptoms of this type worsen when it rains.

Mold extracts are extremely helpful in controlling allergic responses to mold, both in an infection and in hypersensitivity reactions. The specific mold or molds causing the problem must be included in the extract, as well as for the treatment in hands-on allergy treatment.

PART IV

Nutrition and Allergies

As an active participant in your own health care, it is essential to understand the relationship between nutrition and good health. Our body contains trillions of cells, each with its own biochemical function and need for very specific nutrients. Numerous enzymes within each cell control its chemical processes, and each enzyme also has specific nutrient requirements.

We receive some of the needed nutrients from our diet. However, much of the food available to us is deficient in vitamins, minerals, amino acids, and fatty acids and cannot supply all of the nutritional needs of our bodies. In addition, many people eat very poor or restricted diets that do not supply their nutritional needs. Supplementation of vital nutrients is necessary to guarantee our bodies an adequate supply. The quality of nutrients that people take is just as important as the quality of food that they eat.

In the chapter that follows you will learn about dietary deficiencies and nutrients, particularly those that are important for people with allergies. Proper supplementation of tolerated nutrients is essential for control of and recovery from allergies.

CHAPTER 19

Why Nutritional Supplementation

is Critical

VITAMINS, MINERALS, amino acids, and fatty acids are the "building blocks" used by all cells and body functions to affect growth, repair damaged tissues, and keep our bodies in a healthy state. When the "right molecules" are in short supply, or are in greater demand, we need to provide additional nutrients through supplementation. This is known as nutritional biochemistry or orthomolecular medicine.

Consider the constant readjustment taking place within each cell for it to maintain adequate numbers of "building blocks." To keep this internal environment functioning properly, correct replacements for damaged or missing parts must be provided. We do not substitute parts from a waffle iron or toaster when a washing machine is broken. Likewise, we must be certain to supply our bodies with the exact nutrients needed by the cells to function and repair. At one time it was thought that a balanced diet provided all the nutritional factors our body required; only the elderly and infants who did not eat a balanced diet needed nutritional supplementation. Whether this was ever true is debatable and certainly it is not true today.

Unless we grow it ourselves or obtain it from special sources, our food is of inferior quality. The way it is grown, shipped, and stored affects food for the following reasons:
• The soil in which it is grown is depleted because of poor agricultural practices.
• High-nitrogen fertilizers are used rather than organic replacement fertilizers that contain essential minerals.
• Some hybrid seeds produce inferior plants with high productivity, but with low nutrient levels.
• Fruits and vegetables are harvested before they are ripe, and may then be ripened artificially.
• Produce is contaminated by herbicides, insecticides, and fungicides.
• Some produce is coated with paraffin (which has a petrochemical base) to slow deterioration.
• Preservatives, colorings, and flavor enhancers are added to foods.
• Many foods are not fresh, because of long periods of storage and transport.
• Some foods are stored improperly often with inadequate refrigeration.

When the food reaches us, its quality is

further degraded because of the way it is cooked and processed. The following practices rob food of its nutrients:

- Foods are overprocessed (heat and chemicals used in processing destroy nutrients).
- Improper cooking methods, reheating, or keeping food warm rob it of nutrients.
- Vitamins and minerals are lost when food is soaked.
- Fast food and refined foods have lost most of their nutrients during processing.

Besides poor food quality, other factors also affect our nutritional status:

- Dietary restrictions may prevent our eating a balanced diet and receiving the needed nutrients.
- Environmental pollution affects the detoxification pathways of the body and increases the need for nutrients.
- Stress causes our body to use extra nutrients.
- Economic status can prevent our being able to purchase needed foods and nutrients.
- Personal food preferences can severely limit dietary choices if there are many foods a person does not like or will not eat.
- Ethnic backgrounds also affect food preference, and in addition, can affect the ability to properly digest some foods.
- Chronic infections prevent the body from functioning efficiently and rob it of nutrients.

It is clear that a variety of factors affect the balance and quality of our nutrition. Nearly everyone needs some supplementation, and those with special health problems or allergies may need extensive supplementation.

Nutritional Deficiency Symptoms

The following symptoms signal the possibility of a nutritional deficiency. If you have many of these symptoms, have your nutritional status evaluated.

Mental and emotional symptoms include:

- constant awareness of your body
- excessive worry
- unhappiness without cause
- depression
- inability to cope with stress
- poor self-image
- lowered mental acuity and memory
- sensitivity to foods, inhalants, and chemicals

Physical symptoms include:

- headaches
- joint pains, swollen, tender joints
- skin problems, such as dry scaly skin or scalp, acne
- poor connective tissue quality
- nail problems such as misshaped nails or spots on nails
- inadequate musculature, muscle soreness
- grooved, scalloped, or reddened tongue
- edema
- dental caries
- poor or diminished eyesight
- ringing in the ears
- no reserve energy
- metabolic insufficiency
- frequent infections
- varying stages of digestive problems, gastric distress
- lowered sexual interest and performance
- poor work output
- no tolerance for noise, flashing lights, or variations in temperature or altitude

Your Nutritional Needs

Dr. Roger Williams, author of *The Advancement of Nutrition*, writes that there are five levels of nutrition: starvation, poor diet, fair diet, good diet, and super nutrition. Super nutrition is the level for which we should all strive. It consists of diet and nutritional supplementation for optimum health and performance.

You should determine your nutritional needs with the help of your physician, a healthcare practitioner, or a nutritional counselor. Because of biochemical individuality, your needs will not be the same as those of your spouse, siblings, children, friends, or environmentally ill people. Each of us has specific requirements or deficiencies that must be addressed, in addition to the basic amounts of essential nutrients that should probably be taken by everyone.

▋▋ FACTORS AFFECTING NUTRITIONAL REQUIREMENTS FOR ALLERGIC PEOPLE

People with allergies and sensitivities have an increased need for nutrients. Supplementation with tolerated nutrients is particularly important, both for helping the body to heal and for controlling allergic reactions.

▋ STRESS

Demand for all nutrients is greater during times of stress caused by allergic reactions; infections; physiological conditions; psychological, emotional, and environmental problems; or disease states.

▋ INCOMPLETE DIGESTION

Many of us who are sensitive to chemicals, foods, or inhalants have low levels of hydrochloric acid in our stomach, low levels of

> ## Importance of Diet *and* Supplementation
>
> *Diet is the most important factor in our nutritional status, but if we have a nutrient deficiency, the highest quality diet will not be sufficient to meet our increased needs. Conversely, even the finest vitamin and mineral supplements cannot compensate for poor eating habits.*

digestive enzymes in our gastrointestinal tract, or low bicarbonate release from our pancreas. This causes incomplete digestion of food, resulting in poor absorption and assimilation of nutrients. This creates a vicious cycle because too few nutrients are available to manufacture adequate amounts of hydrochloric acid, regulating hormones, digestive enzymes, and immune factors.

As offending foods pass through our intestinal tract, they inflame and irritate the intestinal lining. Histamine and serotonin are released in the gastrointestinal tract during an allergic episode, further irritating the mucosal lining. This causes the microvilli to swell and flatten. The villi (microscopic hair-like fingers that line the small intestine) are responsible for enzyme function to help break down food particles, and for nutrient absorption. Loss of this twofold function contributes to vitamin, mineral, essential fatty acid, and amino acid deficiencies.

ALLERGIC REACTIONS

In the leaky gut syndrome, food is not digested properly, and larger molecules of food material are absorbed into the bloodstream, becoming allergens. Systemic inflammatory responses result, requiring additional nutrients to repair the resulting tissue damage.

Lack of nutrients also heightens sensitivity reactions. Magnesium deficiency increases the histamine release during an allergic reaction. Calcium can help to neutralize the effect of histamine, but if body calcium is deficient, excess histamine circulates in body fluids, causing greater damage from the immune cascade. While in the reactive state, our bodies can become overly acidic, and nutrients are lost.

■ RESTRICTED DIETS
Nutrients can be low or unbalanced in the restricted diets of some food-sensitive people, or as a result of personal choices. Rotation diets offer a greater variety of balanced food choices. (See chapter 10, Eating Safely, for more information.)

■ LOWERED ENDOCRINE FUNCTION
Many allergic or sensitive people have impaired endocrine system functioning (pituitary, thyroid, adrenal glands, thymus, pancreas, pineal gland, and gonads). The adrenal and thyroid are always the first endocrine glands to suffer; as they underfunction, our body requires more nutrients. Specific nutrient supplements will help the endocrine system regain much of its normal function.

■ OVERWORKED IMMUNE
FUNCTION
Especially in those with allergies or sensitivities, the body's defenses are overworked. Continued overstimulation leads to an even-

tual dysregulation of the immune system. This situation creates additional demand for specific nutrients to protect against frequent infections and to rebuild defenses against other foreign invaders (allergens, antibodies, debris from inactivated organisms, and toxins).

■ NERVOUS SYSTEM SUPPORT
The nervous system regulates all body functions involved in a reactive state, and it is under assault in a hypersensitive person. Many inflammatory responses affect neurotransmitter functions in the brain. Neural tissue needs amino acids, minerals (calcium, phosphorous, magnesium, potassium), and B vitamins, while neurotransmitter production requires all nutrients. Low neurotransmitter production adversely affects the entire body and all of its functions.

■ ENVIRONMENTAL POLLUTANT
EXPOSURES
Each of us is continually exposed to environmental pollutants. If cell membranes are not protected against these pollutants, tissue damage will occur. Specific nutrients known as antioxidants and free radical scavengers are essential to protect the cells, tissues, and organs against chemical pollutants. These nutrients help the body detoxify after either acute or prolonged exposure to chemicals, pesticides, fungicides, and industrial pollutants.

■■ HOW TO ASSESS YOUR
NUTRITIONAL DEFICIENCIES
Begin with a detailed history, including genetic and hereditary information, your dietary habits and major food intake, chemical

or inhalant exposures, trauma, present symptoms or diseases, and your current nutrient supplement intake.

Carefully observe mental, emotional, and physical signs that indicate nutritional deficiencies. (See Nutritional Deficiency Symptoms, above.)

Levels of many nutrients, however, cannot be determined without laboratory evaluation.

- Blood or urine analysis of amino acid levels determine possible deficiencies of vitamins and minerals required for proper amino acid metabolism.
- Detoxification panels may indicate a need for increased antioxidant/detoxification nutrients and precursors.
- Tests that show functional levels of nutrients confirm nutritional status.
- Hair, serum, and blood analyses for mineral levels are useful. Hair analysis also indicates high levels of toxic metals, which require specific nutrients to reduce them.
- Testing with nitrazine or pH paper determines alkalinity or acidity of saliva and urine, indicating a need for specific nutrients.
- C-stixs indicate spilled vitamin C in the urine. If none is spilled, it may indicate the need for vitamin C supplementation.

If you have or suspect you have specific diseases that increase the demand for specific nutrients, tests should be done to confirm the presence or absence of the disease. All test results should be evaluated along with your history and symptoms. In our body's effort to maintain a homeostatic state (a stable balance), nutrients are moved from one type of tissue to another as needed. Examining only one type of tissue will not give a true picture of our body's state or needs. Hair samples show levels of stored nutrients, blood and serum samples show circulating nutrients, and urine and fecal samples show levels of excreted nutrients.

Guidelines for Nutrient Supplementation

For allergic or hypersensitive people, the entire cell metabolism needs to be supplemented with nutrients. Supplements are an important part of a recovery program that also includes diet changes, moderate exercise, environmental cleanup, immunotherapy, and elimination of infection.

Take nutritional supplements, vitamins, minerals, essential fatty acids, and amino acids throughout the day for best utilization. Choose brands that are free of all common allergens, such as milk, corn, wheat, egg, soy, sugar, and yeast. Pay attention to the form in which they are supplied, as some forms are more readily absorbed than others are.

- *Powders:* Rapidly absorbed and contain no fillers or binders. They can provide a higher potency, and are less expensive than tablets. However, their taste and texture are unpleasant to some people. Powders are an excellent form for those who have difficulty swallowing tablets or capsules.
- *Liquids:* Useful for people who have difficulty swallowing pills and for children. They are rapidly absorbed, but may contain sugars, additives, and coloring agents.
- *Chewables:* Suitable for children, but be

Expensive Urine?

It has been said that people in North America have the most expensive urine in the world. This statement is referring to the fact that many people excrete a large portion of their nutrients in their urine. Some people also pass their nutrients, undigested, in their stool. The tablets have not dissolved and look much as they did before they were swallowed.

These two problems emphasize the importance of taking nutrients in a form that the body can assimilate. Simply taking the nutrient does not guarantee its bioavailability or assimilation. The nutrient's form—liquid, powder, capsule, or tablet (in descending order of assimilation)—must be taken into consideration. The chemical form of the vitamin must also be considered. In general, if vitamins and minerals do not at least partially dissolve in water, they are not going to dissolve in your body.

aware of sugar, additives, and coloring agents.

- *Time-release tablets:* Contain a water-soluble vitamin released over a period of time. Allergic people frequently lack adequate stomach acid to dissolve the tablet coatings to release the vitamin.

- *Tablets:* Have a longer shelf life. Sensitive people should be cautious of the binders and fillers used in tablets. Tablets are not absorbed as rapidly as powders, liquids, or capsules.

- *Capsules:* Easier to swallow than tablets. They generally contain fewer binders and fillers than tablets, but are not absorbed as rapidly as liquids or powders. While most capsules are made from pork or beef gelatin, vegetable-based capsules are available at health food stores.

Each brand of nutritional supplement varies in its bioavailability (absorptive properties) depending on its fillers, coatings, or binders. The quality of the nutrient itself depends on the source material from which it is extracted, the ratio of ingredients, and the chelating materials (substances that aid absorption).

While you should choose hypoallergenic brands of vitamins and minerals as much as possible, there is no such thing as a completely hypoallergenic material for everyone. If possible, have supplements tested to see which you tolerate before you begin using them. Carefully read the labels on the supplements. The presence of many extra ingredients could be a warning sign that tolerance may be a problem for this product. The presence of herbs in some preparations prohibits some sensitive people from taking them.

Sometimes people who need nutrients the most are unable to tolerate them. Allergy extracts or hands-on allergy treatment for the specific nutrients will allow people to safely take and utilize the necessary nutrients. Very pure nutrients that can be administered rectally are now available. Some very sensitive people, particularly chemically sensitive people, are able to tolerate nutrients by this route of administration quite well. (See Recommended Sources.)

It is best to start your nutritional supplementation program gradually. When the body is stressed, it is unable to readily adjust to sudden changes. Introduce one new supplement every four days, unless otherwise instructed. By starting each supplement separately, if you experience any adverse symptoms it will be easier to trace the cause. Most symptoms last only a short time. Drinking more fluids and taking a brisk walk will reduce symptoms quickly. If problems do arise, contact your nutritional counselor or physician so minor adjustments can be made to your program.

Do not become discouraged and discard the whole program if you have problems with one nutrient. Other brands are available that may be more compatible with your metabolism. Take most of your supplements with a meal unless otherwise instructed, since supplements taken on an empty stomach sometimes cause slight nausea or other abdominal discomfort. These nutrients are very concentrated, and mixing with food dilutes their potency. Some people also experience a temporary increase in gas and bloating when a different nutritional program is introduced. This usually subsides in several weeks—however, if it persists, inform your nutritional counselor or physician.

Think of supplements as concentrated food, not as medicine. Just as food is more readily absorbed when eaten in small amounts more frequently, so are your nutritional supplements. Divide supplements into smaller doses taken throughout the day. This ensures adequate absorption and will not overload your digestive system. Since these materials are food substances, they act more slowly, and visible results will not appear in a short time. Nutritional therapy should be given a fair trial of consistent use for at least six months. Use beyond that period will bring continued improvement.

Advantages of Nutritional Supplementation over Pharmaceuticals

There are many advantages to taking nutritional supplements instead of drugs. In fact, Dr. Abram Hoffer states in his book *Orthomolecular Nutrition* that if nutritional deficiencies and biochemical defects are identified and corrected by treating with the proper nutrients, the health of the patient will be restored, and medication will not be needed.

• Nutrients are not taken singly, as are drugs. There are over 40 vitamins and minerals that work together as a team, needed every day in balanced amounts. One nutrient cannot effect a change unless all of the other nutrients are present either in food, reserves, or supplements.

• Vitamins act slowly; drugs act rapidly.

• Vitamins are food; drugs are chemicals.

• Vitamins have a wide action; drugs are narrow in their effects.

• Side effects from vitamins are infrequent, and usually minor and reversible; side effects from drugs are more serious, and sometimes can be fatal. Symptoms will disappear within one to two days after stopping a vitamin supplement.

When our bodies are properly nourished, they function more efficiently and we are healthier. Physical problems improve or disappear. We are better able to withstand stress and resist disease. Allergies are easier to control, and in many cases can be eliminated with proper treatment.

CHAPTER 20

Treating Allergies with Nutrient Supplements

THE FOLLOWING DISCUSSION of nutrients applies specifically to the effects and treatment of allergy and environmental illness. Each of the nutrients listed has many additional functions in our body. Remember that each nutrient functions not as a single unit, but only in the presence of all other nutrients. Our body requires all of these nutrients, operating by multiple interactions.

In *The Advancement of Nutrition*, Dr. Roger Williams states: "If the available amount of any essential nutrient is inadequate, the body as a whole may be afflicted with generalized cytopathy, a condition in which every cell in the body is deficient and the whole body may be said to suffer from 'cell sickness.'"

The importance of adequate nutrition cannot be overemphasized. It is essential for our health, for our sense of well-being, and for personal control over and healing from our allergies.

Vitamins

Vitamins are organic substances that are essential to life. They regulate metabolism and help to release energy from food. They are considered micronutrients because they are needed in small amounts. Most vitamins cannot be manufactured by the body and must be supplied in the diet or by nutrient supplementation.

■■ VITAMIN A

- Drops sharply in serum level tests of chronically stressed people. If adequate supplements are not taken, the body tries to maintain homeostasis by taking vitamin A from mucous membranes, increasing vulnerability to infection and allergies.
- Necessary for proper immune function.
- Used in cells of mucous membranes, which are the first sites of penetration by antigens, viruses, bacteria, fungi, and chemicals.
- Essential to suppressor cell, B-cell, T-cell, and killer lymphocyte activity.
- Enhances our body's immunological response to both DNA and RNA viruses.
- Is needed by the liver to anabolize (build) protein, and stabilizes protein in epithelial structures (skin, mucous membrane).

- Acts as an essential cofactor in the metabolism of essential fatty acids.
- Protects the lipid portion of cell membranes from oxidation. Damage to the cell membrane can also harm receptor sites for hormones and neurotransmitters.
- Protects against pollution.

Dose: 10,000 IU is the usual suggested daily dose. For deficiencies, up to 25,000 IU may be taken. However, if you are pregnant or might be pregnant, do not take over 8,000 IU daily.

▮ BETA-CAROTENE

- Converts to vitamin A, but is not readily converted by diabetics and people with hypothyroid conditions.
- Acts as an excellent antioxidant, especially for free radicals (a highly reactive form of oxygen).
- Prevents damage to cellular components, especially DNA, and cell membranes.

Dose: The recommended daily dose is 10,000 to 15,000 IU. Because beta-carotene has not been recognized as an essential nutrient, there is no official RDA.

▮ VITAMIN B₁ (THIAMINE)

- Maintains normal carbohydrate metabolism.
- Acts as a cofactor in many enzyme functions in the nervous system. In deficiency states, nerve cells become swollen, impairing transmission of messages from one nerve cell to another.
- Stimulates immune function.
- Works with antioxidants, such as vitamin C and cysteine, to combat the effects of acetaldehyde and free radicals.

- Is needed to prevent shrinkage of the thymus and lowered antibody response.
- Is essential to hydrochloric acid production in the stomach.
- Improves muscle tone in the gastrointestinal tract.
- Helps the body absorb and utilize magnesium.
- Needs increase during stress, illness, and surgery.
- Protects the body from the degenerative effects of aging, alcohol consumption, and smoking.

Dose: The recommended daily dose is 50 mg, taken in balance with the other B vitamins.

▮ VITAMIN B₂ (RIBOFLAVIN)

- Necessary for red blood cell formation, cellular respiration, and growth.
- With a group of enzymes, helps to break down proteins, carbohydrates, and some fats.
- Utilizes oxygen to liberate energy within the cell.
- Is known as an electron transfer vitamin.
- Needed for protein, fat, and carbohydrate synthesis.
- Necessary for antibody production.
- Is used by the adrenal glands in cortisol production.
- Transports hydrogen ions by enzyme action.
- Is involved with vitamin A in synthesizing muco-proteins that improve mucous membranes in the digestive tract.
- Need increased by strenuous exercise.

Dose: The daily dose needed by most people is 50 mg. Riboflavin should be taken with a balanced B complex.

▌▌ VITAMIN B₃ (NIACIN/ NIACINAMIDE)

- Operates in coenzyme forms to carry hydrogen ions in all cells. Vitamin B₃ also acts as a coenzyme in the energy cycle of the cell.
- Helps to control blood lipid levels.
- Improves circulation.
- Is essential to all enzyme functions in the nervous system.
- Involved in the production of hydrochloric acid and secretion of bile.
- Increases flow to blood capillaries in epithelial tissue. This function is helpful when niacin is used during detoxification baths or dry saunas because it helps to mobilize toxins from fat cells, and allows more toxins to be excreted in the sweat.
- Helps in glucose metabolism to stabilize blood glucose levels.
- Is needed for histamine production. However, large doses are helpful in controlling histamine release during an allergic reaction.
- Increases energy through helping with the proper utilization of food.
- Deficiency can cause irritation of the entire gastrointestinal tract.
- Necessary for proper brain function.

Dose: For both the niacin and niacinamide forms of B₃, the recommended daily dose is 100 mg, taken with a balance of all the B vitamins.

▌▌ VITAMIN B₅ (PANTOTHENIC ACID)

- Is necessary for antibody production.
- Helps in synthesis of anti-inflammatory substances (cortisol) produced by the adrenal glands.
- Aids in synthesis of cholesterol and fatty acids.
- Stimulates movement of the gastrointestinal tract.
- Helps in production of hydrochloric acid in the stomach.
- Is essential for adrenal support and prevention of adrenal exhaustion during any type of stress.
- Is helpful in large doses in reducing allergic reactions (has an antihistamine effect).
- Has antioxidant properties.
- Is needed for conversion of choline to acetylcholine (an important neurotransmitter).
- Is a precursor for synthesis of coenzyme A (an enzyme needed for various cellular functions).

Dose: The usual recommended daily dose of pantothenic acid is 100 mg. Some people receive relief from allergies by taking 1,000 mg of B₅ with 1,000 mg of vitamin C, with food, morning and evening. B₅ should always be taken with a B complex vitamin.

▌▌ VITAMIN B₆ (PYRIDOXINE)

- Involved in more body functions than any other nutrient.
- Is essential for proper metabolism and utilization of protein.
- Aids in transportation of amino acids across cell membranes.
- Is necessary for proper nervous system function.
- Facilitates magnesium and B₁₂ absorption.
- Regulates sodium and potassium balance (useful in some types of edema).
- Helps with production of protein-based antibodies.
- Facilitates glycogen conversion in the liver.

- Required with high-protein diets.
- Is essential to DNA and RNA synthesis.
- Helps with degradation of estrogen (estradiol) to estriol in the liver. Estradiol is more potent than estriol, and if it is not degraded it causes an increase in estrogen levels in the body.
- Is needed in synthesis of hydrochloric acid.
- Heightens T-cell and B-cell function.
- Increases thymus hormone production. Deficiencies cause immune tissue to shrink, diminishing activity of the thymus and spleen.
- Strengthens the immune system.

Dose: The recommended daily dose is 50 mg, taken in balance with the other B vitamins.

■■ VITAMIN B$_{12}$ (COBALAMIN)

- Helps in formation of DNA and RNA in cells.
- Is essential for maintenance of myelin sheath (lipid covering on nerve fibers).
- Needed to properly utilize fats, carbohydrates, and proteins.
- Is deficient in some vegetarian diets and in people with digestive problems. Hydrochloric acid, pepsin, and the intrinsic factor (a substance produced by normal gastrointestinal mucosa) are all required to extract vitamin B$_{12}$ from food.
- Is necessary for B-cell maturation.
- Helps in histamine production in people with gluten allergies. Used in conjunction with folic acid.
- Is most effective when given as an injection. Although not as effective as an injection, sublingual tablets are more effective than tablets or capsules that are swallowed.

- Is used as an injection with success in some cases of fatigue and unresponsive asthma.
- Needed to prevent anemia.
- Deficiency signs may take more than a year to appear after body stores are depleted.

Dose: The recommended daily dose is 300 mcg, taken in balance with the other B vitamins.

■■ VITAMIN B$_{15}$ (DIMETHYLGLYCINE OR DMG)

- Acts as an antioxidant.
- Enhances immune system function.
- Lessens lactic acid accumulation in muscles.
- Building block for neurotransmitters and hormones.
- Increases tissue oxygenation.
- Improves function of many organs.
- Stimulates glucose oxidation, which increases energy and prevents rapid fatigue.
- Increases antibody production to provide anti-allergenic properties.
- Reduces blood lipids.
- Protects against pollution.

Dose: The daily dose most often recommended is 50 to 150 mg. However, it can be difficult to find B$_{15}$ in retail outlets.

■■ OTHER B VITAMINS

■ BIOTIN

- Essential for normal metabolism of fat and protein.
- Assists in synthesis of essential fatty acids.
- Necessary for synthesis of vitamin C.
- Improves colonization of intestinal flora.
- Acts in cell growth.
- Helps with eczema.

Dose: Biotin is usually included in a B complex vitamin. The usual recommended dose is 300 mcg daily.

❚ CHOLINE

- Helps in transportation and utilization of fats and cholesterol.
- Aids elimination of toxins from the liver.
- Is essential to the integrity of the myelin sheath structure covering nerve fibers.
- Helps in thyroid hormone production.
- Assists the function of vitamin E.
- Is a component of the neurotransmitter acetylcholine chloride.
- Necessary for proper brain function.

Dose: The recommended daily dose is 1,000 mg.

❚ FOLIC ACID

- Is produced in the large intestine if adequate bacterial flora is present.
- Works in conjunction with vitamin B_{12}.
- Is essential for red blood cell formation.
- Stimulates hydrochloric acid production in the stomach.
- Is required for DNA and RNA formation in the cells.
- Is required in larger quantities during periods of stress or disease.
- Is absorbed at a diminished rate with aging.
- Is essential to the metabolism of tyrosine, a precursor for the neurotransmitters dopamine, epinephrine, and norepinephrine.
- Raises blood histamine levels.
- Aids in protein metabolism.

Dose: The recommended daily dose is 800 mcg.

❚ INOSITOL

- Stimulates the musculature of the intestinal tract.
- Metabolizes fats and cholesterol.

A Critical Vitamin

Vitamin B_9, or folic acid as it is more commonly called, is considered a B complex vitamin. Also called folacin and folate, it is named after foliage because it was first identified in leafy green vegetables. A folic acid deficiency is considered to be the number-one vitamin deficiency in the world.

Folic acid is crucial for preventing neural tube birth defects, which affect the formation of the spinal column. If the neural tube fails to close at the base of the spine, the result is a condition called spina bifida—a crippling paralysis of the lower extremities, and a number of associated health problems. Because the majority of pregnancies are not planned, all women of childbearing age should supplement their diet with folic acid. Folic acid levels must be adequate before conception to prevent spina bifida.

- Helps remove fats from liver.
- Aids brain cell function.
- Helps to induce sleep.
- Caffeine can cause deficiency.

Dose: Be certain to take inositol with other B vitamins. The recommended daily dose is 100 mg.

❚❚ VITAMIN C

- Helps to relieve allergic symptoms and prevents local inflammatory reactions.
- Provides an antihistamine-like effect (without the side effects of antihistamines).

- As an antioxidant, it protects our body from the effects of pollutants by joining with oxygen and enzymes to convert toxic substances into nontoxic derivatives (which are then excreted in the urine).
- Assists in the manufacturing of adrenal hormone, needed to combat the stress imposed by allergic reactions.
- Enhances T-cell and phagocyte function.
- Increases immunoglobulin production by the lymphocytes.
- Improves tissue oxygenation.
- Promotes wound healing.
- Acts as a natural laxative when optimum dosage is taken.
- Is used heavily and rapidly expended during any infection.
- Has active antiviral properties.

Vitamin C has many additional physiological benefits, but those mentioned are of the most help to people with food, chemical, or inhalant sensitivities.

Dose: Take bowel-tolerance levels daily. See Vitamin C: A Key Nutrient later in this chapter for directions and further information.

▮ VITAMIN D

- Acts on intestinal mucosa to synthesize enzymes needed to transport calcium and phosphorus into the blood.
- Is necessary for deposition of calcium and phosphorus into bones and teeth.
- Helps the thyroid gland to produce the hormone thyroxin.
- Helps to maintain a healthy nervous system.
- Enhances immunity.

- Aids in assimilation of vitamin A and protects it from oxidation.
- Helpful in intestinal disorders and malfunctions of liver and gallbladder that interfere with absorption.

Dose: The usual recommended dose of vitamin D is 400 IU daily. Do not take vitamin D without calcium.

▮ VITAMIN E

- Prevents oxidation of ingested fats, of lipids in the cell membranes and other cell structures, of the vitamins A and K, and of fat-soluble hormones by joining with the lipid molecule.
- Acts as a free radical scavenger by joining with harmful oil-based chemicals, ozone, and nitrous oxide.
- Protects lungs against air pollution.
- Is found in large amounts in the brain, pituitary gland, and adrenal glands.
- Activates the immune system. Its function is enhanced with the addition of selenium.
- Affects prostaglandin (chemical messenger) functions.

Dose: The usual recommended daily dose is 600 IU. People who cannot tolerate the oil should take the dry, water-dispensable form.

Minerals

Minerals are inorganic substances required by the body in small amounts. They are needed for the formation of blood and bone, proper composition and balance of body fluids, regulation of muscle tone, and healthy nerve function. They also function as coenzymes, enabling enzymes to function, and are necessary for the utilization of vitamins and other nutrients.

▌▌ CALCIUM

- Is essential for the proper function of magnesium and phosphorus.
- Acts as a catalyst for some enzyme synthesis.
- Aids in displacement of lead in tissues and inhibits absorption of lead into the teeth and bone.
- Helps maintain a proper acid/alkaline (pH) balance in tissues.
- Regulates movement of nutrients and waste products in and out of cell membranes in its exchange with magnesium, sodium, and potassium.
- Absorbs excess stomach acid.
- Reduces histamine production.
- Discourages cell uptake of toxic metals such as lead, cadmium, and mercury.
- Is prevented by high sugar intake from being reabsorbed (together with magnesium) in the kidneys.
- Is essential to neuromotor impulses. Acts, together with magnesium, as a natural tranquilizer.
- May contribute to migraines if not metabolized properly.

Dose: Calcium doses are more effective taken in divided doses throughout the day. People aged 19 through 50 should take 1,000 mg daily. Those 51 and over should take 1,200 mg daily.

▌▌ CHROMIUM

- Stimulates enzymes involved in metabolizing glucose, thereby stabilizing blood sugar levels at either end of the spectrum (both hypoglycemia and hyperglycemia).
- Is essential to the synthesis of fatty acids, cholesterol, and high-density lipoproteins (HDL).
- Aids in metabolism and transport of amino acids.
- Is removed from foods in processing.
- Is required in larger quantities if diet is high in sugar and refined foods.
- Moderates effectiveness of insulin.
- Helps reduce hyperinsulinemia.

Dose: There is no official dietary allowance for chromium. However, the recommended daily dose is 150 mcg.

▌▌ COBALT

- Activates a number of enzymes.
- Is needed for proper utilization of vitamin E.
- Works in concert with copper.
- Aids in mucous membrane repair.
- Is a mineral component of vitamin B_{12}.

Dose: Cobalt does not normally need to be supplemented and is rarely found in supplements. When cobalt is deficient, it is usually given as B_{12} (cobalamin).

▌▌ COPPER

- Activates synthesis of a number of enzymes.
- Is essential to synthesis of thyroid-stimulating hormone (TSH) produced by the pituitary gland.
- Is essential to the metabolism and utilization of some amino acids.
- Is a component of superoxide dismutase (SOD), which protects against free radical

damage to the mitochondria (energy-producing portion of the cell).

- Aids enzymes needed for neurotransmitter production in the tyrosine-to-dopamine pathway.
- Is essential to vitamin C utilization in collagen tissue formation.
- Is required for the formation of phospholipids in cell membranes.
- Is required by the liver to degrade estrogen.
- Aids regulation of essential fatty acid metabolism.
- Is required for the movement of calcium from the blood into bone tissue.
- Is crucial to the formation of helper T-cells.

Dose: Copper usually does not need to be supplemented, but if it does, it must be taken in balance with zinc, which is contained in most multimineral supplements. The recommended daily dose of copper is 3 mg.

▮▮ GERMANIUM (ORGANIC)

- Increases serum levels of gamma interferon, which increases killer cells, T-suppressor cells, and macrophages.
- Acts as a free radical scavenger.
- Stimulates and restores immune response.
- Aids in heavy metal detoxification.
- Has oxygen-enrichment properties at the cellular level.
- Raises levels of glutathione (a peptide used in the body's detoxification processes).
- Can "turn off" an allergic reaction.

Dose: Germanium is not normally supplemented regularly. However, Japanese research has shown that taking 100 to 300 mg daily helps to control food allergy. It must always be taken in the organic form.

▮▮ IODINE

- Is essential, along with the amino acid tyrosine, for the formation of thyroxine (a thyroid hormone).
- Keeps mucous lining of the body healthy.
- Affects tone of smooth muscle, including intestinal tract and lungs.
- Facilitates passage of nutrients into the cell mitochondria (energy-producing portion of the cell).
- Helps to thin mucous membrane secretion.
- Improves mental acuity

Dose: The recommended daily dose of iodine is 225 mcg. Supplementation over that contained in a multivitamin/mineral is usually not necessary.

▮▮ IRON

- Binds quickly to protein molecules during an infection in order to prevent bacteria from using it for their growth metabolism.
- Energizes T-cells and macrophages when they are needed for inflammatory processes.
- Is a constituent of chemicals produced by T-cells to destroy organisms.
- Is required for the production of hemoglobin, which carries oxygen in the blood.
- Requires sufficient hydrochloric acid for absorption.
- Deficiency prevalent in people with candidiasis.
- Excess in the blood can promote the formation of free radicals.

Dose: Iron should be taken only if a deficiency (anemia) exists and should be taken separately from a multivitamin/mineral. The daily dose is 18 mg.

> ## Iron Overload
>
> *If you have anemia, make certain it is not due to hemochromatosis, which can cause what appears to be anemia by causing a deposition of iron in the tissues.*

▌▌ MAGNESIUM

- Aids in the production of antibodies.
- Affects permeability of cell membranes to allow for transport of nutrients.
- Is essential to protein metabolism and to the energy cycle of the cell.
- Is an essential component in over 300 enzymatic reactions.
- Is essential for the proper function of calcium by activating the release of parathyroid hormone.
- Maintains the electrical potential of cells.
- Has a calming effect on the nervous system.
- Regulates the body's acid/alkaline (pH) balance. Buffers the acidic stage of an allergic reaction, along with calcium and potassium.
- Is required in converting glycogen (sugar stored in liver and muscles) to glucose (body fuel).
- Helps the body metabolize essential fatty acids into prostaglandins, which regulate many body functions.
- Deficiency causes mast cells to increase histamine secretion.
- Is usually used in a ratio of two parts calcium to one part magnesium. In immunocompromised or hypersensitive people, this ratio often must be 1:1 or greater to alleviate symptoms.

- Is required for many detoxification pathways.
- Necessary for calcium, vitamin C, potassium, phosphorus, and sodium metabolism.
- Known as the anti-stress mineral.

Dose: The recommended daily dose is 750 to 1,000 mg.

▌▌ MANGANESE

- Needed for a healthy immune system.
- Is essential in synthesis of glutathione (a peptide used in the body's detoxification functions).
- Is needed for synthesis of three neurotransmitters (glutamine, gamma-aminobutyric acid, and acetylcholine).
- Aids production of superoxide dismutase (SOD).
- Works in balance with molybdenum.
- Acts as a catalyst for synthesis of fatty acids and cholesterol.
- Aids enzymes used in digestion and absorption of proteins, fats, and carbohydrates.
- Is essential for synthesis of insulin needed for glucose utilization.
- Is essential for production of some hormones.
- Improves memory and reduces nervous irritability.
- Works with B complex to give an overall feeling of well-being.

Dose: There is no official recommended daily allowance for manganese, but 10 mg is the usual suggested dose.

▌▌ MOLYBDENUM

- Promotes normal cell function.
- Enhances the use of sulfur amino acids by

the body. Sulfur is critical to immune system function, to antioxidant activity, and to detoxification pathways.

- Is a component of enzymes that regulate hormone and neurotransmitter functions.
- Is a component of enzymes that detoxify sulfites (chemicals that contain sulfur and oxygen) and aldehydes (a large family of compounds, including formaldehyde and acetaldehyde).
- Is essential for cell utilization of vitamin C.
- Aids in carbohydrate and fat metabolism.
- Promotes general well-being.

Dose: A safe dose of molybdenum is 30 mcg per day.

▮ PHOSPHORUS

- Works in multiple interactions with calcium.
- Present in every cell of the body.
- Is an important component of phospholipids (fats containing fatty acids and a phosphate group) in cell membranes and the brain.
- Is essential to many chemical reactions in the body.
- Leads to calcium loss in the bones if consumed in excess. The most common excess of phosphorus is caused by drinking too many soft drinks (soda pop).
- Essential for normal kidney function and contraction of heart muscle.

Dose: Supplementation is not usually necessary, as phosphorus is found in many foods.

▮ POTASSIUM

- Acts with sodium, calcium, and magnesium on cell membrane permeability to allow the transport of nutrients and waste products in and out of the cells. (Potassium works outside cells, and sodium works inside.)
- Aids many enzyme functions.
- Supports the adrenal glands.
- Is required for synthesis of structural protein within the cells.
- Helps ensure function of smooth involuntary muscles (heart, lung, and intestinal tract). Relieves arrhythmia and intestinal and uterine cramping.
- Is necessary for neuromuscular interaction.
- Hypoglycemia causes potassium loss.
- Aids in allergy treatment.
- Helps dispose of body waste.
- Fatigue can be a sign of potassium deficiency. Coffee causes potassium loss.

Dose: Potassium is in most high-potency multivitamin/mineral preparations. It can also be supplemented separately with 99 mg of elemental potassium, available at health food stores. Larger amounts are available by prescription. Have your potassium levels checked before taking a supplement.

▮ SELENIUM

- Acts as an antioxidant, protecting cell membranes.
- Is synergistic with vitamin E.
- Aids in synthesis of the enzyme glutathione peroxidase to support detoxification pathways in the cells.
- Enhances the function of vitamin C.
- Is essential for protein synthesis and antibody formation.

- Protects the immune system and stimulates immune functions.
- Increases B-cell antibody response.
- Neutralizes the effects of cadmium (a heavy metal).
- Is essential to the production of coenzyme Q_{10}.
- Helps with hot flashes and menstrual problems.

Dose: The usual recommended dose is 200 mcg daily. *Caution:* Dosage must not exceed 500 mcg daily.

∎ SODIUM

- Is essential for cell permeability to provide for nutrient and waste exchange across cell membranes.
- Affects nerve cell excitation.
- Helps nerves and muscles function properly.
- Keeps other minerals in a soluble state.
- Aids in hydrochloric acid production.
- Is necessary, along with potassium, for muscle contraction.
- Is excreted at a greater rate if taken in excess. Excessive consumption also increases potassium excretion, which can lead to adrenal exhaustion.

Dose: Supplementation with sodium is not necessary, as most people consume too much sodium in their diet.

∎ ZINC

- Is essential to protein synthesis.
- Is essential to RNA and DNA production.
- Is an essential ingredient in 90 metalloenzymes (enzymes whose structure contains a metal).
- Keeps mucous membranes intact and aids in their healing.
- Is needed for alkaline phosphotase (enzyme in white blood cells that destroys bacteria).
- Is needed for alcohol dehydrogenase (enzyme that detoxifies aldehydes).
- Is necessary for neurotransmitter synthesis.
- Is necessary for white cell differentiation.
- Promotes a healthy immune system.
- Maintains the balance between fighter and suppressor cells and increases the number of T-cells.
- Is depleted during chronic infections and inflammatory diseases.
- Deficiency can cause loss of taste and smell.

Dose: The recommended daily dose is 50 mg. Taking more than 100 mg per day can suppress the immune system. The zinc-copper ratio should be 10:1 for a healthy balance.

Other Nutrients

The following nutrients do not fit into any of the classes discussed in this chapter, but are important for body function and in the treatment of allergies and environmental illness.

∎ COENZYME Q_{10}

- Is an enzyme normally manufactured in each cell of the body.
- Enhances phagocytosis (foreign matter destruction) by the lymphocytes (type of white blood cell).
- Induces energy in the immune cells, increasing immune system function.
- Reverses cell immunosuppression.

- Acts as an antioxidant to protect cell membranes.
- Increases tissue oxygenation.
- Counters histamine, which helps people with allergies.
- Helps fight candidiasis.
- Essential in the treatment and prevention of cardiovascular disease.

Dose: Most adults need a minimum of 30 mg of CoQ$_{10}$ daily. Up to 1,500 mg may be necessary for people with cardiovascular disease.

▮▮ DHEA (DEHYDROEPIANDRO-STERONE)

- Strengthens the immune system.
- Protects the immune system from damage caused by stress.
- Boosts natural killer cells and T-cells.
- Reduces fatigue.
- Increases cognitive function.

Dose: The doses needed by women and men differ, but 25 mg daily is the usual recommended dose. Have your DHEA levels checked before beginning supplementation.

▮▮ ESSENTIAL FATTY ACIDS (VITAMIN F)

- Is essential for oxygen transport to cells.
- Aids in absorption of fat-soluble vitamins, lipids, and minerals.
- Is an essential part of the lipid layers in cell membranes and other structures.
- Stimulates conversion of beta-carotene to vitamin A.
- Is essential to the formation of enzymes, steroid hormones, and lipoproteins.
- Aids in prostaglandin synthesis. Prostaglandins regulate immunity, cell recognition, and inflammation.
- Helps to slow down peristalsis of the intestinal tract, thereby relieving some cases of diarrhea.
- Suppresses the formation of leukotrienes, which are 1,000 times more inflammatory than histamine.
- Modulates pain, water retention, and mucus secretion in inflamed tissues.
- Helpful for candidiasis.

Dose: Take 1 to 5 Tbsp. of a vegetable oil daily. If taking evening primrose oil, the recommended dose is one to two capsules three times daily.

▮▮ GLUCOSAMINE SULFATE

- Regulates mucus secretion of the respiratory, digestive, and urinary tracts.
- Helps repair damaged joints.

Dose: The usual recommended dose of glucosamine sulfate is 1,500 mg daily.

▮▮ MSM (METHYLSULFONYL-METHANE)

- Is a main source of bioavailable sulfur needed for connective tissue health.
- Reduces inflammation and relieves pain.
- Improves peristalsis.
- Has antiparasitic properties, particularly against *Giardia lamblia.*
- Normalizes the immune system.

Dose: MSM is usually taken in doses of 200 mg daily.

▮▮ PROANTHOCYANIDINS OR ANTHO-CYANIDINS (BIOFLAVONOIDS)

- Marketed as pycnogenol, grape pips, or grapeseed extract.

- Are extremely powerful antioxidants and free radical scavengers.
- Improve capillary activity, strengthen capillary membranes, and restore flexibility to arterial walls.
- Bind to collagen fibers (basic matrix of skin tissue), and help realign these fibers, preventing wrinkling and damage to the skin.
- Retard aging, improve vision, and increase flexibility.
- Stimulate blood circulation and reduce bruising.
- May reduce the risk of cancer, heart disease, and stroke; reduce inflammation in arthritis; and help alleviate a variety of other conditions.
- Moderate allergies and inflammatory response by reducing histamine.

Dose: The usual recommended dose is 30 to 100 mg three times daily.

❚❚ QUERCETIN (BIOFLAVONOID)

- Has a strong affinity for mast cells and basophils. It stabilizes their cell membranes, preventing them from spilling histamine during an allergic reaction.
- Inhibits two enzymes that regulate release of leukotrienes, which are implicated in asthmatic-type reactions.
- Reduces spontaneous bruising, along with vitamin C.
- Taken between meals has a powerful antihistamine action.
- Effective treatment for inflammatory disorders.
- Decreases reaction to certain foods, pollens, and other allergens.
- Powerful anticancer substance.

Dose: The usual recommended dose is 400 mg before each meal. Take 400 to 500 mg between meals two times daily for a powerful antihistamine effect.

Amino Acids

The base components of protein are amino acids, sometimes spoken of as "building blocks." While the importance of these materials in animal studies has been understood for about 50 years, the application of this knowledge to human health has only recently been explored.

Amino acids interact with all of the other groups of nutrients: minerals, trace elements (usually minerals required in very small amounts by the body), fats, vitamins, and carbohydrates. They are involved in most body functions, including:

- building, repairing, and maintaining all cells.
- degrading and excreting damaged protein material.
- aiding all chemical reactions within the cell.
- producing hormones, enzymes, and antibodies.
- serving as neurotransmitters or precursors to make neurotransmitters.
- joining with vitamins and minerals to carry these cofactors to the cells.
- detoxifying cells and protecting them from foreign chemicals.

All 28 of the amino acids are necessary for proper body function. The liver manufactures about 80 percent of the amino acids needed by the body. The other 20 percent come from the diet and are called essential amino acids. The amino acids manufactured by the body are called nonessential

Taking Amino Acid Supplements

When taking amino acids individually to treat a specific problem, take them on an empty stomach so that they will not be competing for absorption with the amino acids in foods. It is best to take them first thing in the morning or between meals, along with vitamins B$_6$ and C to aid in their absorption.

If you are taking a single amino acid, also take an amino acid complex to ensure you are getting adequate amounts of all the amino acids. Amino acid complexes should be taken one half-hour before or after a meal. They should not be taken for long periods of time without a healthcare professional's advice.

amino acids, in reference to the fact that they do not need to be obtained through the diet.

There must be a balance between the amino acids in the body. Taking single amino acid supplements is sometimes desirable in order to correct imbalances or to satisfy a temporary demand, but ordinarily a balanced mix of amino acids should be taken.

Individual amino acids are being used in clinical practice to correct some genetic problems, to repair damaged health, to support metabolism in chronic illness, and to promote optimum health. Individual assessments must be made on the basis of symptoms, diagnosis, diet, genetic factors, nutritional imbalances, and relationships between various amino acids and specific body functions. Diagnostic tests to determine amino acid levels in the urine or blood will aid you in planning therapy with your physician or healthcare practitioner.

Only those amino acids that pertain to treating allergy and environmental illness will be discussed here. All of them have many functions other than the ones listed.

■■ ARGININE

- Can be produced in the body.
- Initiates release of growth hormone, an immune system stimulant.
- Stimulates white blood cell production in the thymus gland.
- Aids detoxification of ammonia in the liver.
- Enhances immune system function.

Dose: Available in 500 mg capsules or tablets. Prescribed doses range from 1 to 30 grams. No more than 20 to 30 grams should be taken in a day, as enlarged bones and joints could result. Do not give to growing children or people with schizophrenia.

■■ ASPARTIC ACID

- Can be produced in the body.
- Helps to detoxify ammonia that results from improperly degraded, damaged, or excess protein in the body. The brain is especially sensitive to ammonia.
- Is beneficial for neural and brain disorders.
- Enhances the production of immunoglobulins.
- Increases stamina and helps reduce fatigue.

Dose: The usual recommended dose is 250 to 500 mg one to three times a day.

▌▌ CYSTEINE

- Can be produced by the body.
- Is a sulfur-based amino acid needed for detoxification in the cell.
- Is a precursor to the peptide glutathione (a reducing agent that protects the body against oxidizing chemicals).
- Detoxifies aldehydes produced by consumption of alcohol or foreign chemicals, or produced by the Candida organism.
- Promotes healing from respiratory disorders.
- Is a component of mercapturic acid, a detoxification end product.
- Protects the liver and brain from damage by alcohol, drugs, and toxic chemicals in cigarette smoke.
- Helpful for stress and allergic disorders.

Dose: Available in 500 mg capsules. The usual recommended daily dose is 500 to 1,000 mg. Must be taken with vitamin C ; does not need to be taken on an empty stomach.

▌▌ GLUTAMIC ACID

- Can be produced by the body.
- Lessens the seesaw effect of fluctuations in insulin production in hypoglycemia or diabetes.
- Helps reduce mental symptoms resulting from some types of allergic reactions.
- Can detoxify ammonia by converting it to glutamine; the only mechanism by which ammonia in the brain can be detoxified.

Dose: Available in 500 mg capsules, but should be prescribed by a physician.

▌▌ GLUTAMINE

- Can be produced by the body.
- Changes into glutamic acid by combining with ammonia, reducing excess amounts of ammonia, which accumulate in people who cannot convert it into urea for excretion.
- Is an important component of the antioxidant glutathione.
- Helps to maintain a healthy digestive tract.

Dose: Available in 500 mg capsules. The usual recommended daily dose is up to three capsules a day, either an hour before eating or two hours afterward.

▌▌ GLYCINE

- Can be produced by the body.
- Helps to reduce excess secretion of hydrochloric acid in the stomach.
- Is an important component of the antioxidant glutathione.
- Proper amounts increase energy.
- Necessary for central nervous system function.
- Is useful for repairing damaged tissues and promoting healing.
- Necessary for the production of other amino acids in the body.

Dose: Available in 500 mg capsules and tablets. The usual recommended daily dose is 3 to 5 grams, but it is best prescribed by a healthcare professional.

▌▌ HISTIDINE

- Is an essential amino acid.
- Is a precursor to histamine, which is released from mast cells during an allergic reaction.

- Reduces excess stomach acid secretion.
- Binds with excess copper when copper levels become toxic.
- Is significant in the repair of tissues.
- Can relieve symptoms of arthritis.

Dose: Available in 500 mg capsules, but does not usually need to be supplemented. People who produce too much histidine genetically can suffer serious problems. Supplementation should be under the direction of a physician, as histidine can increase blood pressure.

▮ LYSINE

- Is an essential amino acid.
- Acts as a deterrent to viral replication while the immune system mounts its defense; must be initiated at the start of infection.
- Is essential to carbohydrate metabolism.
- Is required in increased amounts during periods of stress.
- Aids in the production of antibodies, hormones, and enzymes.

Dose: Available as 500 mg capsules. Take one to two daily half an hour before meals.

▮ METHIONINE

- Is an essential amino acid.
- Offers up a methyl group (CH_3) that combines with free radicals to deactivate them.
- Lowers histamine levels if used together with calcium; detoxifies histamine.
- Is essential to collagen formation.
- Stimulates bile production.
- Is necessary for production of heparin, which can modulate allergic reactions.
- Is used to make choline (a B vitamin), a precursor to the neurotransmitter acetylcholine.

- Is a precursor for all other sulfur-containing amino acids used in detoxification pathways.
- Protects cell membranes against lipid peroxidation.

Dose: Methionine is available in 500 mg capsules or tablets. The usual recommended dose is 500 mg, three times a day.

▮ ORNITHINE

- Can be synthesized by the body.
- Stimulates growth hormone production in the pituitary gland, thereby stimulating the immune system.
- Helpful for people with insomnia.
- Necessary for proper immune system and liver function.

Dose: Available in 500 capsules. The usual recommended dose is several grams a day, taken with arginine. Do not give to growing children or people with schizophrenia.

▮ PHENYLALANINE

- An essential amino acid.
- Affects the tyrosine-dopamine-norepinephrine pathway, which increases vitality, mental acuity, learning ability and attention span.
- Stimulates the production of cholecystokinin, which is helpful in reducing inflammatory responses in allergic people.
- Is effective for controlling pain in the DL form.

Dose: Available in 250 or 500 mg capsules. The usual recommended daily dose is 500 mg. Take 1 hour before meals with juice or water, but no protein. Also available as DL-phenylalanine, which helps with pain control by prolonging the body's natural painkilling ability. Take one or two capsules every four hours, as needed for pain. Do not give to people with phenylketonuria, as they lack the enzyme to convert phenylalanine to tyrosine, or to pregnant women.

▌▌ TAURINE
- Can by synthesized in the body with sufficient B_6.
- Acts as a detoxifying material.
- Combines with bile acids from the liver to aid in absorption and metabolism of lipids (cholesterol and triglycerides).
- Is vital for the proper utilization of sodium, potassium, calcium, and magnesium.

Dose: Available in 500 mg capsules. The usual recommended dose is 2 grams, three times a day.

▌▌ TRYPTOPHAN
- Is a nonessential amino acid.
- Is a precursor to serotonin, required during the sleep process.
- Is necessary to antibody production by the bone marrow (B-cells).
- Raises pain threshold.
- Helps control hyperactivity.
- Converts to niacin in the presence of vitamin B_6.

Dose: Tryptophan is available only by prescription in the U.S. Be sure to take a balanced B complex formula with tryptophan.

▌▌ TYROSINE
- Is a nonessential amino acid.
- Is used by the thyroid gland, along with iodine, to produce the hormone thyroxine (necessary for proper thyroid function).
- Is a precursor to norepinephrine (a neuro-transmitter) and to some adrenal hormones.
- Aids in the function of the adrenal, thyroid, and pituitary glands.
- Promotes healing of respiratory disorders.
- Helpful for stress and allergic disorders.

Dose: Available in 500 mg capsules. The usual recommended daily dose is 500 mg. Take with a high-carbohydrate meal or at bedtime. People on MAO inhibitors should not take tyrosine, as it can lead to a sudden increase in blood pressure. People on medication for depression should discuss dietary restrictions with their healthcare professional.

Vitamin C: A Key Nutrient

Vitamin C is one of the most important, protective, biochemical substances in all life processes. It is essential to a large number of biochemical functions, yet humans, apes, monkeys, and guinea pigs cannot synthesize vitamin C in their bodies. Obtaining adequate amounts of vitamin C from food is difficult, so supplementing this vital nutrient is important. Ascorbic acid and the various forms of ascorbates are all classified as vitamin C. Ascorbic acid and ascorbate are used interchangeably in this discussion.

Vitamin C is found in the following tissues, in order of decreasing concentration: adrenal glands, white blood cells, pituitary gland, brain, pancreas, liver, cardiac muscle, and plasma. Because so many body tissues require it, it is extremely important for the allergic person.

Large amounts of vitamin C will have additional benefits by increasing mental acuity and reducing symptoms of stress. Vitamin C

Allergy Relief

Vitamin C will help to relieve many symptoms that a sensitive person experiences. It will not cure allergies, but it will help to control them and to repair all body tissues.

is also an important component of collagen, the material that "cements" our cells together, and a component of cell membranes throughout the body.

■ SAFETY OF VITAMIN C

Vitamin C is very safe to use; it is one of the least toxic substances known. Even at high levels, there has been no evidence of toxicity. There has been much discussion in the media about the possibility that a high vitamin C intake could cause the development of oxalate kidney stones. Physicians such as Dr. Robert Cathcart of Los Altos, California have found, instead, that the slight increase in acidity and flow of urine prompted by vitamin C use causes the calcium salts associated with kidney stones to dissolve. High concentrations of ascorbate, which are bacteriostatic (inhibit bacterial growth), along with vitamin B_6 and magnesium in adequate amounts have been found to prevent the formation of calcium oxalate kidney stones.

Victor Herbert of the Mount Sinai School of Medicine in New York claimed in 1974 that supplementary vitamin C taken with a meal destroys 95 percent of the B_{12} contained in the food. These claims were researched by two other teams of investigators, who found that improper analysis methods led to erroneous conclusions in the original study.

Small numbers of people with a G-6-PD deficiency (glucose-6-phosphate dehydrogenase) are found in groups of Asian and Mediterranean extraction. Large doses of ascorbate in these people may cause hemolysis (dissolution of red blood cells).

■ VITAMIN C SUPPLEMENTATION— BOWEL TOLERANCE

Because of its action on the immune system, allergic people should take vitamin C daily. Reactivity will be lessened if a daily level of vitamin C is maintained. It is impossible to recommend an exact amount of vitamin C for everyone—the amount needed will vary depending on age, stress, exposure to allergens or infection, absorption rate, and other factors. Bowel tolerance is the best indicator of your need.

As an effective vitamin C requirement indicator, Dr. Cathcart introduced bowel tolerance level. Dr. Cathcart states that the maximum relief of symptoms to be expected with oral doses of ascorbic acid is obtained at a point just short of the amount that produces diarrhea. The individual usually learns to control the timing and amount of the doses.

At bowel tolerance level, diarrhea occurs when adequate amounts of ascorbate accomplish detoxification, free radical scavenging, and repair. The level of vitamin C in the blood then rises, slowing ascorbate absorption from the intestinal tract. The excess reaches the rectum and produces diarrhea.

Diarrhea can also occur when a buffered form of vitamin C is used. This material can be irritating to the gastrointestinal tract and can cause diarrhea because of its magnesium content. (However, the diarrhea usually subsides in a few hours.) This does not represent a true bowel tolerance level—you should try a different form of vitamin C, such as ascorbic acid or ascorbate forms, or ascorbic acid plus a sodium/potassium buffer. (Do not take more than 500 milligrams of potassium per day unless you check with your physician or nutritionist. Some buffered forms of vitamin C contain potassium.)

The degree of toxicity in your body will dictate the amount of vitamin C you can tolerate before bowel tolerance is achieved. We cannot stress enough the importance of consistently taking your bowel tolerance level of vitamin C to improve health. The best results are achieved only if bowel tolerance levels are reached and maintained. Most people err in taking too small rather than too large an amount of vitamin C. Remember, too, that other nutrients in adequate amounts are equally important to balance the vitamin C and to enhance its action in the body.

▮ BEGINNING YOUR VITAMIN C THERAPY

When starting your vitamin C therapy, begin with 1 gram of the ascorbic acid form (non-buffered) per day, taken at mealtime. Increase that amount by 1 gram daily, spacing the doses evenly throughout the day, until you have diarrhea. Then back up 1 gram. This amount will be your maintenance level. Test this level periodically, since exposures may change your need from time to time. For children, start with 500 mg rather than 1 gram (1,000 mg = 1 gram).

If you experience diarrhea when you are taking only 2 to 3 grams daily, try again after a few days to increase your bowel tolerance level. When diarrhea does occur, it will subside in a few hours. Drink additional tolerated water to flush out the excess vitamin C causing the diarrhea. You may experience a small amount of bladder irritation or burning in the stomach when increasing your vitamin C; however, this is not a sign of toxicity or reactivity to the vitamin. These symptoms usually subside if a different form or source is used.

You may also experience gas as you increase your vitamin C consumption to your maintenance level. This may be temporarily uncomfortable, but it usually subsides. If you do develop gas, you may want to time dosage increases to coincide with your days off so that you will be more comfortable at work. You can also divide your doses into smaller amounts and take them more frequently through the day. Patients who have candidiasis may experience more bloating and gas, and sometimes diarrhea, when increasing vitamin C levels. The *Candida* organism ferments the vitamin C in the lower bowel, forming gas bubbles.

When nearing your correct level, you will develop a sense of well-being, your energy level will be high, and you will feel better able to cope. Dosages below this level will not relieve your symptoms. When the sense of well being lessens, it is always a good indicator of the need for more vitamin C. This will become no more difficult to discern than knowing how much water you need to quench your thirst. At first, the mechanics of spacing your intake may seem cumbersome, but in a short while it will become routine.

Another important aspect of vitamin C therapy is consistency. Once you have achieved a daily maintenance level, you should keep your consumption at that level in order to keep inflammation and cell damage caused by allergies to a minimum. If taking more than 20 to 30 grams per day, you should supplement with a balanced multimineral, because vitamin C at that level will act as a diuretic (increase urine flow) and will rinse out some of your minerals.

It is wise to take other nutrients along with vitamin C in order to enhance its action in your body. Each of the more than 40 essential nutrients is linked to all of the others. Because of this, special attention should be paid to providing adequate amounts of all vitamins, minerals, and other nutrients so that your body will have the materials needed for repair and proper cell functioning.

Vitamin C is water-soluble; it is not stored in our body. Excess is usually excreted within two to three hours, so you need to space your intake evenly throughout the day. If you awaken at night, take vitamin C at that time; your body repairs itself most effectively during rest periods. If you have difficulty remembering to take your vitamin C every hour or two, carry a small timer to remind you. Since most of your exposure to allergens will be during the day, it is essential to keep a high concentration of the vitamin in your bloodstream during waking hours.

When you are exposed to unusually high amounts of allergens or to infection, you will need to increase your dosage above your maintenance level as soon as possible after the exposure. Quick action will prevent the cascade effect of adverse symptoms that accompany inflammatory reactions. You may be able to tolerate as much as 3 to 4 grams every half-hour without experiencing diarrhea. Your body will utilize that increased amount of vitamin C in the presence of a virus, an infection, an allergic reaction, or an increased stress level. You will soon learn to reach for vitamin C whenever a sensitivity reaction begins, and the benefits will be evident.

If you have temporarily increased your intake of vitamin C above your maintenance level, return to maintenance dose gradually over a period of several days to avoid a "rebound" effect, which is a rapid return of your symptoms or infection. If your dosage of the vitamin is reduced too rapidly, a scurvy-like condition can result.

▊ FORMS OF VITAMIN C

If you experience problems (other than gas formation) with vitamin C, it is usually attributable to the substance from which the vitamin has been extracted. Problems may also result from the chemicals used in the manufacturing process. Ascorbic acid is currently extracted from beets, sago palm, tapioca, corn, potato, beets, and carrots. (See Recommended Sources and Organizations.) An allergy to any of these substances may prevent you from being able to use vitamin C from that source unless it is highly purified.

Consider rotating vitamin C extracted from different sources so that you will not develop a sensitivity to any one source.

Use only hypoallergenic forms of vitamin C. Some less expensive brands may have allergenic binders, fillers, or coatings, or may not have been adequately refined. Do not use time-released or chewable vitamin C. Most sensitive people do not have enough hydrochloric acid production in their stomachs to properly process the time-released form. Chewables always contain some type of sugar or sweetener as well as flavorings to conceal the "vitamin" taste. Be sure to rinse your mouth after chewing vitamin C to prevent damage to your teeth.

Several different forms of vitamin C are available, but ascorbic acid is the most common. Ascorbic acid is available in both crystalline form (powder) and capsule form. Vitamin C in tablet form is not easily assimilated by some people. The crystals have a "tart" taste and can be added to either juice or water. Each 1/4 tsp. of the crystalline form contains 1,000 mg or 1 gram of ascorbic acid. The capsule form is easier to use, particularly when traveling, but the capsule is made from either beef or pork gelatin, which can be allergenic for some people. Do not add vitamin C to hot liquids; the heat decreases its effectiveness.

Vitamin C is also available as sodium ascorbate and calcium ascorbate, which are considered to be a type of buffered C since they are not acidic. Those on salt-restricted diets should avoid the sodium ascorbate form, using the ascorbic acid form for the major portion of their vitamin C intake. Both the ascorbic acid and ascorbate forms of vitamin C should be rinsed off the teeth, since prolonged exposure can cause damage to the enamel.

▮ BUFFERED VITAMIN C

Several companies manufacture a product called "buffered vitamin C," which is ascorbic acid in combination with a buffer of calcium carbonate, magnesium carbonate, and potassium bicarbonate. Buffered C is very well absorbed by the body, and is an excellent aid for stopping reactions to many substances. (See Temporary Relief During an Allergic Reaction, in chapter 21.)

Take buffered C routinely one hour after meals. During the digestive process, the pancreas releases bicarbonate to neutralize the acidic food from the stomach as it passes into the small intestine; the buffered C will aid in this process. You should not take buffered C less than one hour before or one hour after a meal since the buffers interfere with the stomach acid necessary to start digestion. However, if you are experiencing an allergic reaction and need the buffered C to stop the reaction, take it promptly, regardless of proximity to a meal.

Like ascorbic acid, buffered C is available in both powder and capsule form. The powder acts more quickly than the capsule, and 1 tsp. of powder is equal to about four capsules. One tsp. of buffered C powder usually contains 2.4 g or 2,400 mg of vitamin C. Stir 1 tsp. buffered C into a small amount of water and follow it with a glass of water. Some brands of buffered C dissolve more easily than others do. If you do not like the taste in water, add it to juice—however, the acidity of the juice inhibits some of the buffering action.

If you are experiencing a reaction that is particularly severe, you can dissolve buffered C powder in a very small amount of water and hold it under your tongue. In a situation where there is no water, a capsule of buffered C held under the tongue will dissolve and act in the same way. If the magnesium content of buffered C is irritating to your intestinal tract, you can hold the solution under your tongue for five minutes and then spit out the solution, rather than swallowing it.

When taking buffered C, do not exceed more than 5 tsp. or 20 capsules daily (10 grams) because potassium, calcium, and magnesium intake will exceed safe levels for some people. Each teaspoon contains 450 mg calcium, 250 mg magnesium, and 99 mg potassium. These amounts must also be added to any other calcium, magnesium, or potassium supplements that you are taking. If you feel better with some buffering, and want to increase your intake of vitamin C, you can add some ascorbic acid powder to your buffered C powder, or take one capsule of ascorbic acid and one to two capsules of buffered C.

▌ ESTER-C

Ester-C is a nonacidic mega-molecular complex mixture made up of ascorbic acid molecules fully reacted with calcium, magnesium, zinc, potassium, or sodium, or a combination. This form of buffered C is reported to enter the bloodstream more rapidly, cause higher vitamin C levels, and produce less oxalate excretion.

Some people experience less gas from this form of vitamin C. It is produced from an ascorbic acid that has been extracted from corn. However, it is highly refined and supposed to be safe even for corn-sensitive patients. As with all substances, though, sensitivity is an individual matter, and corn-sensitive patients may or may not tolerate it. This form of vitamin C may benefit some people, while others will not be able to tell a difference between it and other vitamin C preparations.

▐▌ VITAMIN C SUMMARY

1. Take your bowel tolerance level of vitamin C daily. Use mainly an ascorbic acid form.
- To determine your bowel tolerance level, add 1 gram daily until you develop diarrhea.
- When you develop diarrhea, back up 1 gram. This will be your daily maintenance level except when you are experiencing increased stress, infection, or allergic reaction, at which times you should increase your dosage.
- Spread your vitamin C doses throughout the day to maintain a constant level in your body. It is excreted rapidly.
2. Take 1 to 2 grams buffered C one hour after each meal to aid digestion unless you are experiencing an allergic reaction.
3. If you are in reaction, take buffered C immediately, regardless of proximity to a meal.
- Take 1 to 2 grams of vitamin C every 15 to 30 minutes until your reaction clears.
- If taking 2 grams, take 1 gram each of

buffered C and ascorbic acid so that you will not exceed the mineral safety level of calcium, magnesium, and potassium.

• As long as you do not develop diarrhea, your body is using both the vitamin C and the buffers to stop your reaction and to repair and protect your body.

• Because most people think poorly when they are in reaction, instruct your family or friends to give you buffered C whenever they see you experiencing symptoms.

PART V

Taking Steps to Wellness

ALL OF US CAN TAKE measures to improve our health, and every positive step we take is another step toward wellness. Many are self-help procedures and do not require the help of a healthcare professional. Some people must take many steps over many months before they are successful in achieving wellness. Others may have only a few steps to take and will reach their goal of good health quickly. If you have numerous allergies and your health is suffering, consult a healthcare professional, in addition to using any of the self-help procedures that are appropriate.

Those of us with allergies must conquer them so that we can live without being in a state of constant reaction. Sometimes our daily lives become very complicated because of our allergies and the restrictions they impose upon us. Fortunately, there are ways to remove these restrictions. In this chapter, we discuss the steps that will enable you to regain a healthy, relatively reaction-free life. Some of them are quite simple, while others require work on your part. Remember that the prize, optimum health, is worth every step you must take to reach that goal.

Solving Everyday Problems

SOLVING EVERYDAY PROBLEMS is essential for us to feel well and to maintain an enjoyable lifestyle. For people with allergies, whether they have food, chemical, inhalant or microorganism allergies and sensitivities, sometimes the days are so full of problems that a normal lifestyle, let alone an enjoyable lifestyle, seems not to be possible. The simplest, daily maintenance tasks can seem out of reach to the allergic person.

The purpose of this chapter is to give you some constructive hints on how to accomplish an enjoyable lifestyle in spite of your allergies. At first, some of the suggestions may seem too complicated. However, when you become accustomed to them, you will do them automatically, without thinking about it. Many of the modifications suggested will allow you to maintain your independence and to continue your life, within limits, much as you had done before.

Some of you may realize that the modifications you have made are far better than the routines you used to follow and may continue to make them a part of your life, even after you have conquered your allergies and recovered your health. Most of them are commonsense approaches that will allow anyone, with or without allergies, to live a cleaner, healthier life.

Tips for Common Activities

▌▌ GROCERY SHOPPING

Unfortunately, grocery stores can constitute massive exposures for the allergic person because of the thousands of products they carry. These products range from whole foods, cleaning products, and pesticides to hardware and motor oil, depending on the size of the store. Many of these items are a toxic and allergenic exposure, particularly to chemically sensitive people. The suggestions below may enable you to make short trips into stores without reacting. You must avoid long, involved trips, however.

If you are extremely sensitive, wear a charcoal mask when you go to the store. Yes, people will look at you, but enduring stares is better than becoming ill. Remember, do not let what other people think make you sick!

Safest Shopping

Shop from mail order catalogs. There are hundreds of catalogs that carry clothing, ranging from traditional clothing to all-cotton, organic clothing made for the chemically sensitive. The packages will be delivered to your home, and most companies have liberal return policies. You may have to pay some return postage if the garments are not suitable and you must send them back. However, this postage is frequently less than the cost of a shopping trip, and your exposures are negligible. Shopping on the Internet is also a possibility for some people.

Shop from a list, organized according to the layout of the store, to minimize your time and exposures in the store. As much as possible, shop only the outside aisles of the store. In most stores, the fresh produce and meats are on opposite sides of the store and the processed foods, cleaning supplies, and other toxic products are in the middle aisles.

Shop in health food stores or health food supermarkets if they are available to you. While they will not be perfect (some of them carry incense, the odor of which can be very strong), they are usually considerably safer than commercial grocery stores. They will also carry more products that will be safe for you to use. Even so, not all products in this type of store are guaranteed to be safe for your use. Read labels!

If you are too ill to shop, have your spouse, friend, neighbor, or special helper shop for you. Use a personal shopper if there is a grocery store with this service. Frequently in cities you can call in your grocery order and have it delivered. There is a fee, of course, but it may be well worth it to you not to have to go to the store.

▮ SHOPPING FOR CLOTHES

Because we must wear clothes both for warmth and modesty, we cannot give up shopping for clothes just because we have allergies. In all seriousness, this is a difficult task for the chemically sensitive because a store that sells new clothing is "formaldehyde city." Formaldehyde makes colors brighter and surfaces smoother, producing the attractive clothes we like to wear. Dyes, fabric sizing, and in some cases, fire retardant chemicals on clothing can also be a problem. Several methods can be used to assure our continuing ability to clothe ourselves.

Always try to purchase clothing made from natural fabric that is washable. Fabric that has been dry-cleaned must be aired and outgassed for months before wearing. Even so, it may always contain a toxic residue from the dry-cleaning fluid. Also purchase natural colors or white clothing, avoiding the bright or very dark colors, which may have toxic dye residues. Black, brown, navy, and red dyes can be a problem for some chemically sensitive people.

If you shop in stores that carry new clothing, wear your charcoal mask. Plan your shopping tour carefully so that you know exactly which stores you must visit and, if possible, precisely where in the store you want to go. This will limit your time in the store.

In some cases, you may be able to call ahead and have a salesperson have garments ready for you to look at. You may want to avoid shopping in malls because the sheer volume of new merchandise makes them very toxic.

Shop at second-hand clothing stores or thrift shops. The clothing in these stores will have outgassed most, if not all of their formaldehyde. Many times you can find safe clothing at bargain prices in these stores. However, keep in mind that the former owners may have worn perfumes and used other scented products that you may not be able to completely remove from the clothing.

Shopping at garage sales may provide another way to shop for clothing. Most garage sales are held outdoors, which will be safer for you, but your selections may be limited. Again, the former owners of the clothing may have worn or used scented products.

Sewing your own clothes is also a possibility, but shopping for fabric can be difficult as most fabric stores are an enormous chemical exposure. A few catalogs offer fabrics as well as clothing. Most new fabrics will have to be carefully washed before you handle them, to cut out the garment or stitch it on your machine. Have someone else wash the fabric for you if you are unable to do it. Use a baking soda final rinse before drying the fabric.

▌▌LAUNDERING YOUR CLOTHES

Even if you do not own a washer and a dryer or have them accessible to you, you still have several choices for keeping your clothes clean.

Going to a laundromat can involve multiple exposures to scented detergents, fabric softeners, and many different types of anti-static and anticling products. If the dryers are natural gas dryers, this adds another exposure, both for you and your clothes. To survive going to the laundromat, go either late at night or very early in the morning to avoid crowds and increased scents. Try to find out by telephone when they clean the washers and dryers and go shortly after they have finished this task, so that your clothes will absorb fewer odors from the machines.

Take your own laundry products and use only them. Use an unscented laundry detergent or ceramic laundry disks. Some people use baking soda instead of a detergent. Do not use spot removers, fabric softeners, or anti–static-cling products. (See chapter 12, Living Safely, for safe alternatives.)

If the dryers are gas dryers, they may leave a residue from natural gas combustion on your clothes. Consider taking your wash home without drying it and hanging it on your clothesline to dry. Do not take time to fold your clothes if you do use the dryer. Take them home and fold them in the safety of your house.

Hand-washing your clothes in the sink or bathtub is also a possibility. You should wash your clothes in small batches, frequently, to preserve your back and strength. Having a friend or helper wash your clothes either at the laundromat on in their own washer and dryer is another possibility. Some laundromats have employees who will wash and dry clothes for their customers for a fee. Should you have either of these alternatives available to you, furnish your own safe laundry products.

▮ SERVICING YOUR CAR

The care and feeding of a car can be a big problem, particularly for a chemically sensitive person. There probably is no ideal or perfect solution for accomplishing this task, but the following suggestions are helpful for most people.

Patronize a full-service station whenever possible. The employees of these stations will pump the gas for you, check under the hood, and put air in your tires. This will spare you the worst exposures. However, wear a charcoal mask while you are at the station to prevent incidental exposures when rolling down the window to talk to the employees.

At self-service stations, check the wind direction when selecting the pump to fill your car. Pick one for which the wind is blowing from the front of your car toward the rear, or vice versa rather than across the car. Even though this will blow the fumes of the gasoline away from you, wear a charcoal mask. You will have to enlist the help of a friend to check under the hood and put air in your tires unless you can safely do this task wearing a mask and perhaps gloves. If you are very ill, a friend may have to perform all of these tasks for you if a full-service station or cooperative garage is not available.

When you must take your car in for maintenance or repairs, make as many arrangements as possible on the phone before you go to the garage. This will limit the time you must spend when you get to the garage. Talking directly to the shop foreman will usually help you to get safe service. Try to set up the visit so you do not have to go into the garage. Arrange for someone to meet you outside so you can talk there and turn over your keys without going into the garage. Make certain no one is going to smoke in your car while it is at the garage. Ask them to park your car outside when they complete the work.

▮ ATTENDING CHURCH

Sometimes people with chemical sensitivities must forego attending church because of the many exposures they encounter there. Perfumes, fabric softeners, personal care products, and dry-cleaned clothes are among the exposures from other people in the church. In addition, they may be sensitive to the cleaning products used by the church, as well as the carpeting, church fixtures, and other equipment. The following measures will allow some people to continue going to church.

Go to the early church service where there are often fewer people and the building has had a chance to air out overnight. Some churches have a scent-free service or a scent-free room for people with chemical sensitivities. If this is not possible at your church, you may have to attend a church in a different neighborhood or of a different denomination to find a safer environment until your health is better. Explaining your problem to the pastor, priest, or rabbi may enable you to receive cooperation in accommodating your sensitivities.

Sit near an open window, or in the best-ventilated area of the church. Always sit toward the back of the church, so that the majority of the people attending the service are in front of you. Wear your charcoal mask, if necessary. If the exposures become overwhelming, quietly leave. If you are sitting in the back of the church, you can do this without disturbing the worship of others.

If actually attending church is not possible, you can still listen to church services on the radio or watch a service on television. Remember that worship is in your heart and soul, not in the facility.

▮▮ ATTENDING MOVIES

Many movie houses are "chemical cesspools" before the moviegoers even enter the theater. Others are relatively clean and safe before the people arrive. Using the following commonsense measures may allow you to go out to a movie occasionally.

It will be best to rent movies most of the time and watch them in your own home, going only to very special movies that require the large screen and wrap-around sound for complete enjoyment. Go to the early afternoon movie before the theater becomes contaminated with personal care products and before your feet stick to the floor from spilled soft drinks. Bring your own safe water and possibly some refreshments. Movie refreshments are high in sugar, salt, and fat. Most people with food sensitivities will not find any tolerated food to purchase.

Wear your mask if necessary. No one will see you in the dark! Select a theater and a movie that may not be as well attended to reduce your exposures to people and chemicals. Sit toward the back of the theater, where there will not be many people sitting around you. Never sit in the middle of the theater, where you could be completely surrounded by people.

▮▮ TROUBLE-FREE TRAVEL

Traveling, whether for short or long distances, can be a challenge for a person with allergies. However, you *can* travel safely and enjoyably when certain measures are taken. Simple precautions and planning ahead will make the difference between a safe, happy trip, and one in which you struggle or become ill. None of the following travel precautions are difficult to do. Most of them are simple, commonsense measures.

▮ BY CAR

Our usual mode of travel is by car, whether we are going to the local grocery store or across the country. Because new cars abound with chemical exposures from their interior materials, chemically sensitive people should purchase a well-outgased, used car that previously belonged to a nonsmoker. Ideally, the car should be at least two years old, and have outside air vents that can be closed against traffic fumes. Carefully examine a car before purchasing it. Test-driving the car for a few blocks may help identify major incompatibilities, but for more subtle problems, a drive in traffic and an hour or two on the highway are essential.

Determine your tolerance to upholstery fabrics and padding. Leather interiors may be a safe alternative to cloth or vinyl for some sensitive people. If the trunk lining causes a problem because of strong odors leaking in around the back seat, the area between the back seat and the trunk may have to be sealed.

Safe Home on Wheels

A comfortable way to travel is with a travel trailer or camper. Your safe bedroom goes with you, and you have a clean kitchen facility in which to prepare meals. Some models also offer a safe bath and shower. Motor homes are not recommended, however, since engine odors can easily enter the vehicle's interior.

The car's exhaust and fuel systems should be maintained in top condition, as leaks from both systems can find their way to the passenger area, especially in an older car. Leaks of engine oil, transmission fluid, antifreeze, and power brake fluid can also cause serious chemical exposures if they come in contact with a hot manifold or exhaust pipe.

When traveling in the city, keep the windows closed to avoid traffic fumes and operate the air conditioner on its maximum setting to recirculate inside air. Passengers in the front seat are usually exposed to fewer exhaust fumes than passengers in the back. Whenever possible, take less-traveled, open-air routes. When stopping in traffic, try to stay two to four car lengths from the vehicle in front of you.

Using an automobile-model air cleaner will filter out chemicals, and wearing a charcoal mask while traveling is also helpful. Using oxygen while in your car will help some sensitive people prevent exposure to circulating allergens and help to clear reactions.

▮ BY AIR

Air travel presents many challenges. Airports frequently are difficult to endure if smoking is allowed and ventilation is poor. Jet fuel exhaust is always present, as are the odors of the personal care products of workers and travelers, and the cleaning products used to clean the airport. Most airports seem to be continually under construction, which gives passengers and airport employees exposure to building materials.

On board the plane, you are also subjected to the personal care products of the crew and your fellow passengers, some jet exhaust, and the cleaning products used to clean the plane. These exposures are concentrated in a small area where the ventilation is poor and the humidity is too low. Many times, only low amounts of fresh air are added to the ventilation system.

Wearing a charcoal mask is helpful. Being prepared with chemical extracts to gas diesel, smog, perfume mix, fabric softener, ethanol, phenol, formaldehyde, and cigarette smoke will also reduce your allergic load. If the flight is an international one, the plane may be sprayed with pesticide before passengers are allowed to disembark. In some cases, arrangements can be made to deplane before pesticide is applied.

Very sensitive people can fly if they make arrangements ahead of time. Oxygen during the flight can help, but you will need a letter from your physician stating that you need it, and arrangements must be made with the airline well in advance of your flight. Wear your charcoal mask when you are not using the oxygen. Ask for preboarding and to sit by the bulkhead to minimize the number of people sitting around you.

▌ LODGING

When traveling for long distances, it is usually necessary to find safe lodgings. Bed and breakfast establishments may be suitable if you call ahead and inquire about smoking, pets, cleaning products, clothes washing products, room deodorizers, and heating and cooling systems.

It is possible to minimize allergic reactions when staying in a motel or hotel if you ask for the following when you call for reservations:

- a nonsmoking room
- a room in which pets have not been allowed
- a room without a deodorizer
- a room not recently treated with pesticides or redecorated
- a room cleaned with only baking soda in water (if possible)
- airing of the room prior to your arrival
- a room away from the parking lot, pool, laundry area, and heating plant
- a room in which windows can be opened

Air cleaners are essential for the very sensitive; you may need to open a window and run the air cleaner. This will help clear any chemicals in the room, as well as helping with mold. Sometimes hotels, motels, and cabins, particularly in humid climates, may be moldy. A water leak in a room can also cause a substantial mold exposure.

Upon your arrival at the hotel or motel, it is wise to call the housekeeping personnel and reiterate cleaning instructions. Ask the housekeeping staff to make the bed, empty the trash, and vacuum only. Tell them not to clean the bathroom and emphasize that they cannot use any product with a scent, such as a room deodorant.

You may have to take your own linens (sheets, pillowcases, and towels). If you are using your own linens, you will want to advise housekeeping of this. If you use the hotel or motel linens, request no linen changes during your stay to reduce your exposure to detergent, fabric softener, or gas dryer residue.

▌ FOOD AND WATER

Water is often a concern when traveling. You can take your own, buy water after you arrive, carry a water-purifying Thermos or pitcher (available at health stores), or set water aside to outgas chlorine after you arrive. Set the water in a well-ventilated area to avoid having chlorine fumes in your sleeping area.

Those with severe food allergies may need to take their own food to ensure an adequate supply of safe food. Alternatives include contacting the chef either before or just after you arrive to make specific arrangements for your meals. (We have found the majority of chefs to be very helpful and cooperative.) Purchasing safe food at a natural food store or health food store after you arrive is another option.

Natural Remedies for Common Complaints

There are many simple, nontoxic remedies for common complaints. It is usually not necessary to take pharmaceuticals or to undertake complex treatments to relieve the symptoms of common problems that can

379

plague us all. Because of the difficulty that food- and chemically sensitive people have in tolerating medications, it is particularly important for them to be familiar with these natural ways of controlling and relieving symptoms. (For additional information on natural treatments for many conditions and illnesses, see *Finding the Right Treatment* in Recommended Books.)

■ PROBLEMS WITH MEDICATIONS

Many sensitive people cannot tolerate chemical exposures from medications commonly prescribed by most physicians. Many sensitive people also cannot tolerate any over-the-counter medications for relief of minor symptoms. There are a number of reasons for this.

- Medications are chemicals that can cause sensitivities in many people.
- Medications must be processed in our body by detoxification pathways, which process all chemicals (endogenous and exogenous) to which we are exposed. In most sensitive people, one or more of these pathways does not function well.
- Extra nutrients are required so that the detoxification pathways in the liver can process the medications. Adequate amounts of these nutrients are frequently lacking in sensitive people both because they are not present in the diet or because they are not well absorbed by the body.
- Some medications are manufactured from byproducts of mold metabolism. Mold-sensitive people may have difficulty tolerating this type of preparation.
- Fillers, binders, dyes, flavorings, coatings, shellacs, and inks in tablets may be aller-

genic and are poorly tolerated by most sensitive people. Most tablets contain cornstarch as a binder, which will not be tolerated by some food-sensitive people.
- Some liquid medications contain sweeteners, dyes, preservatives, and flavorings that may be allergenic.
- Most injectable medications contain preservatives to which many people are sensitive.
- Medications given to alleviate one condition may create other problems. For example, both antibiotics and birth control pills may cause candidiasis to flare up.

A sensitive person should be tested for their tolerance to any medication before beginning a course of treatment. Medications taken regularly should be tested periodically to be sure an intolerance has not developed.

■ HOMEOPATHIC AND HERBAL REMEDIES

Homeopathic remedies can be used to treat many common complaints. Two types of remedies are available – classical and complex. Classical remedies contain one substance only and are usually purchased as pellets. The 30C strength is generally best for treating most uncomfortable symptoms. If 30C is not available, you can purchase an X potency.

The pellets can be taken dry, under the tongue. Alternatively, one pellet can be dissolved in 4 ounces of distilled or filtered water, with 1 tsp. taken twice daily. Some homeopaths feel the "wet" remedies work more deeply and more effectively. Only a few of the possible remedies will be given for each condition included in this section, and all of the symptoms that a given remedy can treat will not be listed.

The complex remedies are usually available as both tablets and liquid. These preparations contain all of the remedies that will help a given condition. The body selectively uses the one that will help. Sometimes this is referred to as "shotgun therapy." The liquid remedies will contain ethanol, to which some people are sensitive. However, many sensitive people tolerate these remedies in spite of the ethanol. Putting a dose of the remedy in hot water, or simply allowing it to sit in a glass of water will allow most of the ethanol to evaporate.

Herbal remedies are very effective treatment for many conditions. However, many sensitive people do not tolerate them because of their phenolic and terpene content. If you are sensitive to phenolics and terpenes, it would be wise to be tested for a given herb before trying it. Some herbs, such as goldenseal, are not safe for use by pregnant women. Sensitive people should have all herbs checked and okayed by their healthcare practitioner before using.

▮▮ RELIEF FOR AN ALLERGIC REACTION

The following remedies are intended to help provide immediate relief of the symptoms accompanying an allergic reaction, whether it is caused by food, chemical, or inhalant exposures. These remedies do not, of course, address the specific underlying causes of an allergic reaction.

None of us thinks clearly during an allergic reaction. You may want to post this section so that you and your family can find

it quickly. If you feel ill and are thinking poorly, it is a good idea for another person to check whether you are taking the proper substances at the proper times.

▮ ALLERGY EXTRACTS

If you know what substance is causing your reaction and you have extracts for that substance, take your recommended dosage immediately. The extracts you may possibly need include extracts for foods, pollens, chemicals, mold, dust, dust mites, and microorganisms. Then use the following methods to further aid in clearing your reaction. Even if you have had hands-on allergy treatments, the following methods will be useful to stop any reactions you may have. Speed of treatment is the most important factor in stopping an allergic reaction. Some reactions cannot be reversed if there is a delay in starting treatment.

▮ CONTROLLING PH

Some people become acidic when they react, and others become basic, or alkaline. This can be determined by taking the pH of the urine or saliva. Knowing the body pH is important in determining which of the treatments below will best stop your reaction. Normalizing pH is the first step in reversing an allergic reaction.

Use pH paper, nitrazine paper, or litmus paper (available at pharmacies) to test both your saliva and urine to determine your pH. Take the appropriate material to stop your reaction.

▮ *Vitamin C*
• Buffered C is the most effective form of vitamin C for stopping reactions. It works because allergic reactions may cause our bodies to become acidic; a substance that

---

Exercise as First-aid

A brisk walk or other moderate exercise will sometimes clear an allergic reaction. The adrenalin produced during exercise helps to turn off the reaction.

---

reverses this condition will help stop the reaction. The buffer (calcium carbonate, magnesium carbonate, and potassium bicarbonate) will aid in eliminating excess acidity, restoring the proper pH balance. The vitamin C content also aids in reversing or stopping allergic reactions, but by a different mechanism.

- Many reactions can be "turned off" with buffered C if it is taken promptly, before the reaction progresses to the point where the cascade effect makes it no longer reversible.

- Some people become more alkaline when they have an allergic reaction. Take the ascorbic acid form of vitamin C to stop this reaction.

- For dosage amounts and additional information, see Vitamin C: A Key Nutrient in chapter 20. Taking bowel tolerance vitamin C daily will help to reduce reactions.

▌*Magic Brew*

- "Magic Brew" helps to stop reactions by reducing acidity and correcting pH imbalance. You may alternate Magic Brew with buffered C.

- To make Magic Brew, mix 1 tsp. salt and 1 tsp. baking soda with 1 quart water. Take 2 to 4 ounces (two to four large mouthfuls) at least every 15 minutes the day you have the reaction, and every hour the next day. (It

will taste better cold until you become accustomed to it.)
If you have high blood pressure, you will want to take this preparation in very limited amounts because of its sodium content.

▌*Alka Seltzer Gold*

- The "Gold" version of Alka Seltzer has a buffering action to reduce acidity; however, it does contain corn. Corn-sensitive individuals should not use this remedy.

- A dose of Alka Seltzer Gold may be repeated every 45 minutes to an hour until symptoms lessen.

- Alka Seltzer Gold is available only in the U.S., or through Miles Consumer Healthcare Division. (See Recommended Sources and Organizations)

▌*Tri-Salts*

- Cardiovascular Research Ltd. produces this formula, which contains carbonate and bicarbonate sources of calcium, magnesium, and potassium. (See Recommended Sources and Organizations.) It is the same buffer used in buffered Vitamin C.

- Take 1/4 tsp. of Tri-Salts with each gram of vitamin C. You may stir Tri-Salts into water or juice, but because juice is acidic the buffering effect will be reduced.

- This is an excellent buffer to combine with nonbuffered vitamin C (ascorbic acid), or to use alone.

▌*Bi-Carb Formula*

- Vital Life produces this formula, which is a combination of sodium and potassium bicarbonates. (See Recommended Sources and Organizations.) It is an excellent buffer and will help to lower acid levels.

- Take two to four capsules at a time. This dose may be repeated every 15 to 30 minutes if necessary, depending on your symptoms.

- You may combine Bi-Carb Formula with any nonbuffered vitamin C (ascorbic acid) that you can tolerate, to make your own buffered vitamin C.
- If you have high blood pressure, you will want to take this preparation in limited amounts because of its sodium content.

▌ OXYGEN

- Oxygen is an excellent aid in clearing many allergic reactions even when there is no breathing problem. In reactive or inflammatory processes, hemoglobin releases more oxygen to the cells actively involved in combating foreign substances. This creates a greater demand for oxygen. By providing an increased supply of oxygen to these active cells, energy in the form of adenosine triphosphate (ATP) is increased to help maintain proper cell function and accelerate the metabolic process of detoxification.
- Oxygen can be used in conjunction with the alkaline salts found in buffered C, Tri-Salts, or Bi-Carb Formula. Most people tend to be acidic during reactions, and in this medium the hemoglobin has less affinity for oxygen.
- You can obtain an oxygen tank for emergency use by prescription from a physician familiar with your condition. Ceramic masks and special tubing are available for people who do not tolerate plastic masks and tubing. (See Recommended Sources and Organizations.)
- Organic germanium increases oxygen utilization at the cellular level, and is helpful during allergic reactions. Two to three cap-

sules will help to clear a reaction, and may be repeated if necessary.

- Cellular Oxygenator by PHP (homeopathic division) facilitates increased transport and absorption of oxygen into the cell. It contains homeopathic remedies and homeopathic dilutions of vitamins and minerals to help repair the damage of oxidation and free radicals that occurs in allergic reactions. This preparation is more for repair than for stopping an acute reaction.
- A stabilized oxygen product such as Aerobic 07 or Dioxychlor will help to increase oxygen at the cellular level. Use the recommended number of drops for each product.

▌ ENEMAS

- Plain-water enemas are very helpful for stopping food reactions. Removing the food from the bowel eliminates the source material for the reaction.
  —Use plain, tolerated, warm water in the enema bag.
  —Lubricate the nozzle with vitamin E or a tolerated cooking oil. Do not use Vaseline, as it is a petroleum product and is toxic.
  —Hang the bag 24 to 36 inches from the floor.
  —Lie on the floor in the knee-chest position, face down, supporting your weight on your knees and upper chest.
  —Insert nozzle into the rectum and start the flow.
  —At the first urge or cramp, remove the tube and allow elimination.
- Coffee enemas (low volume) are most helpful for stopping chemical reactions, as well as encouraging the detoxification of chemicals. The caffeine in the coffee will cause

the liver and gallbladder to release the toxins they are holding, allowing them to detoxify more chemicals. Coffee enemas are tolerated by most people, even those who are allergic to coffee and caffeine.

To prepare a coffee enema:

—Boil 1 quart tolerated water in a stainless steel or glass pot.

—Add 2 Tbsp. organic caffeinated coffee and boil for 5 minutes.

—Turn off the heat and add 1 Tbsp. molasses (if tolerated).

—Leave on the burner and allow to cool.

—Pour half of the mixture into an enema bag.

—Administer the enema and retain for 10 minutes.

—Empty the bowel and take the other half of the enema.

—There will be a sensation of squirting under the right ribcage if the bile duct empties. When this happens, the liver and gallbladder are releasing their stored toxins to be excreted through the bowel.

Do not exceed the recommended volume for the enema. If you are a small person, you may need to reduce the volume even more. This is a low-volume enema that stays in the sigmoid colon (the S-shaped lower portion of the large intestine), which has a special circulation route to the liver that allows the caffeine to go directly to the liver without getting into the general bloodstream.

▌ PROTEOLYTIC ENZYMES

• Proteolytic enzymes, such as papain from papaya, bromelain from pineapple, and pancreatic enzymes, can be used to reduce the inflammatory processes that accompany allergic reactions. Inflammatory reactions, when allowed to proceed unchecked, will cause damage to mucous membranes, arteries, capillaries, brain tissue, and other organ tissue. Take two tablets/capsules three times per day between meals.

▌ OTHER REACTION STOPPERS

• Histamine, serotonin, and ACC (acetylcholine chloride) extracts, as well as heparin and adrenalin, are all very effective in stopping allergic reactions, but a physician familiar with your condition must prescribe them.

• Adaptosode RR, the American Rescue Remedy, made by HVS Laboratories, is a homeopathic preparation of classical homeopathic remedies and flower essences. One capful will clear most allergic reactions and can be repeated if needed. It can be taken in conjunction with vitamin C. It will also relieve acute stress. This preparation does not contain ethanol as a preservative.

• Bach Flower Rescue Remedy will help stop many types of allergic reactions, as well as relieve stress, but some people do not tolerate the ethanol. This remedy can be added to water and set aside for a period of time to allow the ethanol to evaporate.

▌▌ COMMON COMPLAINTS

The following are some simple, nontoxic remedies for relief of common symptoms. The dosages listed are adult dosage suggestions only. Do not use all remedies listed for any one condition; use only the remedies that will be helpful for you. Check with your physician or healthcare professional for recommendations for children.

■ ANXIETY (SIMPLE)

Take the following:

- Take buffered vitamin C, if your pH is acidic, to stop an allergic reaction that might be causing part of the anxiety. (See Vitamin C: A Key Nutrient in chapter 20.)
- Take Anxiety Control from the Pain and Stress Center. (See Recommended Sources and Organizations.) You may take up to two capsules a day, morning and evening, to help control anxiety. This preparation is specially balanced for proper neurotransmitter balance in preventing anxiety. Anxiety Control contains amino acid precursors for neurotransmitters, two herbs, and vitamin B$_6$. It is tolerated well by most people.
- Take Balanced Neurotransmitter Complex from the Pain and Stress Center. It contains amino acid neurotransmitter precursors, alpha-ketoglutaric acid, vitamin C, and vitamin B$_6$ and chromium picolinate as activating agents. Up to two capsules twice a day will help balance your neurotransmitters and make your emotions more stable.
- Take 1,000 mg calcium and 500 to 1,000 mg magnesium daily. These minerals are natural tranquilizers that help relieve anxiety and tension.
- Take 250 mg evening primrose oil up to three times daily, to aid proper functioning of the brain.
- Take BHI Calming, a complex homeopathic tablet for promoting calmness.
- Take the appropriate classical homeopathic remedy: *Aconite* for acute panicky

fear with restlessness; *Arsenicum album* with anxiety worse after midnight, springing out of bed to catch the breath; *Lycopodium* when the person is anxious and doubts abilities; *Rhus toxicodendron* for anxiety and inability to be comfortable unless moving about.

- Take a capsule of valerian root or skullcap at bedtime to promote sleep and to prevent anxiety during the night.
- *Kava kava* promotes relaxation and helps you get a good night's sleep. Take 10 to 30 drops in juice or water.
- St. John's wort calms anxiety. Take 10 to 15 drops in water daily.

Do the following:

- Use a breathing exercise like the one suggested by Dr. Andrew Weil in his book, *Natural Medicine, Natural Health: A Comprehensive Manual for Wellness and Self-Care.* Put your tongue on the area of flesh behind your upper front teeth. Breathe in through your nose to the count of four. Hold your breath for the count of seven, and release your breath through your mouth to the count of eight. You will make a noise as you do so. Do this four times to complete one cycle. Do as many cycles as necessary to relieve the anxiety.
- Learn relaxation techniques, such as meditation or progressive relaxation where you tighten and relax major muscle groups one at a time, starting with your feet and working up to your head.
- Get regular exercise, engaging in an activity that fits your lifestyle. Most people notice an improvement in their anxiety levels after several weeks.

▮ ASTHMA

See Wheezing and Tight Chest at the end of this section.

▮ BAD BREATH

Take the following:

- Place 1/2 tsp. acidophilus powder underneath your tongue and allow the sweet liquid to trickle down your throat. This will help to recolonize the oral mucous membranes with "friendly" bacteria. Undesirable bacterial growth in your mouth or esophagus can cause bad breath.
- Take 500 mg daily of a high-quality magnesium supplement to correct a magnesium deficiency, which can be the cause of bad breath.
- Take one chlorophyll tablet or capsule three times a day.
- Take digestive enzymes with each meal to increase efficiency of digestion.
- Take niacin, 50 mg two times a day, for canker sores that can contribute to bad breath.
- Take *Kreosotum,* a classical homeopathic remedy, if your mouth is offensive from inflamed gums or decayed teeth.

Do the following:

- Maintain proper dental hygiene with brushing and flossing. Keep your toothbrush disinfected so as not to reinfect your mouth. Use hydrogen peroxide or Zephiran (benzalkonium chloride, a germicide and disinfectant) soaks for your brush. Rinse the brush well afterward and allow it to thoroughly dry. Buy a new brush every one to two months, or more often if you become ill.
- Investigate and treat food allergies, which can be the cause of bad breath.
- Candidiasis can also be the cause of bad breath. See chapter 17, Fungi, Yeast, and Mold, for a discussion of treatments.
- Chew on a fresh parsley sprig to freshen your breath.

▮ BEE OR INSECT STINGS

After an insect sting or bite, consult a physician if any of the following systemic reaction symptoms occur:

- Wheezing or difficulty breathing
- Constriction in the throat and chest
- Difficulty swallowing
- Dry, hacking cough
- Drop in blood pressure
- Thickened speech
- Numerous hives
- Nausea, vomiting, and abdominal pain
- Dizziness
- Severe itching

Whether or not you are sensitive, consult a physician immediately if the insect sting is in the throat, face, nose, or eye area. Acutely sensitive people who have life-threatening reactions to insect venom and bites should be carefully desensitized with extracts or hands-on allergy treatment, and they should always carry insect bite kits containing adrenalin.

If you do not have systemic symptoms, take the following:

- Take a combination of 1,000 to 2,000 mg vitamin C, 99 mg potassium, and 50 mg zinc to help alleviate systemic reactions from a sting.
- Take histamine, serotonin, ACC (acetylcholine chloride) and/or heparin extracts to reduce systemic effects of the sting.
- Take the appropriate classical homeopathic remedy: *Ledum,* for any insect bite

or sting, but particularly for bee stings or when the sting area feels cold and is relieved by cold applications; *Apis* when there is marked redness and swelling.

Do the following:
- Apply a paste made of a small amount of papain meat tenderizer and water.
- Mix proteolytic enzymes (papain, bromelain, pancreas) in a small amount of water and apply to the sting site.
- Apply baking soda paste or witch hazel.
- Apply buffered Vitamin C paste to the sting.
- Rub a drop of lemon juice on a bee or insect sting to relieve the irritation.
- Place a raw, cut onion on the sting site to help draw out the venom.
- Place cold compresses on the sting to keep toxins and inflammatory byproducts from spreading to a larger area, and to reduce the pain.

▎ BURNS (MINOR)

Take the following:
- Take 600 IU of vitamin E daily to aid in healing.
- Take vitamin C, 10,000 mg immediately and 2,000 mg three times a day, until the burn is healed.
- Take 50 mg of zinc daily for healing.
- Take the appropriate classical homeopathic remedy: *Cantharis*, which relieves the severe pain following a burn and helps to promote healing; *Urtica urens* can be used for first- and second-degree burns, and in tincture topically.

Do the following:
- Apply ice or cold running water to the burn as soon as possible.
- Apply apple cider vinegar to burns to help reduce pain.
- Use Calendula homeopathic ointment to relieve the pain of burns and speed healing.
- Apply aloe vera to lessen the pain and aid in healing.
- Apply vitamin E to lessen pain, aid in healing, and prevent scarring.

▎ COLDS

Take the following:
- Take vitamin C, 1,000 to 2,000 mg every 30 minutes to an hour, to speed recovery.
- Take Viricidin or Monolaurin, and lysine. (See Viral Infections, below, for additional help).
- Use zinc lozenges at the first sign of a cold to prevent it from developing, and to relieve a sore throat.
- Take BHI Cold (complex homeopathic tablet) to help relieve symptoms.
- Take the appropriate classical homeopathic remedy: *Belladonna*, when the face is dry, flushed, and red from high fever, accompanied by leaping pulse: *Allium cepa* when the cold causes a clear, burning nasal discharge that irritates the nostrils and upper lip, and the profuse tearing of the eyes does not cause skin irritation; *Euphrasia* if the watery nasal discharge is nonirritating, and the copious tears burn.
- Cayenne tea helps relieve discomfort caused by colds and helps warm the body when there are chills. Use 1 tsp. dried herb in 1 cup hot water.
- Ginger root, lemon juice, and cayenne in hot water also makes a healing–and tasty— drink. Honey may be added to taste.
- Drink goldenseal powder mixed with warm water to relieve congestion and soothe mucous membranes. Put 1 tsp.

goldenseal powder in 1 pint boiling water. After it cools, take 1 to 2 tsp. up to six times daily as needed. *Caution:* Do not use goldenseal if you are pregnant.

Do the following:

- Begin treatment as soon as symptoms appear to prevent the virus from attaching to and growing in body cells.
- Drink lots of water, regardless of whether you are thirsty.
- Take vitamin C nose drops to ease a drippy or stuffy nose.
- Use NaSal or Ocean Spray (saline nose sprays) to help clear clogged nasal passages and keep mucous membranes moistened. You can make a homemade spray using 1/2 tsp. salt in 8 ounces of water. Do not use medicated nasal sprays, which can cause cause rebound swelling of the nasal passages.
- Sleep with your head elevated on pillows or a wedge, or with your head down and your feet elevated so your nasal passages will drain more easily.
- Do not consume dairy products during a cold because they tend to thicken mucus.
- Eat chicken soup, which has mild antibiotic and decongestant properties as confirmed by the *New England Journal of Medicine.*

■ CONSTIPATION

Take the following:

- Prevent constipation by taking vitamin C to your bowel tolerance level every day. One gram of vitamin C every 30 minutes to an hour will eventually loosen bowels.
- Take extra magnesium to help relieve constipation. One 500 mg capsule of magnesium citrate at bedtime will prevent constipation for many people.

- Take BHI Constipation (a complex homeopathic tablet) to relieve constipation.
- Take the appropriate classical homeopathic remedy: *Alumina* when there is no urge to pass stool; *Bryonia* with large, hard, dry stools and difficulty expelling them; *Nux vomica* when there is constant, ineffectual urge to pass stool, but the feeling of never being finished; or *Silicea* when there is a "bashful" stool that is partially expelled but then slips back into the rectum.
- Take the herb *Cascara sagrada* in capsule form; do not exceed recommended dose.

Do the following:

- Obtain increased fiber and fluid from dietary sources. Dehydration is a large contributor to constipation.
- Add psyllium seed to your diet. Use 1 tsp. in 1 cup of water or juice and drink two to three times a day along with eight glasses of water.
- Exercise as much as possible. Walking is an excellent form of exercise to promote good bowel function.

■ COUGH

Take the following:

- Take lemon juice with enough honey to cut the tartness, to soothe the cough. Use hot or cold; sip slowly.
- Use slippery elm lozenges, available at health food stores.
- Dissolve vitamin C crystals in a small amount of water and sip slowly.
- Take BHI Cough (a complex homeopathic tablet) to control a cough.
- Take Cough Drops by PHP (complex homeopathic drops) for temporary relief of cough attacks.
- Take the appropriate classical homeo-

pathic remedy: *Aconite* for a dry, barking cough; *Phosphorus,* if the cough is dry and hard and the person holds the chest; *Bryonia* for dry and spasmodic cough, worse with motion, breathing deeply, drinking, and eating; *Spongia,* for a croupy, harsh cough.

- Take mullein tea for a dry, nagging cough. Put 1 Tbsp. dried herb in 1 cup hot water. Drink up to 2 cups daily.

Do the following:

- Breathe steam from hot water in a basin or bowl to help relieve coughing spasms.
- Do not eat dairy products as they can increase and thicken mucus, which can increase the need to cough or cause a stuffy nose.
- Do postural drainage to reduce bronchial congestion. Lie across a bed on your stomach with your head, shoulders, and chest bent downward at the waist over the edge of the bed. Rest your elbows on a pillow on the floor. While in this position, force yourself to cough. Hold this position for five minutes, three to four times daily.
- Remember to cough often enough to keep your throat clear of mucus.

█ DIARRHEA (IF OCCASIONAL)

Take the following:

- Take small amounts of buffered vitamin C over several hours to help stop diarrhea. A small amount of buffering—containing calcium, magnesium, and potassium (Tri-Salts)—taken at the same time may also help. The buffering will help replace minerals lost during excess bowel evacuation. Mix the buffered vitamin C in a small amount of water and hold under your tongue for five minutes so the minerals

will be absorbed; then spit out the remainder of the solution.

- Take BHI Diarrhea (a complex homeopathic tablet).
- Take the appropriate classical homeopathic remedy: *Veratrum album* for violent diarrhea with watery, sometimes greenish stools forcefully ejected; *Podophyllum* with large volume, profuse, offensive-smelling stools; *Arsenicum album* when diarrhea is accompanied by abdominal pain and is worse at night, particularly after midnight.
- Take catnip tea to relieve diarrhea. Use 1 Tbsp. dried herb in 8 ounces hot water and sip.

Do the following:

- Replace water and electrolytes during a bout of diarrhea since fluid is being excreted at a greater rate. Warm water or liquid will help to slow peristaltic bowel action. Pedialyte and Ricelyte may be used to replace fluids and electrolytes.
- Check to see if your diet includes any sorbitol, an artificial sweetener. It has a strong laxative effect.
- Adopt a temporary liquid diet during a bout of diarrhea to prevent bowel irritation.
- Eat a grated, raw apple (with the skin) or three grated raw carrots.
- Call your physician if your diarrhea persists. Dehydration can occur and the cause of the diarrhea should be identified with the help of a physician.

█ ECZEMA

Take the following:

- Take 25,000 to 50,000 IU vitamin A daily for smooth skin and to prevent dryness.
- Take vitamin B complex, 50 to 100 mg

three times daily. It is needed for healthy skin, aids in the reproduction of all cells, and increases circulation.

- Take extra vitamin B_3, 100 mg three times daily. Do not exceed this amount and do not take if you have high blood pressure.
- Take extra vitamin B_6, 50 mg three times daily. Deficiencies have been linked to skin disorders.
- Take extra vitamin B_{12}, 200 mcg daily. It helps with cell formation and longevity of cells.
- Take 300 mg biotin daily. Deficiencies have been linked to skin problems.
- Take 400 IU vitamin D daily to aid in healing.
- Take 400 IU vitamin E daily to relieve itching and dryness.
- Take essential fatty acids, as directed on the label of your product, to promote lubrication of the skin.
- Take 50 mg zinc daily to aid healing.
- Take the appropriate classical homeopathic remedy: *Arsenicum album*, for eczema with dry skin and intense burning and itching, itching made worse by scratching; *Graphites,* when the skin is unhealthy, eczema oozes a thick, yellow, or "honey-like" fluid that dries into golden crystals on the skin, eruptions itch, worse from heat of the bed, scratches to the point of bleeding; *Psorinum* for eczema with tremendous itching that is worse at night, worse from being overheated and heat of the bed, scratches until bleeding, yellow, offensive discharges from the skin; *Sulphur* when the eczema is unusually moist and itches tremendously, itching is worse

from heat and heat of the bed, worse at night, from bathing, and from wearing wool.

- Alternate between dandelion, goldenseal, myrrh, Pau d'arco, and red clover capsules or tea. Do not take goldenseal daily for more than a week, or if pregnant.
- Take one chickweed capsule up to three times daily and use chickweed ointment as needed.

Do the following:

- Have allergy testing and treatment for food and chemical sensitivities. Food allergy, in particular, is a big offender in eczema.
- Avoid processed and fried foods.
- Do not use bubble bath or any scented products on the skin.
- Be sure to include fiber in the diet to keep the colon clean.

▌ EDEMA, OR SWELLING (IF INTERMITTENT)

Take the following:

- Take vitamin B complex, 50 to 100 mg one to two times daily.
- Take extra vitamin B_6, 50 mg three times daily, as a natural diuretic.
- Take extra vitamin B_1, 50 mg three times daily, if your hands and feet swell. Swelling of hands and feet may be caused by a vitamin B_1 deficiency.
- Take 400 IU vitamin E daily, for its diuretic action.
- Take bowel tolerance level of vitamin C, a natural diuretic.
- Take 1,000 mg calcium and 500 to 1,000 mg magnesium daily to replace lost minerals when edema is corrected.

- Take 99 mg potassium daily if taking a diuretic.
- Use Lymphomyosot tablets or liquid by BHI (a complex homeopathic tablet and liquid) to enhance lymph drainage, which can help reduce edema.
- Take Lymph Liquescence by PHP (a complex homeopathic liquid) to support lymphatic regeneration and fluid movement, reducing edema.
- Take the appropriate classical homeopathic remedy: *Apis* for swelling of the face or extremities; *Colchicum* for edema when there is nephritis or the urine is dark or "ink-like;" *Medorrhinum* with great swelling of the ankles; *Terebinthina* for swelling of the extremities.
- Take alfalfa tea or tablets.
- Mix 10 to 20 drops of juniper berry extract in 1 cup of liquid. Can be repeated two or three times a day, as needed.

Do the following:

- Exercise followed by a 20-minute rest, lying down, will help ease edema. The kidneys work more efficiently when the body is at rest.
- Eat foods high in potassium (bananas, watercress, strawberries, spinach, chicken, and tuna) to help lessen edema. Potassium supplements are another alternative, but do not exceed daily dosage recommendations.
- Reduce salt (sodium chloride) consumption in heart disease, pregnancy, and premenstrual edema.
- See your physician if edema is prolonged. A physician should diagnose causes of prolonged edema.

▌ EYE FATIGUE OR EYESTRAIN
Take the following:

- Take extra vitamin A with your nutrients for a total of 25,000 IU daily. Do not exceed 8,000 IU daily if you are pregnant. Deficiencies can cause eye fatigue.
- Take vitamin B complex, 50 to 100 mg daily.
- Take additional vitamin B_2, 50 mg three times daily. Deficiencies can cause eye fatigue.
- Take the appropriate classical homeopathic remedy: *Onosmodium* for blurry vision, with eyes feeling strained; *Ruta graveolens* when there is general stiffness about the eyes caused by and worse from doing fine work; *Senega* with eyestrain accompanied by inflammation of the eyes and eyelids.
- Take eyebright (*Euphrasia officinalis*) for eyestrain, 1 capsule three times daily.

Do the following:

- For a quick refresher while reading for prolonged periods: move your eyes to the extreme left, hold for 30 seconds, then close your eyes and relax for 10 seconds. Repeat, moving them to the extreme right, hold, then close and relax them again.
- Vitamin C eye drops soothe tired or itchy eyes.

▌ FEVER BLISTERS (COLD SORES)
Take the following:

- Take neutralizing doses of fluogen or *Herpes simplex* extract to relieve the pain of fever blisters.
- Take lysine, 1,000 to 1,500 mg daily, and Monolaurin, one to three capsules daily, to lessen your tendency toward cold sores.

When sores first appear, immediately increase dosages of both substances.

- Take coenzyme Q_{10}, 90 mg daily, and organic germanium, 150 mg daily, to prevent fever blisters.
- Take Herps by Vibrant Health (a complex homeopathic liquid) for *Herpes* infections.
- Take Viral Immune Stimulator or Virox by PHP (complex homeopathic liquids) to assist in eradicating a viral infection.
- Take the appropriate classical homeopathic remedy: *Rhus toxicodendron* for cold sores around the mouth with intense burning and itching; *Arsenicum album* when the herpes sores burn but feel better with warmth; *Hepar* for lesions sensitive to touch or cold; *Natrum muriaticum* when the blisters contain a clear liquid and appear like little pearls about the lips.
- Raspberry leaves (*Rubus idaeus*) are soothing for fever blisters. Mix 1 tsp. of the herb in 1 cup of warm water. Drink daily.

Do the following:

- Apply ice before a blister forms to shorten its duration and lessen pain. Use the ice 10 minutes on and 5 minutes off. Repeat as needed. Wrap the ice in a cloth to minimize dripping and either discard or wash the cloth in hot water afterward.
- Apply tea tree oil to the tingling area before the actual outbreak.
- Apply buffered C paste to a fever blister to lessen pain and encourage healing.
- Apply vitamin E directly on the lesions to reduce pain and to speed healing.
- Apply aloe vera directly to the blister to aid healing.
- A virus (*Herpes simplex*) causes fever blisters. See also the suggestions under Viral

Infection, below, and Treatment of Viral Infections in chapter16.

◼ FOOT ODOR

Take the following:

- Foot odor accompanied by chocolate craving can be a sign of magnesium deficiency. Take 500 to 1,000 mg magnesium daily.
- Take the classical homeopathic remedy *Silicea* for offensive and profuse foot sweat that may be corrosive, causing wearing of the skin and holes in the socks.

Do the following:

- Fungal infections of the feet are often a cause. Wear shoes that "breathe," such as canvas, leather, or sandals. Wear only cotton or wool socks and avoid plastic or rubber footwear. Change socks frequently.
- Some brands of anti-odor shoe liners contain activated charcoal to destroy odor and absorb perspiration. Some products may also contain antibacterial agents. Do not use these products unless you have a bacterial infection.
- Wash feet daily and soak in a mixture of $1/2$ cup vinegar in 2 quarts water.
- Place powder (talc) or baking soda in the socks to help absorb some moisture.

◼ GAS AND BLOATING

Take the following:

- Buffered vitamin C (1 tsp. dissolved in water and held under the tongue) will be absorbed rapidly and will help stimulate intestinal tract peristalsis to expel the gas.
- Take the appropriate classical homeopathic remedy: *China officinalis* when the abdomen is bloated or distended, but there is no relief from belching or expelling gas; *Colchicum* where there is tremendous abdominal distension, trapped gas; *Carbo*

vegetabilis for tremendous bloating with frequent belching which helps the stomach.

- Drink basil tea made from 1 tsp. dried herb in 1/2 cup warm water. Strain and drink 1 to 2 cups daily.
- Fennel tea relieves gas and cramps. Mix 10 to 20 drops of fennel extract in 1 cup warm water. Sweeten with a small amount of honey if desired. Drink up to 3 cups daily, as needed.

Do the following:

- Bloating pain is caused by a stretching of the bowel, and can be relieved if you move some of the gas forward. Gently press on the lower right abdomen, and gradually work your finger pressure up to the ribcage. Move your hand across the upper abdomen and proceed downward on the left side. Repeat this procedure several times until the gas "bubble" moves forward.
- A hot water bottle (placed on the abdomen), a heating pad, or a hot bath will help relieve intestinal spasm and allow the gas to move.

■ HEADACHE (SIMPLE)

Take the following:

- Take white willow bark (available at health food stores), which contains salicin, a mild pain remedy similar to aspirin, and without its cornstarch filler.
- Use the buffering action of Magic Brew (see Relief for an Allergic Reaction, above) to reduce acidity and correct pH imbalance, which often causes headache.
- Take two to three capsules organic germanium to help relieve a mild headache.
- Take two 500 mg DLPA (DL-phenylala-

nine) capsules every four hours, alone or with a pain reliever, to help reduce or eliminate headache pain. DLPA causes the body's endorphins, as well as the painkiller, to be metabolized more slowly.

- Take vitamin C, alternating between buffered C and ascorbic acid.
- Use BHI Headache (a complex homeopathic tablet).
- Take the appropriate classical homeopathic remedy: *Belladonna* for people whose headaches are intense with violent throbbing pains; *Bryonia* when the headache is worse with motion; *Nux vomica* for headaches of irritable people, frequently brought on by overeating; use of alcohol, coffee, or drugs; or staying up too late and missing sleep; *Gelsemium* for headaches beginning at the back of the head and extending to the rest of the head—feels as if a band is around the head.
- For tension headaches, use rosemary tea or 15 to 60 drops of passionflower extract in a glass of water as needed.
- Use feverfew herb (a member of the chrysanthemum family) as a pain reliever. Be sure you tolerate this plant material before using it.

Do the following:

- Apply an ice pack or a heat source (hot water bottle or heating pad), depending on your response.
- Avoid any offending substance that triggers your headache.
- Eat regular meals in order to avoid fluctuations in blood sugar levels.
- Massage therapy can be very effective in relieving headaches caused by muscle tension.

▌ HEADACHE (MIGRAINE)

Take the following:

- Take 2 to 4 grams of buffered C at the first sign of a migraine to prevent a headache. 2 to 4 grams of vitamin C in ascorbic acid form every 15 to 30 minutes, as bowel tolerance will allow, will also help clear a migraine. Alternate with buffered C on the half-hour or hour.
- Take six to ten capsules organic germanium. This will sometimes stop a migraine if taken when the aura or warning symptoms first appear.
- Take six to eight Bi-Carb Formula capsules (see Relief for an Allergic Reaction, above) at the first sign of a headache, followed by two to four capsules every 15 to 30 minutes to prevent a headache.
- Sip Magic Brew (see Relief for an Allergic Reaction, above) every 15 minutes the rest of the day, to help re-establish your body's proper pH.
- Take two 500 mg capsules of DLPA every four hours to help control the pain.
- Take BHI Headache II (complex homeopathic tablet) to relieve migraines.
- Take the appropriate classical homeopathic remedy: *Bryonia* for left-sided migraines over the left eye that are worse with motion and when coughing; *Iris vesicular* when the headache is right-sided, accompanied by changes in eyesight, and by nausea and vomiting, made worse by vomiting; *Phosphorus* for migraines that are better with sleep and cold, open air; *Melilotus* for throbbing headache of the greatest severity; *Ipecac* for severe migraine with severe nausea and vomiting; *Lachesis* for bursting, pulsating migraine headaches.
- Take peppermint tea to help reduce the sick feeling of a migraine headache.
- If you tolerate the herb, take feverfew to prevent migraine headaches and to reduce anxiety of migraine symptoms including nausea, vomiting, and pain.

Do the following:

- Initiate treatment methods immediately when the first signs of migraine appear. Very aggressive treatment is necessary to abort a migraine.
- Avoid any offending substances that trigger your migraines.
- Avoid foods containing tyramine (wine, beer, cheese, avocado, nuts, chicken livers, and pork).
- Avoid foods containing monosodium glutamate (MSG, a flavor enhancer), or dyes.
- Eat more fish or take omega-3 fatty acid supplements. The fish oil inhibits prostaglandin secretion, which occurs during a migraine episode.
- Apply either an ice pack or a heat source (hot water bottle or heating pad), depending on your response, to help relieve migraine headache pain.
- Sleep for an hour or more with a heating pad (set on low) over your head to relieve the pain. Some people prefer cold; an ice bag can be substituted.
- For some people, hot baths will reduce the pain of a headache. Take a bath, as hot as you can tolerate, to reduce head pain. Be sure your hands and feet and as much of your body as possible are submerged. Soak until the water cools; repeat several times. Each soaking will lessen the pain.

▌ HERPES

Take the following:

- Take all of the substances listed above for Fever Blisters, which are caused by *Herpes simplex I.*
- Take 50,000 IU of vitamin A daily to aid healing and prevent the infection spreading. Do not exceed 8,000 IU daily if you are pregnant.
- Take bowel tolerance vitamin C daily to inhibit the growth of the virus.
- Add 30 to 60 mg of bioflavonoids daily, as they work in conjunction with vitamin C.
- Take 50 to 100 mg of zinc daily in divided doses to boost the immune system. For genital herpes, take a chelated form.
- Take essential fatty acids to help protect cells, in the amount recommended on your product.
- Take 600 IU of vitamin E daily. It is important in healing and helps prevent spread of the infection.
- Take the appropriate classical homeopathic remedy: *Dulcamara* for genital herpes with eruptions between the scrotum an thighs; *Graphites* with herpes eruptions of genitalia, and upper, inner thigh; *Lycopodium* when the herpes is right-sided and extends down the thigh; *Medorrhinum* with genital herpes or genital warts; *Petroleum* for herpes spreading to anus and thighs, eruptions and moisture of genitalia, scrotum, and inner thighs, herpes lesions between the urethral opening and anus, raw irritated lesions; *Sepia* for genital warts, herpes of the genitalia or area between urethra and anus, or around the anus.
- Take cayenne, echinacea, myrrh, red clover, or St. John's wort in capsule or tincture. Follow the directions on your product.
- Take goldenseal capsules or tea, but not for

longer than one week. Do not use goldenseal if you are pregnant.

Do the following:

- You can do any of the things listed above for Fever Blisters.
- Consider taking acyclovir, available by prescription from a physician.
- Apply black walnut or goldenseal extract to the herpes lesions.
- Use the natural antiseptic tea tree oil on the lesions. You may have to dilute it with water or cold-pressed vegetable oils.
- Use ice packs on the genital area to ease swelling and reduce pain.
- Take warm Epsom salts or baking soda baths to help itching and pain.
- Keep lesions dry and wear cotton underwear.
- Should you develop a herpes lesion on your eye, see your physician immediately. It can cause serious eye complications.
- If you are pregnant, be certain your physician is aware that you have genital herpes.

▌ INDIGESTION, HEARTBURN, NAUSEA, OR STOMACHACHE

Take the following:

- Take digestive enzymes with meals, in the amount recommended on the product, to increase the efficiency of your digestion and lower the possibility of developing heartburn, gas, and bloating.
- Use papaya tablets for indigestion, taking one tablet up to three times daily.
- Take a buffered vitamin C dose, containing 500 to 1,000 mg of vitamin C. Both the buffers and the vitamin C will help stop the heartburn.
- Take Magic Brew (see Relief for an Allergic Reaction, above). Drink 2 to 4 ounces, sip-

ping slowly. For this problem, it may be more soothing warm than cold.

- Take two to four Bi-Carb Formula capsules to help ease indigestion, heartburn, nausea, or stomachache.
- Take BHI Stomach or BHI Nausea (complex homeopathic tablets) to help relieve stomach pains, cramps, indigestion, and nausea.
- Take the appropriate classical homeopathic remedy: *Causticum* for acid indigestion: *Sepia* for acid indigestion and abdominal bloating; *Lactic acid* when there is burping, heartburn, and nausea; *Ipecac* for nausea and vomiting with loathing of food and the smell of food; *Nux vomica* for nausea and vomiting that are worse with anger, accompanied by abdominal pains; *Arsenicum album* when there is stomach pain ameliorated by drinking milk; *Sanguinaria* with marked heartburn, reflux, and acrid belching; *Magnesia phosphorica* when there is stomach pain, better with pressure and bending over double.
- Take aloe vera, which helps heartburn and is particularly soothing to the gastrointestinal tract. Take 1/4 cup aloe vera juice on an empty stomach twice a day.
- Use caraway for indigestion. Mix 3 to 4 drops of extract in 1 cup of liquid. Drink three to four times a day as needed.
- Chamomile tea relieves indigestion and calms the body. Drink 1 cup nightly.
- Ginger root or peppermint tea will relieve nausea.

Do the following:

- Drink a glass of warm water. Many times this dilutes stomach acid and stops the pain.
- Limit your intake of legumes, which can inhibit enzymes and contribute to heartburn.

■ INSOMNIA

Take the following:

- Take 1,000 to 1,500 mg of tryptophan at bedtime to help induce sleep (currently available in the U.S. by prescription only).
- Take two to three calcium/magnesium supplements at bedtime to help you to relax. These can be repeated during the night.
- Take melatonin (currently available at health food stores in the U.S., or can be ordered from the U.S. to Canada for personal use only.), 1.5 to 5 mg two hours before bedtime.
- Take 1 tsp. powder or two to four capsules of buffered C (containing calcium, magnesium, and potassium). This may be repeated during the night.
- Take two 500 mg capsules of ornithine (an amino acid available at health food stores) at bedtime.
- Use a serotonin extract or tincture. These preparations are available from physicians and some homeopathic and nutritional suppliers.
- Take PHP Insomnia Drops (complex homeopathic drops).
- Take the appropriate classical homeopathic remedy: *Nux vomica* if insomnia is due to abuse of coffee, alcohol, or drugs of any type; *Pulsatilla* when fixed ideas will not let you go to sleep; *Arnica* for physical overexertion physically or mentally that will not let you go to sleep; *Chamomilla* for physical pains that will not let you sleep; *Ignatia* when grief accompanied by sighing and yawning keeps you from sleeping.

- Take a capsule of valerian or skullcap up to three times a day, or drink a cup of valerian tea at bedtime.
- Drink a cup of lemon balm or peppermint tea daily.

Do the following:

- Check any medication or beverages you may be taking to see if they contain caffeine, which can cause insomnia.
- Establish a schedule and go to bed at the same time each night.
- Avoid tobacco and alcohol. They may seem to be relaxing at first, but will stimulate you later.
- Also avoid nasal decongestants and other cold medications late in the day.
- If you snore, elevate your head.
- Do deep breathing and other breathing techniques. (See Dr. Andrew Weil's breathing technique under Anxiety, above.)

▌ MENSTRUAL CRAMPS

Take the following:

- Take neutralizing doses of hormone extracts—progesterone or estrogen—to help relieve or control cramps.
- Take two calcium/magnesium capsules every four hours to help relieve cramps.
- Take essential fatty acids, such as evening primrose oil or black currant oil, in the amount recommended on the product, to help lessen menstrual cramps.
- Take vitamin B_6 (100 to 150 mg per day) to help relieve cramps and PMS symptoms. It should be taken in addition to a nonyeast source of B complex vitamins.
- Increase your buffered vitamin C intake to 5 tsp. daily about three days prior to your period. The increase in calcium, magnesium, and potassium will encourage

smooth uterine contraction rather than spasmodic, cramping contractions.

- Take BHI Female (a complex homeopathic tablet).
- Take Ovarian Drops, Female Liquescence, or Female Endocrine Axis (complex homeopathic drops) from PHP.
- Take Female+ by Vibrant Health to assist in production and flow of female hormones.
- Take the appropriate classical homeopathic remedy: *Belladonna* for acute pain that begins suddenly and ends suddenly; *Magnesia phosphorica* when cramps are relieved by pressure, warmth, and bending forward; *Colocynthis* if there is irritability and cramps are relieved by pressure, warmth, and bending over double; *Cimicifuga* when cramps that dart from side to side in the abdomen make the woman double over with pain and marked lower-back pain.
- Several herbs relieve menstrual cramping, including false unicorn, valerian, dong quai, pennyroyal, and vitex. They are available in easy-to-use form at health food stores.

Do the following:

- Do pelvic strengthening (Kegel) exercises daily to help relieve cramping during menses.
- Use castor oil packs on your lower abdomen at least three times per week for several months. This helps increase circulation, which will ease cramps, as well as aiding in detoxification. Soak a cotton cloth in cold-pressed castor oil and place the cloth on your abdomen. cover with plastic and put a heating pad or hot water bottle over it. Leave in place for 30 to 60 minutes.

Clean your skin with a baking soda and water solution afterward. You can reuse the cloth three to five times before washing it.

▌ MUSCLE AND JOINT PAIN

Take the following:

- Take two 500 mg DLPA (DL-phenylalanine) every four hours, with a tolerated painkiller, for greater and longer-lasting pain relief.
- Increase your vitamin C intake to bowel tolerance level.
- Take 500 to 1,000 mg magnesium daily to help relieve muscle spasms and pain.
- Take 99 mg potassium daily to help to relieve muscle cramping, especially premenstrually.
- Take 1,000 mg to 1,500 mg tryptophan for chronic pain (currently available in the U.S. by prescription only).
- Take two to four 500 mg capsules MSM (methylsulfonylmethane) daily. It is a natural, utilizable sulfur source that helps control pain and heal the joints.
- Take one to three 150 mg capsules organic germanium daily as needed, with pain medications, to enhance their effectiveness.
- Take 500 to 2,000 mg glucosamine sulfate and chondroitin sulfate daily. These nutrients strengthen connective tissue and joint integrity. They act as building blocks for connective tissue and other cementing materials that pack cells together.
- Take BHI Arthritis, (a complex homeopathic tablet) for the relief of pain.
- Use Large Joint or Small Joint Pain Drops (complex homeopathic drops) by PHP to help relieve discomfort in the joints.
- Take the appropriate classical homeopathic remedy: *Apis mellifica* when joints sting and burn with pain that is worse with warmth; *Bellis perennis* for pain from deep muscle injuries or injuries to the joint; *Bryonia* for muscle and joint pain made worse by motion; *Kali bichromicum* when joint pains alternate with digestive problems, diarrhea, or respiratory difficulties.
- Take 10 to 20 drops of fennel extract in warm water with honey, if desired, for joint pain. Use daily. Fennel oil can be rubbed on the painful joints.
- Take white willow bark, a natural source of salicin and a mild pain remedy similar to aspirin.

Do the following:

- Apply heat to help lower pain levels. Hot baths, heating pads, or wet towels can be used.
- Use Zeel, a BHI homeopathic cream, for soothing joint pain.
- Use Traumeel, a complex homeopathic cream that will help muscle pain.
- Exercise regularly, focusing on "range of motion" exercises to reduce pain and keep joints mobile.
- Exercise in water to remove the weight-bearing aspects of exercise.
- Use castor oil packs on painful joints and muscles to increase circulation and detoxify the joints.

▌ MUSCLE PULLS AND MILD SPRAINS

Take the following:

- Take *Arnica*, a classical homeopathic remedy, to heal bruises and injury from trauma.

Do the following:

- Apply ice immediately to help reduce

swelling. Continue using ice packs for 36 to 48 hours, depending on the severity of the injury.

- Use Traumeel, a complex homeopathic cream, to help reduce muscle pain or trauma.
- Use *Arnica* ointment to heal bruises and injury from trauma. *Caution:* Do not use *Arnica* on broken skin.

▌ SINUS PAIN AND CONGESTION

Take the following:

- Take 10,000 IU of vitamin A daily for the health of mucous membranes.
- Take 400 IU of vitamin E for speeding healing.
- Take BHI Sinus (a complex homeopathic tablet) to drain sinuses and relieve pain.
- Take PHP Sinusitis Drops (complex homeopathic drops) for temporary relief of sinus congestion and irritation.
- Take the appropriate classical homeopathic remedy: *Kali bichromicum* for sinus pain and congestion when the pain or pressure is worst above the root of the nose and when the discharge is extremely thick; *Pulsatilla* when sinus pain is worse at night, in a warm room, or with standing, stooping, or raising the eyes; *Silicea* when sinus pain is distinctly improved with pressure and warm applications; *Spigelia* when sinus pain begins after exposure to cold or cold, wet weather, or when pain is worse with stooping or bending the head forward.
- Goldenseal, 1 to 2 capsules up to three times daily, has an anti-inflammatory action that soothes irritated mucous membranes of sinusitis. *Caution:* Do not use goldenseal when pregnant.

Do the following:

- Apply heat to soothe sinus pain. Apply wet heat or a heating pad on low setting directly to the sinus area.
- Use vitamin C nose drops to reduce sinus congestion.
- Use Euphorbium Compositum nose drops (a homeopathic mixture by BHI) to drain the sinuses and relieve pain.
- Use NaSal or Ocean Spray nose drops to moisturize the nasal passages.
- Exercise regularly to keep nasal mucus flowing so it cannot back up, creating congestion.
- Use a salt water rinse, adapted from *The Yeast Syndrome* by Dr. John Trowbridge, to help moisturize dried nasal passages, reduce nasal mucous secretions, and relieve sore throat caused by post-nasal drainage. The mixture is inexpensive, and can be used throughout the day as often as needed, since it has no side effects.

1. Mix a solution of 1/2 tsp. sea salt or table salt to 1 cup warm water. Cool the solution to body temperature.
2. Fill an infant bulb syringe (available at pharmacies) with the solution.
3. Insert the narrow tip of the syringe into your right nostril first. Lean over a sink with your face downward and gently and slowly squeeze the solution well back into the nostril. Do not take a breath while the solution is in your nose. Gently blow out the solution into a tissue.
4. Gently sniff the solution remaining in your nose well back into the sinuses.
5. Repeat steps 3 and 4 with your left nostril.
6. The remaining solution can be kept refrigerated for later use, or can be used as a gargle to relieve a sore throat.

▊ SORE THROAT

Take the following:

- Take bowel-tolerance vitamin C daily.
- Take 600 IU of vitamin E daily to promote healing and tissue repair
- Take BHI Throat (a complex homeopathic tablet) to reduce pain and aid in healing)
- Take the appropriate classical homeopathic remedy: *Belladonna* when the throat is very red, accompanied by fever and flushed skin; *Rhus toxicodendron* for a painfully sore throat made better by warm drinks and warmth in general; *Lycopodium* when the sore throat is worse or begins on the right side and spreads to the left; *Argentum nitricum* for splinter like pain in the throat; *Mercurous* for a sore throat with tendency to salivate and drool, when throat is red and swollen, and there is pus or other white material on the tonsils or walls of the throat.
- Take fenugreek as a gargle to relieve a sore throat and swollen glands.
- Raspberry tea eases the pain of a sore throat.
- Ginger root and lemon steeped in hot water makes a soothing drink. Honey may be added to taste.

Do the following:

- Gargle with warm saline solution every 30 to 60 minutes to help ease sore throats. (Use the proportions listed under Salt Water Rinse, above.) Keeping the throat moist is the best way to soothe pain.
- Place acidophilus powder under your tongue and allow it to trickle down your throat to ease sore throat pain.
- Suck on zinc lozenges to reduce pain.
- Contact your physician for diagnosis and treatment if your sore throat becomes more severe or continues for longer than two or three days.

▊ TENSION AND STRESS

Take the following:

- Buffered vitamin C contains two ingredients (potassium and vitamin C) that aid in adrenal gland repair. The adrenal glands are overworked during episodes of stress and demand extra nutrients. Use 1 tsp. of powder dissolved in water.
- Take 100 mg of pantothenic acid (vitamin B_5) daily, which is also important for proper adrenal function. Take this in addition to a B complex vitamin.
- Take at least 500 mg of magnesium daily. Magnesium reduces muscle tension and is used by neurotransmitter pathways in the brain. During stress, mental activity is usually very active, and magnesium can be calming.
- Take Balance Neurotransmitter Complex (from Pain and Stress Center) to help relieve stress. Balancing neurotransmitters helps balance emotions and the perception of stress.
- Take Anti-Stress Drops by PHP (complex homeopathic drops), which stimulate rejuvenating and relaxing mechanisms.
- Take hops, a relaxing herb. Mix 1/2 tsp. in 1/2 cup water and drink daily.
- Use 1 tsp. of dried skullcap in 1 cup of hot water for tea.
- Mix 15 to 60 drops of passionflower extract in water. Drink daily.

Do the following:

- Running water helps reduce tension. The negative ions given off by water movement restore your body's electrical balance. The rhythm and sound of moving water (a stream, a fountain, rain, surf) is very soothing to the nervous system. Taking a shower or running water over your lower arms and hands are simple aids to reduce tension.

- With your fingertips, gently stroke your forehead from the center outward toward a point above the ears. Repeat in a slow rhythm.
- Use relaxation techniques daily, such as meditation or progressive relaxation, in which muscles are tightened and relaxed, starting with the feet and working up to the head. Remember that the body perceives repeated allergic reactions as stress.
- Practice deep breathing and exercise frequently during the day to help your body cope with both exogenous and endogenous forms of stress. Exercise releases endorphins, chemical that helps relieve stress.
- Talking with an understanding person helps put any problem into perspective and releases stress.
- Crying is a good physiological tension release. The tears release endorphins, which help our body cope with the stimuli of stress, as well as releasing chemicals that are produced during times of stress.

▌ VIRAL INFECTIONS

Take the following:

- Take six to eight capsules of Viricidin (lauric acid) per day to help control a viral infection, and continue this for two weeks beyond the end of the infection. If taken when symptoms first appear, infection can sometimes be prevented. Viricidin will at least reduce the infection's duration and severity.
- Take three to six capsules of Monolaurin per day to help control a viral infection, but it also must be continued for two weeks after the infection subsides. If taken when symptoms first appear, the infection can sometimes be prevented. (Take either Viricidin or Monolaurin, but not both.)
- Take 3,000 to 4,000 mg of lysine in divided doses during the day to help control a viral infection.
- Be certain to take bowel-tolerance vitamin C daily.
- Oscillococcinum (a homeopathic preparation available in health stores) to stimulate the body's natural defense mechanism and help relieve flu symptoms such as fever, chills, body aches, and pains.
- Use Engystol, tablets or injectable (an immune system stimulator made by BHI). It will abort viral infections if taken promptly, and will reduce the severity and length of the infection.
- Take V'rus (a complex homeopathic remedy made by Vibrant Health) for flu and viral conditions. It aids in immune support.
- Take the appropriate classical homeopathic remedy: *Gelsemium* for flu characterized by chills, which run up and down the back, in people who do not want to be disturbed; *Rhus toxicodendron* when very restless with influenza, and muscles are stiff and achy when lying still for any time; *Eupatorium perfoliatum* when there is severe aching and pain deep inside the bones, with bruised soreness all over the body; *Arnica* when it feels as if the person has been "run over by a truck."
- Take one capsule of echinacea, or liquid echinacea in the dosage recommended on

the product, three times a day to fight a viral infection.

- St. John's wort, 10 to 15 drops in a glass of water daily, helps the body fight viral infections.

Do the following:

- Use neutralizing doses of fluogen extract to help relieve flu symptoms.
- Drink larger amounts of water.
- Cut back on foods containing arginine. Arginine feeds viruses and is contained in nuts, chocolate, barley, corn, gluten, oats, and coconut.
- See Viruses in chapter 16, for additional help.

▍ WHEEZING AND TIGHT CHEST

Take the following:

- Take repeated doses of vitamin C, alternating buffered C and ascorbic acid, for wheezing or a tightening in your chest caused by an allergic reaction.
- Take 1,000 mg magnesium daily in divided doses, in oral, sublingual, or intramuscular preparations, to help reduce wheezing. Magnesium relaxes smooth muscle.
- Take 10,000 IU vitamin A and 10 mg manganese daily to strengthen mucous membranes and enhance cilia function in the bronchial area. Do not exceed 8,000 IU vitamin A daily if you are pregnant.
- Take pyridoxine (vitamin B_6), about 100 to 200 mg daily for four weeks, to help reduce bronchospasms. Take a high-potency B complex vitamin along with vitamin B_6.
- Take Mucolytic Drainage Formula by PHP (complex homeopathic drops) to aid in dissolving the mucus that can be present in chest congestion and wheezing.

- Take BHI Asthma or Bronchitis (a complex homeopathic tablet) to help relieve wheezing.
- Take Asthma Drops by PHP (complex homeopathic drops) for temporary relief of asthma.
- Take the appropriate classic homeopathic remedy: *Arsenicum album* when there is fear, restlessness, weakness, and aggravation of symptoms after midnight; *Pulsatilla* for wheezing that begins or is worse in the evening or at night, with an accumulation of phlegm that must be coughed up; *Ipecac* for wheezing with much rattling of mucus in the chest; *Spongia* when breathing is labored and noisy sounding, like whistling or sawing.
- Steep the chopped leaves and stems of parsley in hot water and drink daily as needed to soothe asthma.
- Mullein oil or 1 Tbsp. of the dry herb in 8 ounces of warm water will reduce irritation due to bronchitis and asthma.

Do the following:

- Avoid the offending allergens as much as possible. In many cases, wheezing is triggered by an allergic reaction.
- Sip warm liquids to help relax your throat and bronchial muscles.
- Make a conscious effort to relax your throat and chest muscles. Breathe deeply and exhale completely in a slow rhythm; this helps alleviate the sensation of panic associated with breathing difficulties.
- Avoid breathing cold air. Wear a scarf that can be quickly pulled up over your nose and mouth when you are suddenly exposed to cold air.

CHAPTER 22

Finding Safe Healthcare

A LL OF US need medical attention from time to time for illnesses and emergencies that we cannot handle on our own. This need for medical help can become difficult to obtain for people with allergies. Most physicians are aware only of the pollen allergies that trigger coughing, sneezing, wheezing, and runny nose. They do not acknowledge food allergy unless it causes immediate asthma, hives, or anaphylactic shock when the food is consumed. They also do not acknowledge or accept chemical sensitivity. Some do accept that infection with microorganisms can have a minimal allergic component.

In addition, most physicians treat with pharmaceuticals, which people with food and chemical sensitivities have difficulty tolerating. Although there are many natural alternatives, as discussed in chapter 21, most physicians are not aware of them. Their belief system and training is such that they prefer to depend on drugs to treat the health problems of their patients. Certainly there are many instances in which the pharma-

ceutical indicated is necessary, in spite of possible side effects. However, for the allergic person, for the majority of the time, alternatives must be of primary consideration, and drugs secondary.

These beliefs of physicians regarding allergies and sensitivities and pharmaceuticals complicate receiving medical care in which there is an adequate understanding of basic allergies, in addition to a knowledge of nontoxic methods to treat illnesses. However, with investigation, you can locate a caring, understanding, and knowledgeable physician. Even if the physicians available do not understand allergies, if they will listen to you respectfully and truly hear what you say, a working relationship in which both of you can learn can be established.

This chapter contains information that will help you select a physician, both a primary care physician and, if necessary, a surgeon. It has helpful hints for surviving a hospital stay, as well as a section on choosing a dentist and information on dental materials.

> ## Know Your Tolerated Medications and Alternatives
>
> *Be aware that any physician who is not an environmental medicine physician will want to treat you with standard pharmacological medications. People with chemical sensitivities frequently do not tolerate these medications because of poorly functioning detoxification pathways. Those with food allergies or sensitivities may also have difficulty with some medications. It is important for you to become knowledgeable about tolerated alternatives in order to avoid a medication crisis.*

Choosing Your Physician

We all need a primary care physician to monitor our health, to care for us when we are ill, and to turn to in case of emergency. In addition, the sensitive person needs a physician who has training in environmental medicine. Ideally, your physician should be both a primary care and an environmental medicine physician; however, this is not always possible because of the limited number of physicians practicing environmental medicine.

If there is not an environmental medicine specialist in your community or in a town near you, you will have to choose a local doctor to be your primary care physician. Ask your friends, relatives, and other health professionals to determine whether there is an open-minded, innovative physician available in your area. You will want this person to be willing to continue as your primary care physician even if you receive care from physicians in other facilities or cities.

Once you find a likely candidate, go to the office to make your appointment. This will give you the chance to determine whether you will be able to tolerate the exposures there. If you are chemically sensitive you will need to determine the following.

- Is the office clean and well-maintained?
- Does it have an odor of cleaning supplies?
- Is there a strong smell of personal care products, room deodorizers, or other substances generally used in medical offices?
- Is the doctor approximately on schedule, or is the waiting room full of people? This could mean you would have more exposures if you must stay in the office for longer periods of time.
- Is smoking allowed in the building?

If the office seems tolerable, make an appointment for a consultation with the doctor. Ask the receptionist if the doctor treats other patients with chemical sensitivities. If so, this will be a help to you. If not, the interest and sympathy expressed by the reception staff may indicate whether this office will be cooperative.

When you have your consultation, explain that you need a primary care physician to oversee your routine medical care, and to care for you when you are ill. It would also be helpful if you have a brief letter from your environmental medicine physician, outlining the pertinent details of your condition. Invite the doctor to call your environmental medicine physician at any time to receive additional information to help with your care.

You will need to pay particular attention to determining whether you can easily talk to this physician. Is he or she truly listening to what you say? You want the doctor to treat you with courtesy and to be open enough to accept what you say about your condition as true. If the physician immediately refutes your statements, argues with you over your present treatment, or appears uninterested in cooperating, you will know that this person is not the right physician for you.

A physician with whom you can talk freely and develop a rapport is the person who can best help you. Even if he or she knows little about allergies or chemical sensitivities, you can, over time, share information so that the doctor can learn more about helping you.

■■ CHOOSING AN ENVIRONMENTAL MEDICINE PHYSICIAN

Your environmental medicine physician should be able to answer your questions about your condition, the treatment he or she can offer, and possible outcomes. This type of physician will take a lengthy, detailed history, in addition to asking you to fill out a comprehensive questionnaire, which is very important in helping to make a complete diagnosis and to identify all of your health problems.

In addition, you should be given educational literature to help you learn about and understand your condition. Your environmental medicine physician should provide suggestions to improve the quality of your life, as well as referrals to any support groups that might be helpful to you. This type of physician will consider you to be a partner in your treatment, and you will be assuming equal responsibility in your health

care. No one can offer a "magic pill" that will instantly cure you, and it will take effort on your part to get well. However, with a caring and competent physician to help and encourage you, your health can be improved to levels you might not have thought possible!

The organizations listed in Recommended Sources and Organizations can help you locate a physician who will have a treatment philosophy similar to the one described in this book. These organizations can refer you to a physician in your area (if there is one) who can diagnose and treat food, chemical, and inhalant sensitivities. As with any organizations, these groups are composed of people with widely differing personality types, areas of interest, and skill.

The Allergic Person's Guide to Surgery

Surgery is a traumatic physical and psychological experience for everyone. Those with allergies must be concerned about many additional aspects of the surgical experience. Since sensitivities vary greatly in type and severity, the amount of preparation you need depends on your situation. Be sure to take an active part in your care, as successful surgery is always a team effort.

If your primary care physician does not perform surgery, you will have to find a surgeon. Your physician may be able to recommend a surgeon to you, or you may have to make your own investigation. Talk to people whose opinion you trust, or who have had positive surgical experiences. Investigate the procedure you are to have at a medical library so that you will be familiar with the possible techniques the surgeon might use.

Also investigate the credentials of the surgeons available to you.

Make a consultation appointment with the surgeon and ask about the following concerns. As with a primary care physician, ease and clarity of communication are important.

- How many times the surgeon has successfully performed this particular operation. Ten or more times tends to guarantee the safest results.
- Ask about the technique this surgeon prefers to use and the possible complications for this particular type of surgery.
- Find out the usual symptoms resulting from the surgery, the usual recovery period, and the likelihood of the need for a transfusion.
- Because you are likely to need some type of pain control, inquire about the surgeon's philosophy and which pain control medications are likely to be prescribed.
- Also find out which anesthesiologist and hospital the surgeon prefers to use.

Unless your surgery is an emergency, get a second opinion. Most physicians do not mind patients getting a second opinion. This step may prevent unnecessary surgery, and will reduce your anxiety regarding its necessity. However, do not solicit the second opinion from your surgeon's partner, as they will have a similar philosophy.

▌▌ SURVIVING THE HOSPITAL

If you are unfamiliar with the hospital where the surgery will be performed, you should make an inspection tour. During your visit, observe the following to help you determine your ability to tolerate the hospital.

- Is the building well maintained?
- Are the emergency exits, fire extinguishers, and smoke detectors clearly visible?
- Are the patient rooms clean and adequately furnished?
- Can windows be opened?
- Are the rooms air-conditioned? (In some climates, this is a necessity.)
- Is there a thermostat in each room?
- Does each room have a private bathroom?
- Are there grab bars in the bathroom?
- Do the rooms and halls smell of cleaning products, sterilizing solutions, perfumes, or room deodorizers.
- Can the call buttons be reached easily?
- Are fresh fruits and vegetables served?
- Will the kitchen accommodate special diets?
- Do the visiting hours seem reasonable?
- Does the staff seem friendly?
- Are there enough nurses, nurses' aides, and orderlies on duty?
- Is the staff cleanly and neatly dressed?

When you talk to hospital admissions personnel, ask for a no-smoking room. If it is available and affordable, request a private room. If you have to share a room with another person, you will be exposed to their personal care products as well as those of visitors. Obviously, you will have no control over the gifts, flowers, or books your roommate will receive. If you have to share a room, however, you can insist that your roommates be nonsmokers, and that they not be allowed to use scented products. When you meet your roommates, either you or a family member should explain your problems tactfully so that they will understand and cooperate.

Before your surgery, you should also inform hospital housekeeping personnel about your chemical allergies, if any. Ask that room deodorizers, disinfectants, detergents, soaps, and bleaches not be used in your room during your stay. Suggest that clear, hot water or baking soda be used instead, or you may want to provide a "safe" cleaner for use in your room.

If you plan to take an air cleaner with you, ask if someone on the staff needs to see it first. Some hospitals require that the wiring and plug type be inspected by the hospital engineer ahead of time. If you need to take your own bedding, you must also notify the housekeeping staff.

Discuss your major food allergies, if any, with the hospital dietitian, keeping this list as brief as possible. Do not give the dietitian a list of 50 foods to which you are sensitive if only 6 cause significant reactions; you do not want to cause confusion and disbelief. Ask only that the major foods to which you are allergic be omitted. It may be necessary to educate the dietitian about the contents of prepackaged foods and about reading labels.

Suggest that whole, unprocessed foods be served, and inspect each meal tray to be sure that the foods you want to avoid have not inadvertently been served. If it is possible or advisable, with your physician's approval, arrange to have food brought in for you by relatives or friends. Some hospitals may be less willing or able to help.

▮▮ SURVIVING THE SURGERY

Make a list of your questions about the surgery, and make an appointment well in advance of the operation to talk with your envi-ronmental medicine physician, surgeon, anesthesiologist.

Your environmental medicine physician may want to test you for sensitivity to surgical scrub, tape, suture materials, and local and general anesthetic, if you do not already have this information. You also need to find out which vitamin and mineral supplements you should take or increase, as well as any other nutrients you might need.

After you have discussed your sensitivities with your environmental medicine physician, you need to talk about the following specific items with your surgeon:

- any other medical problems you have (such as asthma or diabetes)
- any past severe allergic (anaphylactic) reactions you have experienced
- your specific chemical, food, or inhalant allergies and their symptoms
- your medication sensitivities
- your IV intolerance (lactose IVs are milk-based but also contain some D5W (5% dextrose in water); dextrose IVs are corn-based)
- your allergies to surgical scrub (Betadine), tape (paper tape is usually tolerated), or suture materials (nylon or silk are generally used)
- present medication that you need to continue during your hospital stay, including your allergy extracts (you will need your surgeon to write the order for you to be able to take these while you are in the hospital)
- vitamin/mineral supplements and other nutrients you need to take during your hospital stay (you will need your surgeon to write the order for you to be able to take these while you are in the hospital)

Acupuncture and Hypnosis

Acupuncture has been used for centuries in other countries to aid in the control of pain caused during surgery. It is sometimes used alone, and at other times it is used in conjunction with more standard anesthesia. If your surgeon and anesthesiologist are willing, and if there is a competent and cooperative acupuncturist in your area, you may want to investigate the possibility of using a combination of acupuncture and anes-

thesia for your surgery. This could lessen the volume of pharmacologicals necessary to perform your surgery.

Hypnosis can be helpful in preparing the patient for more extensive surgery. In some cases of repair or removal of skin lesions, local anesthetic may not be required when hypnosis is used. A combination of acupuncture and hypnosis may also be helpful in many surgical cases.

- the possibility of the need for a blood transfusion and your desire to donate your own blood for that purpose. These arrangements need to be made well in advance, as your body needs several weeks to recover from giving blood before undergoing surgery.
- the availability of oxygen in your room for treatment of your allergy symptoms (such as wheezing and chest tightness). Oxygen will aid in clearing almost all allergic reactions. You will need your surgeon to write an order stating that you may use the oxygen to clear a reaction. You may also need to take your own ceramic mask if you have difficulty tolerating plastic oxygen masks.

It is also very important that you talk to your anesthesiologist well in advance of your scheduled surgery. Although you will meet with the anesthesiologist when you have your presurgery blood work done, because you may need special considerations it is important to have discussed them well ahead of time. Be certain to be totally honest about

your weight and height, as medication and anesthesia doses are computed on this basis.

Several anesthesia medications can cause allergic reactions and the anesthesiologist needs to be aware of your allergies. Be certain to speak to the person who will be administering your anesthesia. Discuss the following items that apply to your situation:

- any history or present condition of asthma or throat swelling
- your medication allergies
- your specific chemical, food, or inhalant allergies and their symptoms
- your present medications

The anesthetic formula that works well for most allergic people is 100 percent oxygen for five minutes, followed by a bolus of Pentothal or Brevital to induce anesthesia. Anectine or Curare can be administered to paralyze muscles during the surgery. Sublimaze can be used to obliterate memory, and Innovar or Demerol are usually well tolerated. Of course, known allergies to any of these medications would prevent their use. A new anesthetic, Diprivan (propofol), is being used by many anesthesiologists. It has a rapid onset, and the patient eliminates it more rapidly, minimizing aftereffects. However, propofol is an emulsion, which contains soybean oil, glycerin, and egg lecithin. People with allergies to soy, egg, or glycerine may react to this anesthetic.

❚ PREPARING FOR SURGERY

For as long as possible before your surgery, reduce your total allergic load. Strictly avoid all exposure to the foods, chemicals, and inhalants to which you are allergic so that your immune system can be as strong as possible before the stress of surgery. Also increase your intake of vitamin C, as it strengthens your immune system, promotes wound healing, lessens post-surgical pain, and detoxifies your body of medications and anesthesia—but do not take it the night before surgery because it reduces the effectiveness of the anesthetic. Vitamin C supplements can be resumed as soon as you can tolerate something by mouth, if approved by your surgeon.

Vitamin E should be stopped two weeks prior to surgery and should not be resumed until two weeks afterwards, because it has anticoagulant properties and can result in excessive bleeding during and after surgery. Begin taking coenzyme Q_{10} if you are not already doing so. Both it and organic germanium act as buffers against the effects of hypoxia (oxygen deficiency in body tissues) during surgery and combat the free radicals produced by damaged tissue.

Make a list of special items you need to take to the hospital, such as soap, shampoo, nutritional supplements, allergy extracts, charcoal mask, air cleaner, bottled water, bedding, bathrobe, and pajamas or nightgown that are "safe" for you.

Once you have been admitted to the hospital—and before surgery—talk to the nurses at your station. They need to know if you have allergies to flowers, plants, or molds so that live plants will not be placed in your room. You must also inform them of your medication allergies, to prevent accidental administration of a medication that could cause a serious reaction when your immune system is already weakened by surgery. Some extremely sensitive people may also need to ask the nurses and aides not to wear perfumes, scented hand lotion, or scented hair spray.

Support from your family and friends during this time is especially important. They can watch for and prevent exposures that might cause a reaction when you are unable to be vigilant. You may want to have someone sit with you during the first two days and nights after your surgery, but be sure they are aware of the foods and other substances you need to avoid.

❚ FOLLOWING SURGERY

After the surgery, you can do several things to speed your recovery. Move around as soon as possible, within the limits set by your surgeon. This prevents fluid from collecting in your lungs, causing further complications such as pneumonia. Muscles, nerves, and many body functions begin to suffer from just a few days of inactivity, so you should exercise as soon as your condition permits. Begin your exercise program slowly and increase as tolerated; walking is a good starting point. Do only what is permitted by your surgeon and what feels comfortable to you.

Exercise, increased water intake, vitamin C, organic germanium, and coenzyme Q_{10} help to detoxify the medications and anesthesia in your body. Increase your vitamin C intake until you reach your bowel tolerance level, then take a maintenance dosage just slightly below that amount. These nutrients promote healing of your surgical wound, help reduce pain, and increase your sense of well-being.

Your diet is another important factor in your recovery. Once you are at home you can avoid allergenic foods easily. Stay away from high-sugar and "empty calorie" foods; focus on fruits, vegetables, meats, fish, and whole grains.

Finally, allow yourself to get plenty of rest and do not push yourself to recover too quickly. Each person's body recovers at its own rate. Give your body and immune system the time they need to rebuild after the stress of surgery.

While these suggestions are a good starting point, there may be additional problems or situations for you to consider. With careful planning and patience, however, you can manage well, even with allergies, in a hospital setting.

Dental Care for Allergic People

Our teeth are living structures—even their enamel, which most of us think of as a white, hard, inanimate casing, is alive. Our teeth are intended to last us for a lifetime. If we do not care for them properly, however, they can become a source of pain, and can adversely affect our overall health. Diseased teeth can become a focus of infection. Improper grinding surfaces can result in poor digestion, which can lead to food sensitivity. Materials used in teeth restoration can be toxic. Regular dental care and personal dental hygiene are imperative for good health.

▌▌DENTAL HYGIENE

Good dental hygiene should include brushing and flossing after each meal and at bedtime. Chemically sensitive people should use a natural bristle toothbrush with a bone handle. Purchase a new toothbrush when you are sick, as this may help you to recover more quickly. Bacteria and yeast that can continue to live on your toothbrush for up to one month can extend the length of your sickness. A study done in the 1980s by the University of Oklahoma in Oklahoma City found that the organisms causing pneumonia, stomach ulcers, strep throat, sinus disease, upset stomach, and diarrhea are commonly found on toothbrushes. Store your toothbrush in a dry place to keep toothbrush contamination to a minimum.

Baking soda is a good substitute for toothpaste, although there are a few health store toothpastes that are acceptable (most commercial toothpastes contain glycerine and corn syrup, plus flavorings, coloring, and artificial sweeteners). Sodium lauryl sulfate, contained in most toothpastes, causes canker sores in some people. This substance is not necessarily listed on the toothpaste label.

A good mouthwash is a capful of 3 percent food-grade hydrogen peroxide, several pinches of baking soda, and a little bit of water. Vitamin C (ascorbic acid) dissolved in water also makes an effective mouthwash; use three times per day. Follow with a water rinse to prevent damage to the tooth enamel.

Proper nutrition also will contribute to your health and aid in maintaining gum and tooth quality. Vitamin C, organic germanium, and coenzyme Q_{10} are important in restoring and preserving gum integrity. Calcium and magnesium are also essential for healthy tooth enamel and strong root and bone structure.

Taking proper care of your teeth is important, not only for your general health, but in order to avoid the exposure of restoration materials used in fillings, crowns, bridges, and dentures. Good dental hygiene will help protect your teeth.

■ CHOOSING A DENTIST

Choosing a healthcare professional is often difficult, and when allergies and chemical sensitivities must be considered, it becomes even more complicated. Most medical and dental offices are loaded with chemical exposures, and many health professionals and their staff have minimal or no understanding of allergies.

If you do not have a suitable dentist, perhaps the best person to ask for a recommendation is the physician treating your sensitivities. You may also check with friends and acquaintances who have similar problems; their dentists may be appropriate for you.

When you are considering a dentist, go to the office rather than calling to make your appointment. Observation will help you determine whether the office is safe for you.

- Does the office appear to be clean and well maintained?

- Can you detect chemical odors, strong perfumes, or tobacco smoke?
- Does the staff seem interested in what you have to say, and do they appear to be cooperative after you explain your limitations?
- Is the staff wearing scented personal care products?
- Does the dentist appear to be on schedule, or is the waiting room full of people?
- How many treatment rooms does the dentist use? Generally, you will spend less time in an office with fewer rooms.
- Is the atmosphere one of disorganization and stress, or of calm, efficient functioning?

Introduce yourself to the receptionist, and ask for an appointment for an examination/consultation. Explain that you have chemical sensitivities and may need some special help, but do not go into extreme detail. The receptionist may not know about chemical sensitivities, and you do not want to seen antagonistic so that the office staff will be unwilling to help you. Simply say that because of your chemical sensitivities, some common materials and exposures can make you ill.

Make it clear that your physician has recommended that you receive your dental treatment:

- in the absence of aftershave; perfume; fabric softener; scented hair sprays, hand lotions, and deodorants; and tobacco odors on the dentist and assistants.
- with a minimum of chemical exposures within the office.
- after the dentist has talked with your physician (a simple letter from your physician may be helpful).

If the staff's initial response seems favorable, make an appointment for the examination/consultation. The first appointment on a Monday may be best for you, since the office will have aired out over the weekend.

If, after you leave the office, you decide that the exposures are too great, or that you will not receive the cooperation you need, cancel your appointment. It might be wise to wait a day or two to be sure of your decision.

During your first examination appointment, you can discuss your specific problems with the dentist, as well as the proposed treatment plan. If it seems that there are too many exposures, or that the dentist is not cooperative, you will need to look for another dentist. If everything seems to be acceptable, and you make more appointments, space your visits far enough apart to give you time to recover from the exposures you do encounter.

During your discussion with the dentist, explain the type of symptoms you generally experience, and indicate that your physician is willing to answer any questions. While you want your dentist to understand your problems, you do not want him or her to be afraid to treat you.

▮▮ CHEMICAL EXPOSURES IN DENTAL OFFICES

In addition to general office exposures, you will have to consider the exposure to dental materials used in your mouth. There are five chemicals indigenous to most dental offices: formaldehyde, acrylic, nitrous oxide, phenol, and mercury. Mercury is the most toxic of these substances. There are literally thousands of materials a dentist may use, how-

ever. Some people tolerate the majority of these, while more severely ill people may have difficulty with many of them.

The dentist will examine your teeth and will probably need to take X-rays unless you have recent X-rays you can give him or her. A lead apron should be provided to cover your vital organs as a precaution, although today's X-ray equipment is relatively safe. The X-ray film is wrapped in vinyl, which may be a problem for severely sensitive people. X-ray film wrapped in paper is available.

Professional cleaning (prophylaxis) by the dentist or hygienist is an important part of dental care. Plaque which has hardened to calculus is impossible for you to remove with home dental care. The final step in prophylaxis is polishing the teeth with a paste made of pumice, water, flavorings, and colorings. You can request an alternative material, made of flower of pumice moistened with water.

Many dentists now use fluoride treatment for both children and adults. This is a controversial measure. Some authorities feel it has no benefit after age 11, while others feel it is beneficial for all ages. Still others regard fluoride treatment as administering a poison because of its toxicity.

People sensitive to fluoride should avoid this treatment. The fluoride solutions commonly used all contain a flavoring agent to mask the taste of the fluoride compound, and some also have a coloring agent. In addition to the toxicity of the fluoride itself, the flavoring and coloring agents may also cause reactions in sensitive people.

If study models are necessary, the dentist must make an impression of your teeth. The impression material usually used contains alginate, flavorings, and colorings. There are no problem-free alternatives, so it is best to avoid study models unless they are necessary for making crowns, partial plates, or dentures.

Local anesthetics used during dental procedures are frequently a problem for people with chemical sensitivities. If testing is available, it would be wise to have local anesthetics screened for tolerance before dental work is begun. Hypnosis and acupuncture can be safe alternatives to local anesthetic. (See The Allergic Person's Guide to Surgery, earlier in this chapter.)

▮▮ PROBLEMS WITH AMALGAM FILLINGS

Amalgam fillings (silver fillings) contain approximately 50 percent mercury and 20 to 30 percent silver, with zinc, copper, and tin making up the balance. Amalgams release mercury in minute amounts, especially during chewing. Mercury is also released when amalgams are polished as the final step in prophylaxis. The mercury itself may cause problems for many people, or may contribute to a toxic overload phenomenon. For a person with numerous sensitivities, those fillings should be removed and replaced with a tolerated alternative.

While the American Dental Association, the Canadian Dental Association, and most dentists believe that amalgam fillings are safe, debate over the fillings and their mercury content has flourished since the 1930s. In the 1990s, amalgam studies done on sheep at the University of Calgary's Faculty of Medicine in Alberta showed that labeled mercury from amalgam fillings appeared in organs and tissues within 29 days after the fillings were placed in the mouths of the sheep. Whole-body scanning revealed three absorption sites: the lungs, gastrointestinal tract, and jaw tissue. Once absorbed, high concentrations of mercury from the dental amalgams were found in the kidneys and liver of the sheep.

According to Dr. Anne O. Summers of the University of Georgia at Athens, Georgia, the release of mercury from dental fillings increases the mercury resistance and antibiotic resistance of common mouth and intestinal bacteria. In this study, performed on monkeys, the mercury-resistant bacteria were also resistant to such antibiotics as ampicillin, erythromycin, streptomycin, kanamycin, chloamphenicol, and tetracycline.

Other studies have demonstrated that mercury does leach out of amalgam fillings. The American Dental Association admits this fact, but maintains that the mercury levels are too low to be harmful. However, mercury is considered a hazardous material even before it is put into the mouth. When amalgams are removed, they must be disposed of by the dentist as hazardous waste.

▮ AMALGAM REMOVAL

Some dentists will remove and replace amalgams with safer materials. You should choose a dentist who is experienced in mercury removal. The amalgam fillings must be removed in the proper order because of the "charges" that build up on them. The filling with the largest charge, whether positive or negative, should be removed first. The "charges" are the result of the "battery effect"

Detoxifying from Mercury Amalgams

It takes several months—sometimes years—for the body to completely detoxify from mercury after amalgam fillings have been removed and replaced. Beta-carotene; vitamin C; vitamin B$_1$; vitamin B$_2$; vitamin E; glutathione, cysteine, or methionine; manganese; magnesium; selenium; and zinc all aid in detoxification. Taking detoxification baths or dry sauna treatments will speed the detoxification process. (See Detoxification, chapter 23.)

Many people improve dramatically after having their amalgams removed; others see little or no improvement. Some people require a chelation material, DMPS (2,3-dimercaptopropane-1-sulfonate), to remove the mercury in their tissues. An environmental medicine physician can order tests to determine if chelation with DMPS is needed. This procedure is totally safe unless the person is sensitive to DMPS.

of dissimilar metals in the mouth in the presence of saliva. Continuous exposure to small currents, such as these on the amalgams, stresses the endocrine glands and decreases immune system activity.

Other precautions should also be taken when amalgam fillings are removed. Using a rubber dam in the mouth (if latex sensitivity is not a problem) and maintaining an oxygen supply during amalgam removal reduces the absorption of mercury released as the filling is drilled out. Vitamin C should not be taken for 24 hours before your appointment, as it reduces the effectiveness of the anesthetics used.

■■ ALTERNATIVE FILLING MATERIALS

Restorations or fillings should be carefully considered, since they become a permanent part of your teeth. To be considered an acceptable restoration material, a substance must be:
• nonallergenic
• durable

• biologically inert
• soft enough to fit into the cavity preparation, and then harden
• stable, able to withstand chewing forces
• able to expand and contract similarly to the tooth
• a poor heat conductor, so it does not damage the tooth pulp
• able to seal the cavity preparation to prevent decay

Composite fillings and gold restorations (used mainly in back teeth) are alternatives to amalgam fillings.

Silicate fillings are used in front teeth and contain silver, alumina, calcium or sodium phosphate, calcium fluoride, sodium aluminum fluoride, phosphoric acid, and aluminum and zinc phosphate.

Composite fillings may be used for both front and back teeth. They bond well with enamel and make the tooth more resistant to decay at the margin between the tooth and the filling. Composites are basically ground glass powder with quartz fillers in a plastic binder. Other ingredients may include methylmethacrylate or aromatic dimethacrylates with additives of urethane, diacrylate, vinyl silane, benzoyl peroxide, and benzophenone ether. Composites may be either light cured or chemically cured, depending on their formulation. Sensitive people tolerate the light-cured form better than the chemically cured form.

Gold alloyed with palladium, silver, and trace amounts of copper, iron, indium, tin, and zinc is used in cast restorations. Crowns, inlays, and bridgework are all cast restorations. Non-precious metal crowns and bridges are an alternative, but nickel should not be used—it has both toxic and allergenic properties. The cement used to put cast restorations in place can be a problem for the sensitive person, and it may be necessary to test different brands.

Porcelain, composed of minerals in a glass matrix, may be used for crowns. Gold restorations are an alternative.

Temporary fillings are used while crowns and bridgework are being prepared. They contain zinc oxide, eugenol, and trace amounts of alcohol, acetic acid, and silica. There are no substitutes with less toxic properties.

People who need dentures are subjected both to the impression materials and the denture materials. Acrylic is the most popular material used in the construction of dentures. Most acrylic denture materials contain methylmethacrylate, benzoyl peroxide, butyl phthalate, hydroquinone, and ethylglycol dimethacrylate. Any of these ingredients can be allergenic and trigger contact dermatitis and respiratory problems.

■ OTHER DENTAL PROCEDURES

Recent evidence points to the possibility that root canals may also be a problem for some people. Bacteria remaining in the tubules of the tooth are anaerobic (can survive without oxygen) and produce toxins. If these toxins seep out of the tooth and into the body, they can overload the immune system. A variety of symptoms and seemingly unrelated problems can be produced by these toxins. A gradual decline in health after a root canal signals a problem, and EAV testing can confirm the diagnosis.

Cavitations are another source of dental problems. They are a hole in the jawbone, containing necrotic bone and usually resulting from an extraction that did not heal properly. Bacteria become trapped in the bone after the extraction and remain in the jaw as a chronic infection. As many as 20 to 30 species of bacteria have been isolated from cavitations. Toxins from these bacteria can cause numerous health problems. Cavitations may also develop around the root of a root canal tooth, particularly if the root canal was performed on an abscessed tooth.

A thin, hard layer of bone over the area prevents these areas from showing on X-ray. The best way to diagnose cavitations is by EAV testing. Surgical intervention to remove the necrotic bone is currently the available treatment for cavitations, although injection therapy and other methods are being researched. The existence of cavitations, their significance, and treatment is a source of controversy in dentistry.

CHAPTER 23

Detoxification

A NEW AND MORE EFFECTIVE approach to medicine has been emerging in recent years. It is slowly and carefully identifying and correcting the underlying causes of inferior health. Many people have been treated with "band-aid" approaches, and the use of masking drugs such as antidepressants, tranquilizers, calcium channel blockers, muscle relaxants, painkillers, vasodilators or vasoconstrictors, and many others. Instead of helping, these drugs have added to an already heavy body burden of toxic substances.

Many of these people are burdened with so many symptoms that they are unable to separate one from another, or to trace any single symptom to a single cause. Early warning symptoms have been ignored or suppressed for so long that vital body functions start to deteriorate. Underlying this complicated end result is a complicated cause.

One of the insidious causes of symptoms is an overload of toxins, chemicals, and biochemical debris that our body is unable to properly detoxify and excrete. This cumulative toxicity has developed as a direct result of society's demands over the past 50 years for "better living through modern chemistry."

The adaptive of our biochemistry is amazing, but it has limits. When the detoxification pathways in our body are too heavily bombarded, they are unable to complete their task, and the remaining chemical load will damage the normal functions of each cell, leading to end organ damage (disease).

As the body becomes increasingly burdened with both exogenous (external) and endogenous (internal) chemicals, it becomes more reactive to smaller and smaller amounts of a greater variety of foods, chemicals, and inhalants. The person's allergies and sensitivities become worse and worse. This eventually leads to a condition called pan-reactivity, in which the person will react to almost all substances. Depending on one's genetic target organs and individual susceptibility, a wide variety of symptoms or syndromes are possible. Unless the person

Fat Cells Are Chemical Repositories

Over 300 chemicals have been identified in human fat tissue. Fat molecules are very mobile when our body is stressed. The molecules, along with their toxic burdens, are released from the fat tissue and cell membranes into the bloodstream to circulate freely, causing damage and symptoms. If our bodies are unable to detoxify and excrete these chemicals, they return to be stored in the fat cells and cell membranes. They will continue to be released and restored periodically unless we undertake detoxification procedures.

Fat cells can be mobilized by heat exposure, exercise, emotional stress, illness, and fasting (including the fast during sleep). This mobilization during sleep may explain the severe morning symptoms experienced by some sensitive people. The intermittent, internal release of chemicals can also account for "unexplained" worsening of symptoms during recovery, even while the sensitive person is minimizing exposures to external chemicals and receiving treatment for chemical sensitivity.

is treated for allergies and sensitivities and undergoes detoxification procedures, organ damage and serious health problems will result.

In her book *Tired or Toxic*, Dr. Sherry Rogers of Syracuse, New York, compares the detoxification pathways to a janitorial service, which has the job of ridding our body of daily accumulations of unwanted dirt and stains (biochemical debris). When the janitorial service works properly and efficiently, the debris is swept along a biochemical transformation pathway, changed into a less toxic form, and prepared for dumping (excretion). We are all familiar with our body's excretion areas— liver, lungs, gastrointestinal tract, kidneys and bladder, and skin. When the workload for the janitorial service is too great, some of the debris (toxins or chemicals) is not transformed properly, and more potent toxic chemicals are created. The new chemicals will continue to damage our

body, causing intoxication (too high a level of chemical debris).

Xenobiotic is a term coined to describe foreign chemicals in the body. These undesirable foreign materials enter our body through direct skin contact, through the lungs as we breathe, and through the gastrointestinal tract as we eat and drink. After entry, they are absorbed through the capillaries into the bloodstream. Those that are water-soluble, or that can be converted by the body to be water-soluble, are excreted through the kidneys. Those that are fat-soluble are deposited in the fat tissue and cell membranes.

However, external sources of injurious chemicals are not the only problem that overloads our detoxification system. Our own bodies also add to the load when processing chemicals produced by normal metabolic functions, attempts to fight off acute or chronic infections, the malfunction of any body system, and the release of chemicals from amalgam fillings. Water-soluble chemicals are not difficult to excrete. However, fat-soluble chemicals pose a real threat to our health. All fat-soluble chemicals, both exogenous and endogenous, accumulate in our fat cells and cell membranes, where they remain indefinitely. This is known as toxic bioaccumulation, occurring in most organs and body systems, including all cell membranes, the brain, nerve sheaths, endocrine system, and even in human breast milk.

How Our Body Detoxifies

The detoxification system works to convert toxic chemicals into less toxic metabolites, and to excrete them as quickly as possible. Several mechanisms of detoxification in our body have been identified. The first occurs on the cellular level in a "ripply" network of fibers known as the endoplasmic reticulum. This processing of chemicals, known as Phase I, is accomplished by a system (cytochrome P-450) using specialized liver enzymes. The enzymes aid in destroying or transforming harmful chemicals by several types of oxidation (loss of an electron) and reduction (addition of an electron) reactions. One or more of these reactions takes place before the end product (metabolite) is prepared for excretion. The enzymes that catalyze these functions are greatly dependent on specific vitamins and minerals.

The second stage of detoxification, known as Phase II, is also performed within the cell. Phase II is accomplished by coupling two molecules—the xenobiotic molecule and an amino acid (protein) molecule or a portion of an amino acid molecule. This process is called conjugation. The resultant, larger molecule is more electrically charged, more soluble in water, and easier for our body to excrete in either bile or urine. Several substances that the body needs for conjugation are cysteine, glutathione, glycine, glucuronic acid, and methionine. The combining of glutathione (glutathione conjugation) with a xenobiotic forms a less toxic compound that can be excreted more easily. Many of these conjugation substances contain sulfur, and when joined to another chemical, the process is called sulfonation. Another form of coupling takes place when an acetyl group is joined to a xenobiotic (acetylation) to prepare the chemical for excretion through the kidney. When glucuronic acid is coupled, the process is called glucuronidation. Methionine donates a special group called a methyl group during methylation. Acylation utilizes glycine.

Sometimes detoxification can give rise to new chemical compounds that can injure our body. When these compounds are formed, it is more properly called a biotransformation (changing a chemical structure) than a detoxification (creation of a less toxic material). These new toxic compounds circulate in the bloodstream and lodge in various body tissues, where they can cause irreparable damage. The formation of these harmful chemicals can occur when the two detoxification phases are either overloaded, nonfunctioning, or blocked, or when the first phase is faster than the second.

■■ DETOXIFICATION INHIBITORS

Nutritional deficiencies, poor diet, infections, chemical overload, heavy metal buildup, and genetic factors can disrupt or cause a malfunction in the various detoxification pathways. Many chemicals that make their way into our body are transformed into alcohols in the first phase of detoxification. A problem can occur in the subsequent change of alcohols to aldehydes. The enzyme required in this biochemical exchange, alcohol dehydrogenase, is dependent upon an adequate supply of zinc. The next step in the process is initiated by another enzyme, aldehyde oxidase, which is dependent upon an adequate supply of molybdenum and iron. This enzyme changes the aldehyde into an acid that can be excreted in the urine.

The aldehyde detoxification system can also be overloaded with a high intake of sugar or alcohol, exposure to chemical aldehydes (such as formaldehyde), or the formation of acetaldehyde caused by Candida overgrowth in the intestinal tract. We can begin to see the end result of deficiencies of vital minerals and vitamins coupled with a chemical overload. If there is a breakdown in these two chemical transformations, the resultant free radicals, highly reactive chemicals, can damage our cells, including those of the immune system. Damage to the DNA of the cells can initiate cancer.

In the cytochrome P-450 pathway, a deficiency of nutrients (cofactors) essential for the synthesis of critical enzyme components can severely inhibit our body's detoxification efforts. Damage can be done to the cytochrome P-450 system by the direct action of specific chemicals entering the body. Dry-cleaning or copy machine fluid (trichlorethylene) and plastics (vinyl chloride) are two

such common chemicals. Vinyl chloride overexposure is a known cause of angiosarcoma (a type of cancer) of the liver. This chemical also damages cell membranes and enters cells to further damage the mitochondria (the energy-producing portion of the cell). Highly reactive unstable molecules are also formed when an oxygen molecule is added to some of the ingested chemicals. These molecules (epoxides) are very damaging to cell membranes.

Heavy metals such as cadmium, mercury, or aluminum can cause damage to detoxification enzymes. The sheer volume of chemical intake can overwhelm our body's detoxification systems, as well as the intermittent release of chemicals stored in the fat tissues of the body. Our detoxification systems often cannot process this deluge of material.

Because detoxification enzymes have specific affinities for specific chemicals, they cannot substitute in other pathways that may be overburdened. Metabolites can build up to toxic levels if a person is missing specific enzymes because of genetic or hereditary factors. Clinical studies by Dr. Jean Monro and Dr. Jonathan Brostoff in England have shown that inefficient or defective enzyme systems are a major cause of food intolerance.

Nutrients for Detoxification

The food we eat supplies nutrients for the detoxification function of our bodies. However, pesticide and fertilizer residues; artificial colors, flavors, and sweeteners; preservatives; and other chemicals from processing, packaging, and storing food can add chemicals to the food that, in turn, add to our toxic load. Sugars and salts in processed foods further increase the problem and the need for nutrients. A clean diet of organic and unprocessed foods will supply many of these nutrients without adding toxins to our bodies. It is essential for detoxification and for our health that we eat a balanced diet of clean, nutritious, unprocessed food.

Sometimes, in spite of our best efforts to have a nutritious diet, our food is sadly lacking. It is grown on depleted soil, picked before it is ripe, shipped long distances, and stored too long. Pesticide and fertilizer residues add to toxicity. If it is processed, more chemicals are added to our food, including preservatives, artificial flavors and colors, and many other ingredients.

Our bodies detoxify naturally every day. When they become too overloaded with toxins, however, we must undertake detoxification methods to help them. If our diet does not supply enough nutrients for the detoxification systems to function properly, we must take nutritional supplements. Some of the vitamins, minerals, and amino acids essential for the detoxification system to function properly are listed below.

Vitamins:
• vitamin A
• vitamin B_2 (riboflavin)
• vitamin B_3 (niacin)
• vitamin B_5 (pantothenic acid)
• vitamin B_6 (pyridoxine)
• vitamin C
• vitamin E

Minerals:
• copper
• iron
• magnesium
• manganese
• molybdenum
• selenium
• zinc

Amino Acids:
• cysteine
• glutathione
• taurine

Many of these nutrients are attached to foreign chemicals during the detoxification process and are lost when the resulting metabolite is excreted. It is important to replenish these nutrients continually with diet and nutritional supplements so that body systems can continue to function adequately. Many of these nutrients are also essential for repairing damaged cell components.

Testing for Detoxification Effectiveness

When any one of the detoxification mechanisms is malfunctioning, the chemicals that should be detoxified are then free to circulate in our bloodstream and wreak havoc on cell membranes and tissues. Biochemists and physicians working together have developed sophisticated diagnostic procedures to determine the detoxification status of the body. Blood, urine, tissue, and hair analyses can now determine levels of specific chemicals (pesticides, heavy metals) in our bodies. Urine and saliva tests can determine the effectiveness of our detoxification systems. Blood, urine, and hair analyses are done to measure levels of vitamins, minerals, and amino acids.

When mercapturic acid, a metabolite of

glutathione conjugation, is found in the urine, it indicates that organophosphate pesticides, benzene, and toluene are being detoxified. Low levels of the enzyme superoxide dismutase (SOD) indicate the possibility of damage by free-radical, reactive chemicals, because SOD is a free-radical quencher.

Elevated urine levels of D-glucaric acid signify that liver pathways for detoxification are actively working, and that significant levels of xenobiotics are present in the body. If the D-glucaric acid levels are low, this indicates that the cytochrome P-450 enzyme system is exhausted and almost ready to shut down. In contrast, standard liver function tests will show an abnormal result only after about 70 percent of the liver is damaged.

Lipid peroxides are breakdown products of cell membranes. Increased lipid peroxides in the blood are a sign that free radicals and chemicals are damaging cell membranes.

If formic acid levels are normal or low, this indicates that the detoxification pathway for aldehydes is functioning. If elevated, this is evidence that there is a backlog of this formaldehyde metabolite and that the detoxification pathway is either overloaded or failing to function adequately.

In addition to lab tests that define the body's detoxification status, a careful, detailed history and close monitoring of changing symptoms and progress are also important tools. All of this information—laboratory test results, history, and symptoms—will help in diagnosing the competence level of the body's detoxification systems, the extent of your past and present chemical exposures, and your total body burden.

Detoxification Programs

Nearly everyone needs to detoxify at least occasionally. The supervision of a physician or healthcare practitioner can be very helpful, as during even a moderate detoxification regimen, your symptoms can worsen temporarily when chemicals are released from storage in fat tissue and cell membranes. As these chemicals circulate in the bloodstream being readied for excretion, they will once again cause a variety of symptoms.

For a complex detoxification program and when there are serious health problems, do not attempt detoxification without the help of a physician who is knowledgeable about the biochemistry of detoxification pathways, nutrient and electrolyte management, and symptoms accompanying detox procedures. *Caution:* Pregnant women and people with kidney or heart problems should not undertake detoxification.

▌▌ GUIDELINES FOR DETOXIFICATION PROGRAMS

Follow these measures when starting a detoxification program. Be sure to consider and carefully follow the suggestions in each category.

▌ PREPARATION

- Evaluate present and past exposures to xenobiotics. Then clean up your present environment (work and home) as much as possible in order to lessen your toxic body burden. (See Keeping a Chemically Clean Home Environment in chapter 12.
- Drink large amounts (eight to ten 8-ounce

glasses) of water each day to flush detoxification waste products into the urine for excretion.

- Reduce and manage stress. This will reduce the number of metabolic byproducts and is an important part of any detoxification process. Stress also creates additional demand for nutrients needed in the detoxification process.
- Start a mild exercise program depending on your limitations. Exercise in a "clean" environment.
- Monitor cardiovascular levels during exercise sessions in order to avoid risk and stress. Take increased doses of niacin (vitamin B_3) before each exercise session to increase skin capillary activity, enhancing toxin excretion. Take only the short-acting form of niacin.
- Maintain a proper electrolyte balance with the use of potassium and sodium salts. Your physician should regulate the dosage.
- Maintain proper bowel function. At least two semi-soft stools per day are necessary to rid your body of accumulated toxins. Take adequate water, fiber, and vitamin C to accomplish this. If excreted toxins are not continually moved through the bowel, they can be reabsorbed into the bloodstream and add to the already loaded detoxification pathways. Maintain bowel tolerance levels of vitamin C. (See Vitamin C: A Key Nutrient in chapter 20)
- Use a liver support and drainage remedy to help the liver in the detoxification process. PHP Liver Liquescence, a homeopathic aid, supports liver function and repair.
- Take Kidney Liquescence, a homeopathic preparation from PHP that aids in kidney

repair and detoxification of protein wastes by supplying needed tissue nutrients.
- Do an organ cleansing program for the kidneys and liver before beginning a detoxification program. (See Organ Cleansing in *Natural Detoxification;* more information in Recommended Books.)

▌ DIET AND NUTRIENT SUPPLEMENTATION

- Adjust your diet to remove all sugars, and eat a balance of proteins, vegetables, and whole grains. As much as possible, eat chemically uncontaminated foods in a diversified rotation diet. (See chapter 10, Eating Safely.)
- Include 3 Tbsp. of unsaturated oils daily in your diet. Use cold-pressed oils from nuts, vegetables, fish, evening primrose, black currant, flaxseed, or borage. The oils slow down the assimilation of toxic chemicals from the intestinal tract.
- Get help in evaluating your vitamin and mineral levels and designing a supplement program to include all of the antioxidants and specific minerals that stimulate detoxification pathways.
- Take a high-quality vitamin/mineral supplement or plan a detailed supplement program with your physician.

▌▌ DETOXIFICATION METHODS

- Take detoxification baths to begin the mobilization of chemicals from fat cells, bringing them to the skin for excretion. Directions for these baths are discussed below.
- Use a dry sauna—but only with extreme caution, starting with five-minute sessions and increasing gradually to 20 to 30 min-

Detoxification Centers

Environmentally ill people with severe symptoms may want to consider using the services of detoxification centers. Presently, there are detox units in California, Texas, South Carolina, Florida, and Washington. Their programs are very carefully monitored, and some of the centers have been specially constructed for environmental safety. Periodic laboratory tests and evaluations are performed. (See Recommended Sources and Organizations.)

You may consider this concentrated approach if:

- *you have severe, debilitating symptoms of environmental illness.*
- *you continue to experience acute symptoms after receiving standard treatment from an environmental medical specialist and cleaning up your environment.*
- *you have a high exposure to toxic chemicals, now or in the past.*
- *you have continued high levels of toxic chemicals in your blood, urine, fat tissue, or sweat.*
- *you have continued malfunction of detoxification pathways.*

utes. Scrub your skin well before and immediately following the sauna. (See the preliminary instructions for detoxification baths, in this chapter.) Saunas at health clubs are usually wet saunas or are too hot. They also have inadequate levels of available oxygen, and are made of environmentally unsafe materials. Sauna temperatures should not exceed 150°F. Use saunas only on the advice and under the direction of your physician, as the resulting detox symptoms can be severe and uncomfortable.

- Use your shower to help you detoxify if you do not have access to a bathtub or a sauna. See detailed instructions below.
- Obtain regular massage from a physiotherapist, massage therapist, or rolfer. Massage supports detoxification by increasing circulation in the blood and lymph systems, which carry processed toxins to the proper organs for excretion.

■ DETOXIFICATION BATHS

Detoxification baths are very helpful for those who have toxic, chemical bioaccumulations and do not have access to a sauna or sauna program. The hot bath water increases blood capillary action near the skin surface for faster release of toxins. Although filtered water is preferable for these baths, detoxification will still take place with chlorinated city water.

Heat expands the pores in the skin and increases perspiration carrying toxins to the skin surface. Heat also raises pulse rate (an indicator of increased blood circulation). Substances added to the bath water act as counterirritants on the skin to increase blood supply and activate fluid movement in the tissues. These solutions also change the pH on the skin surface, which also tends to facilitate fluid movement. Substances that promote sweating are also helpful.

However, do not attempt detoxification

baths unless your healthcare professional prescribes them. You may experience detoxification symptoms during and after your bath. If your chemical load is extremely high, the baths can make you feel very ill, and an alternative treatment may be necessary.

Caution: Do not undergo a detoxification program unless you are certain that you are not pregnant.

If you have been advised to take a detoxification bath, follow your healthcare professional's instructions carefully. Do not try another method on your own. Be sure someone is in the house with you when you take your detoxification bath, as you may need assistance if your symptoms become severe. Terminate your bath early if symptoms—which can include dizziness, headache, exhaustion, nausea, weakness, and fatigue—become too uncomfortable.

❚ *Preliminary Bath Instructions*

Your bathtub should be spotlessly clean for a detoxification bath. Clean it with your tolerated cleaner. (See chapter 12, Living Safely, for suggestions.)

- Take your tolerated dose of buffered vitamin C before and after each bath to help removal of toxins released into your bloodstream. If you are using antioxidant therapy, take these vitamins before your bath.
- Drink an 8-ounce glass of water before and during all detox baths.
- Before beginning detox baths, take a trial series of plain hot water baths three times per week. For these baths, follow the detox bath instructions, but do not add the detoxification materials. When you can stay in a

tub of plain hot water for 30 minutes with no symptoms, you may begin the detox baths as directed by your healthcare professional.

❚ *Bath Instructions*

- Wash thoroughly with tolerated soap in the tub or shower before your detox bath to remove excess body oil. Scrub your skin with a loofa sponge or a rough washcloth to stimulate capillary action, while removing a layer of dead skin and excess skin oils. This will allow closer contact with the substances added to the bath water to aid in detoxification. Rinse thoroughly.
- Fill your tub with water as hot as you can tolerate without burning your skin and high enough so you can immerse your body up to your neck. (Overflow drain covers can be obtained at a hardware store to allow for deeper filling of your tub.)
- Soak in the hot bath for only five minutes for the first bath. You may experience delayed detoxification symptoms the following day. Over a period of several weeks, gradually increase the time for subsequent baths to 30 minutes.
- If immediate symptoms become intolerable, release the stopper and allow the water to drain from the tub. Sit until you feel you can safely get out of the tub. If you feel weak, you can easily fall. Ask for assistance if you feel dizzy.
- Scrub your skin thoroughly afterward in a tub of clean water or in a shower to remove any accumulated toxins deposited on your skin during the detoxification bath. Toxins left on the skin will be reabsorbed if you do not remove them.
- If you continue to perspire, repeat a cleans-

ing bath or shower to remove the toxin-filled perspiration.

- Take a detox bath every other day or three times weekly.
- Continue to take detox baths until your general health has improved significantly. Then use the baths once or twice weekly.
- If you have an unusual chemical exposure, take your baths more frequently, but not more than once a day. These baths can help to clear a chemical reaction.
- Detoxification baths may need to be repeated in several series because detoxification in some people occurs in a cyclic fashion, sometimes with months between episodes.

❚ *Detoxification Bath Materials*

When you can take plain hot water baths for 30 minutes with no symptoms, add one of the following materials for your detoxification bath. Rotating them will give you better results, as some of them may lose their effectiveness with repeated use.

Epsom Salts. The sulfur component of Epsom salts is a good detoxifying agent. (Sulfur springs throughout the world are well known for their palliative properties.) Epsom salts work as a counterirritant, activating fluid movement in the tissues and increasing perspiration.

Begin with 1/4 cup of Epsom salts in a full tub of hot, clean water. Over time, gradually increase the Epsom salts until you are using 4 cups in a tub of water. Do not increase the Epsom salts should you experience symptoms at a given level. Stay at that level until you can soak with no symptoms for 30 minutes.

Baking Soda. Baking soda (sodium bi-carbonate) restores acid/alkaline balance through osmosis. Use 8 ounces baking soda to a full tub of hot, clean water.

Soda and Salt. Baking soda baths with sea salt added will help detoxify X-ray and radiation exposure. Use equal amounts of baking soda and noniodized sea salt, building up to 1 pound of each over time.

Apple Cider Vinegar. Apple cider vinegar works as a counterirritant, increasing blood supply to the skin and changing the pH of the skin. Start with 1/4 cup apple cider vinegar in a full tub of hot, clean water. Increase to 1 cup as symptoms permit.

Clorox. Use the Clorox brand of liquid bleach only. (Other brands may contain contaminants.) Its oxidizing properties aid with detoxification. Add 2 Tbsp. Clorox to a full tub of hot, clean water. Chlorine-sensitive people should not use Clorox.

Herbal Tea. Diaphoretic herbs (herbs that promote sweating) added to a detoxification bath aid in eliminating chemicals. Catnip, yarrow, peppermint, boneset, blessed thistle, pleurisy root, chamomile, blue vervain, and horsetail are useful. Add 1 cup of brewed tea per tub of hot, clean water. Use only one of these teas for each bath. Some sensitive individuals may not tolerate these teas.

❚ DETOX SHOWERS

If you do not have access to a bathtub or a sauna, you can use your shower to help you detoxify. Your progress will be slower, but over time you will gradually detoxify. You will need to purchase a bath chair or stool to put in your shower so you can sit under the spray of hot water. With this method you will not be able to use any of the substances listed above for the detoxification baths. However, if you tolerate the herb, you can drink a cup of one of the herbal teas before beginning your shower.

Follow as many of the Preliminary Bath Instructions and the Bath Instructions as are applicable for a shower. Sit in the shower for only five minutes the first time, and gradually increase your time to 30 minutes. You will detoxify if you sweat. Be sure to take a cooler cleansing shower afterward to remove any excreted toxins from your skin.

After Detoxification

After you complete a detoxification program, you will want to maintain your new, improved health. It is important that you continue a careful lifestyle. Keep your home environment chemically free, and be certain your workplace does not contain serious occupational exposures. Continue the measures you have taken to improve your diet, nutrient supplements, and other treatments for environmental illness, and maintain your general lifestyle and health habit improvements.

Together, these factors should enable you to continue on your journey to optimum health. (For more information on detoxification and detoxification programs, see *Natural Detoxification* in Recommended Books.)

CHAPTER 24

Body, Mind, and Spirit

ALL ILLNESS HAS AN EMOTIONAL and psychological impact. The body, mind, and spirit are involved in allergies, sensitivities, and environmental illness in unique ways that are not present for other health problems. It is impossible to have allergies and sensitivities severe enough that environmental illness results without there being an emotional and psychological impact on the person. Perhaps more than any other illness, environmental sensitivity graphically illustrates our body, mind, and spirit interrelationship.

Affected people suffer a great amount of emotional and psychological stress as they react to nontoxic, common substances that healthy people tolerate. The environment becomes painfully different and threatening. This chapter explores the range and complexity of this impact, as well as suggesting positive action for lessening and removing the symptoms and problems caused by it. It further discusses the involvement of the spirit and its role in contributing to complete recovery—or preventing it.

The Emotional and Psychological Impact of Environmental Illness

Environmental illness can masquerade as virtually any type of physical or psychological disorder. The healing process draws attention to the subtle, complex interplay between our body, our mind, and our spirit. The more severe the environmental illness, the more important this relationship becomes.

▌▌CHEMICAL CHANGES

Chemical changes, which occur in our body when we experience an adverse reaction to something in our environment, are one cause of the emotional and psychological dimensions of environmental illness. During a reaction, histamine, endorphins, neurotransmitters, hormones, leukotrienes, or enkephalins (all chemicals produced by the body) are either released in excess, suppressed, or altered, and these changes affect normal brain functions, causing symptoms.

Symptoms that signal a change in brain function include alterations in thought, feel-

Stress-Related Food Reactions

One woman professed that she had allergic symptoms to nearly every food she ate. Test results for the foods to which she felt she was having symptoms were frequently negative. Earlier in her life, this woman had had a life-threatening food reaction in a restaurant. After that time, over a period of years, her allergies and symptoms had magnified to the point that she had very few "safe" foods and was reacting to many other substances, including chemicals and pollens.

After much ineffective treatment the woman finally realized the restaurant incident had to be of importance, and she and her counselor were able to determine that she had a form of post-traumatic stress syndrome that was directly related to her response to foods and other substances.

ings, behavior, mood, and personality. These symptoms vary from one person to the next depending on the severity of the sensitivity and the degree of allergen exposure. People who are mildly affected may feel only some degree of anger or depression, while more severely ill people may experience the entire range of symptoms.

A number of environmental medicine physicians have demonstrated conclusively that behavioral and emotional disturbances can result from adverse reactions to toxic and nontoxic substances found in our everyday environment. Symptoms may include anger, depression, confusion, anxiety, panic attacks, cognitive malfunctions, perceptual disorders, suicidal feelings, hyperactivity, and lethargy.

This same range of symptoms can also occur with illnesses such as Epstein-Barr virus, *Candida albicans*, and parasitic or bacterial infections. A person may react to the organism itself, to the toxins it releases, to debris left by the dead organism, or to the immune response to the organism. The presence of these organisms in an environmentally sensitive person can complicate diagnosis.

■ EFFECTS OF DIAGNOSIS

Some emotional and psychological problems for the environmentally ill are directly related to the diagnosis of the illness. Hearing the diagnosis triggers a cascade of changes that affect every aspect of the person's life, as well as everyone whose life touches theirs.

The health history often reveals a prolonged, gradually deteriorating picture before an accurate diagnosis of environmental illness is made. Usually, after a variety of medical specialists have been consulted, resulting in thick medical files and high costs, the person is labeled a hypochondriac. Friends and family become weary of hearing the various incessant complaints. The severely ill person becomes exhausted, financially depleted, dependent on society, worried that perhaps there is no explanation or treatment, or frightened that this disease will prove totally disabling or fatal. All of these factors place enormous stress on an already burdened psyche.

When the diagnosis of environmental illness is made, the response may initially be one of relief that the problem is not "all in the mind." These feelings may be mixed with feelings of anger that it took so long to arrive at a diagnosis. The person may also feel angry toward the physician making the diagnosis—a type of "kill the messenger" phenomenon.

The diagnosis of severe environmental illness often precipitates a major life crisis. Hard realities must be faced regarding lifestyle changes, changes in workplace, disruption of employment, financial burdens, and pressure caused by lengthy, often complicated allergy and other treatments. Even the treatment of mild sensitivities necessitates some changes. Often, friends and family are critical of the sufferer's need for change, and even small changes can upset others. The person may feel guilty for causing these problems, and also feel unsupported or, at times, like a social outcast.

RESPONSE TO ENVIRONMENTAL ILLNESS

Sources of emotional and psychological stress that are similar to those imposed by any chronic illness are imposed on people with environmental illness. Responses to the illness are many and varied, and in part depend on the innate emotional stability and spiritual health of the person.

FRUSTRATION

You will encounter frustration as you and your clinician try to determine causes in the complex puzzle of this illness. Frustrations and uncertainties build as you temporarily become more ill when offending substances are withdrawn (withdrawal syndrome), or when invading organisms are eliminated (die-off symptoms). Responses of anxiety, depression, anger, or fear are understandable in the face of such an array of frustrations.

Frustrations can arise from the process of the illness itself. At first, everything may appear to be "off limits," and for a long while, it may seem that every step forward necessitates giving up something familiar and important. Every hour of the day can be filled with changing symptoms, depending on various exposures. Being unable to count on your own ability to think clearly, make decisions, or perform physically or sexually is extremely frustrating. You may no longer feel in control of your life.

All environmentally ill people are temporarily overwhelmed by the need for dietary and environmental changes. You may experience feelings of rebellion, disbelief, and denial that such a problem really exists. Some reject, for a time, the measures that must be followed to attain good health. Added frustration ensues when an overnight cure cannot be offered. You may strongly resent that your lifestyle has been so rudely interrupted with health problems.

ANXIETY OR FEAR

The unknown or uncertainty about the future are sources of apprehension for many of us. This is particularly true for the environmentally ill person. During illness, this tendency easily becomes accentuated because of compromised coping skills. You may feel fearful of the consequences of changes in lifestyle, occupation, living accommodations, or financial status imposed by your illness.

These uncertainties create severe stress if they are not addressed. If you dwell on negative possibilities, they can multiply insidiously into energy blocks that can lead to worsening of physical and emotional symptoms.

▮ IDENTITY CRISIS

An identity crisis may also surface at some time during the illness and recovery process. Having to change your self-image from a productive, functioning person to a chronically ill person can be devastating to the ego. This challenge has to be faced by anyone experiencing a chronic or debilitating illness. Fear of doing "irreversible damage" to your body accompanies this change in self-concept. Losing your ability to cope with the everyday environment can also damage your feeling of self-worth.

In our society, a person's identity is strongly associated with career. When your career is terminated or changed because of environmental illness, self-pride and identity are assaulted. As your self-awareness increases, the patterns that have contributed to a state of overload become apparent. Many of us are forced to re-examine fundamental beliefs and goals, to reconsider our life values, and to reassess our talents and skills.

▮ SELF-PITY

A feeling of entrapment can affect your approach to life, if you succumb to the idea that you are a "victim" rather than a "victor." You may be tempted to blame the environment, the government, physicians and staff, fam-ily, friends, time of day or night, world affairs, or the weather. If this outlook continues, progress toward health will be impeded. The "poor me" approach includes:

- repeatedly reviewing symptoms and past history
- indulging in negative thinking and wallowing in self-pity
- projecting anger and blame onto other people or circumstances
- bemoaning your fate
- creating internal stress with dispirited or hopeless thoughts and self-defeating beliefs or fears
- searching for "miracle" cures
- isolating and insulating yourself from every perceived threat

In *Chronic Fatigue Syndrome*, Dr. Jesse Stoff of Tucson, Arizona, claims that "if you argue for your disease and its limitations—they are yours." A "poor me" attitude can indeed make the disease yours forever, unless you take charge and reclaim your life and health.

▮ SHAME

Some people feel deeply ashamed when they cannot solve their own problems or direct the course of their lives. Shame also occurs for some when they become preoccupied with themselves as a result of environmental illness. In response to this temporary awkward feeling, they will hide their emotions, only to have them surface later in anxiety and confusion. As true awareness is gained, illusions and assumptions about oneself and one's weaknesses also become apparent, and there may be a temporary loss of self-esteem.

▮ RELATIONSHIPS

The environmentally ill person needs stable,

constructive, unconditional support. Often that personal network of support is lost when family and friends fail to understand the sufferer's fluctuations in personality and health.

The stress of changes in interpersonal relationships creates another burden on your psyche at a time when you most need nurturing, acceptance, and understanding. Expectations of permanence and predictability in relationships are sometimes shattered.

■■ AFTER TREATMENT BEGINS

The steps that follow diagnosis also place a strain on emotional and psychological stability. The treatment of environmental illness is not like that for any other illness. It requires more effort and participation on the part of the patient and his or her family. The physical, mental, emotional, and financial efforts required sometimes are above the ability of those involved.

■ SELF-EDUCATION

Self-education is an important part of controlling environmental illness. Well-thought-out decisions need to be made to make the environment as safe as possible and conducive to healing. Practitioners in environmental medicine can provide a wealth of information so that you can make choices. Your choices should be acceptable to family and employers, involve the least risk, require the least financial commitment, and provide the greatest health benefits. This major life reorientation requires a great deal of attention and communication, and constitutes an enormous stress.

■ INCONSISTENT RESULTS

When treatment begins, you may find it baffling that progress toward recovery is not always upward. One day you feel quite well and see improvement from treatment. Another day, you react severely to an allergen exposure and fear once again that you will never be well. Another hour or day passes, the allergen is removed, the reaction clears, and improvement begins again.

This "bouncing" toward recovery is a continuing stress, and others around you are often confused by these shifts in health and mood. Reactions of others may range from sympathetic curiosity to disbelief, from sincere offers of help to anxious avoidance, and from warm acceptance to personal blame. In order to test the validity of your illness, others may even deliberately initiate exposures that can cause debilitating reactions.

■ RESPONSIBILITY

Responsibility for much of the treatment for environmental illness falls on the patient. This approach seems foreign to most people in an age where responsibility for disease control is placed on the healthcare practitioner. A mental struggle often ensues between a desire for improved health and an aversion to taking on so much responsibility. This is complicated by the fact that the sufferer is already exhausted and severely stressed. At this point, it may take time for the sufferer and the family to accept the realities of the illness.

If you are unable to accept responsibility for your own health improvement, an unfortunate state of dependency may result, causing a large psychological impact. You may become unnaturally dependent on society, spouse, friends, or healthcare. practitioners, and be "stuck" in a mode of recounting symptoms, laying blame on others, and making unrealistic and unnecessary demands on the people involved with your care. You may give up trying to help yourself, become rebellious and withdraw into despair and isolation, or reject treatment.

▐ GIVING UP

The late Dr. Hans Selye, formerly the director of the Institute of Experimental Medicine and Surgery at the University of Montreal, in Quebec, concluded after 50 years of research that the factors that cause stress are not as important as the way we react to the stress. Fortunately, only a few people view their illnesses as hopeless. Unfortunately, these people believe that neither they nor anyone else can do anything about their problem. They respond with negativity to any suggested form of therapy:

"I tried that and it didn't work."

"My body tells me that I can't stand this treatment."

"I tried the diet for a week and it didn't do anything."

"It is impossible for me to give that up because...."

These people may try a form of treatment but stop it within a few days because "they are reacting to the treatment." This is usually not a valid assessment; in almost all cases, reactivity symptoms are those the sufferer had before treatment began. In other cases, reaction symptoms will generally subside within a few days.

With such a negative attitude, such people will withdraw further from others and will eventually retreat into a shell. This mechanism, known as conservation/withdrawal, is a maladaptive emergency coping system used when adverse stimuli are too great.

▐▐ STAGES OF LOSS

Interwoven with the emotional and psychological impacts of environmental illness is an added burden of loss—the loss of health and well-being, including the loss of various aspects of our roles (worker or parent). These losses make us aware of our human frailty, and cause changes in us and in the course of our lives.

Dealing with the loss of health is similar to coping with the loss of a loved one. There is a series of stages, outlined by Dr. Elizabeth Kubler-Ross of Escondido, California, in her book, *On Death and Dying*, which a person must experience to properly address the grief associated with a loss. The following process has been paraphrased to describe the loss of health in environmental illness.

The grieving process is very complex—there is no strict sequence for these stages. You may experience fluctuations between the stages, and one can occur before another. Each stage must be accepted and experienced to progress toward improved health. If movement from one phase to another does not occur, you may become "stuck," and the process of recovery may be delayed.

▐ SHOCK

Even though you are aware of all of your symptoms, the shock of knowing that they are part of a larger, more complex picture can be temporarily overwhelming. A period of numbness may set in, during which you cannot act on the information you receive about this type of illness and treatment.

DENIAL AND ISOLATION

Since the course of environmental illness varies from day to day, depending on exposures to allergens or on the overload phenomenon, it is very easy to deny the existence of a long-term problem. Denial is readily reinforced by both popular and medical opinion, since treatment for environmental illness is unorthodox, unfamiliar, and often misunderstood. You are confronted with making a decision to accept treatment involving lifestyle changes and unconventional therapy at a time when decision-making is difficult and stressful.

The easier road may seem to be to deny the existence of a health problem or to search for another type of therapy. Some people remain in the denial stage by isolating themselves in remote areas in order to avoid exposures. They hope that the problem will magically disappear, rather than pursuing the causes of illness and subsequent treatment. Others maintain denial by hiding under a canopy of psychotherapy, concluding that they would rather accept a diagnosis of mental illness than one of environmental illness.

ANGER

It is not difficult to understand an angry response to environmental illness. Sometimes the anger is suppressed or mixed with liberal doses of self-pity. At other times, anger is expressed as blame against those who try to help, or as rejection of those who express love or support.

It is important that the person affected by environmental sensitivities fully experiences this stage of anger before more progress can be made. You must acknowledge and express anger in constructive ways, rather than suppressing it, even if it is upsetting and volatile. Be assured that this phase is inevitable, expected, and an acceptable part of the grief process. You have real cause to be angry and resentful. Learn to recognize your envy of people who enjoy good health as unexpressed anger, and work at accepting yourself as you are right now. Ineffectual and unexpressed anger is damaging to your body's homeostasis.

BARGAINING

This stage involves making secret deals with fate, with God, with a higher being, or with yourself. When indulging in a known allergen, you may promise that if you can be free of reaction from the offending substance, you will "be good" for a week or a month. If your allergic load is light enough at the time of the indulgence, you may not experience a reaction, and the bargaining may appear to have worked. This reinforces your actions and you will be apt to try this behavior again until the cumulative effect becomes overwhelming.

Another form of bargaining occurs when you fantasize that your physician can magically dispense good health in exchange for cooperative behavior. How marvelous it would be if this were true. The fantasy is dispelled, however, when you finally realize that this type of thinking is erroneous and manipulative, and that the final responsibility for good health lies with you.

DEPRESSION

Depression can be a primary physical reaction to an allergenic substance. It can also be a psychological response to the complexities of environmental illness. Your coping skills will be tested to the limit at this stage. Discouragement and even despair result whenever there is a setback. The question "Will I ever be well?" is followed by "Can I accept the limitations imposed by this illness?"

This stage will weave throughout every other stage of loss, haunting the ill person with unresolved questions. Responses may vary from sadness to despair, from crying to numbness, from slowed responses to weakness, from withdrawal to apathy, from loneliness to self-imposed isolation, and from forgetfulness to feeling out of touch with reality. Again, this phase will pass if it is accepted and dealt with properly. This is a good time to accept help and support from your physician, friends, and relatives.

GUILT

Guilt is always lurking in the background for the environmentally sensitive person. "If only I had . . . " becomes a frequent thought. Guilt can become a special psychological burden, and self-forgiveness is imperative. However, it is usually easier to forgive others than to forgive yourself for real or imagined offenses. You may feel that if you had done more, felt more, and been more of everything that this illness would not have occurred.

LONELINESS

Loneliness can develop when severely sensitive people change their lifestyle by giving up or changing employment or residence, when they are rejected by family or friends because of their "different" lifestyle, or when they isolate themselves from others to prevent reactions to normal, everyday substances. Some people feel that they are the only person with their type of problems, which increases their feeling of isolation and loneliness.

ANXIETY AND PANIC

Anxiety is understandable when you must face the possibility of lifestyle changes. These changes not only affect you, but also others in close personal relationships. In addition, the stress of these stages of grief places a great demand on your adrenal glands. Continued stress will temporarily exhaust the adrenal system and a physical state of anxiety can result.

Another factor that can provoke temporary anxiety occurs when an environmentally ill person becomes acutely aware of situations or substances that cause reactions. Until you learn that steps can be taken to avoid or relieve reactions, you will probably feel threatened and anxious. If this anxiety is not alleviated, it can become a conditioned response.

NEEDING TO BE ILL

Another trap that sometimes develops in environmentally ill people is learning to manipulate others through chronic illness, which can occur when there are unresolved psychosocial or relationship problems. Illness can be an attention-getting or controlling device, a way to cope with rejection, or a method of extracting love from another.

Some people use their illness to escape from unpleasant circumstances with which they can no longer cope.

For others, being ill gives the person a feeling of importance and purpose in life. They are unwilling to give up being ill because in their subconscious mind, it would be giving up their "reason for being." Their illness allows them to feel protected, to live in a world where they dictate the terms, and do not have to accept many of the responsibilities of life.

Some people continue to be ill because they have very low self-esteem and feel they are worthless and do not deserve to get well. Many feel that they are terrible human beings because of real or imagined transgressions for which they cannot forgive themselves. These people tend to sabotage their treatment. They will often try a treatment for a short time, then drop it with a flimsy excuse as to why they cannot continue it. In many cases, the treatment was beginning to help. They tend to go from treatment to treatment, each time hoping for a "magic pill" or "magic cure"—but deep inside they believe they do not deserve to be well and happy.

Even after working hard to recover physical health, and professing frequently that they want to get well, many people with allergies and environmental illness recover to a point and then do not improve further. They continue to have symptoms, and to bemoan their poor health even though physically they look healthy. They do appear to experience symptoms and have low energy, but there will be inconsistencies in their condition that point to unresolved problems. These people may have a spiritual injury that prevents their complete recovery.

Spiritual Injury

Spirit is difficult to define, but it is that quality that makes us who we are and that connects us to a higher being, energy, or faith system. Some people refer to it as the soul or psyche. This quality can become damaged, even in childhood, and result in an ongoing illness in adulthood that seems to have no cure or solution. When physical symptoms improve to a point and then there is no more progress toward health recovery, the issue of spiritual injury, or a damaged spirit, must be addressed.

Many things can damage the spirit, including lack of nurturing as a child; abuse, whether sexual, physical, or emotional; frightening and terrifying experiences in which the person felt isolated and alone; mugging or rape; and other emotionally stressful events. If the person does not have coping skills to handle and recover from these events, or is not given special help to allow them to adequately recover, the spirit will be damaged. This damage will manifest itself later in life as physical symptoms that appear to have no cure.

Traumatic experiences can have a profound effect on brain chemistry. In the 1990s, studies at Emory University School of Medicine in Atlanta, Georgia showed that women who were physically or sexually abused in childhood showed exaggerated physiological responses to stressful events. If the women also had clinical depression, their abnormal stress response was especially pronounced. Dr. Dennis Charney, chief of the research program on mood and anxiety disorders at the National Institute of Health in Bethesda, Maryland, states that "We are born with a certain genetic constitution to handle many things, including stress. If the developing animal or human is faced with an extraordinary amount of stress, those systems are going to be changed in how they develop."

This is consistent with the time-dependent sensitization model for illness from low-level chemicals proposed by Dr. Iris Bell of the University of Arizona Health Sciences Center in Tucson. In time-dependent sensitization, the response of the brain to low-level environmental chemicals is changed, in turn affecting behavioral, neurochemical, endocrine, and immunological responses when exposed to these chemicals.

Many people with a spiritual injury will turn totally inward, focusing only on themselves and their physical and psychological problems. They are unable to reach out to other people except to take from them, and no amount of energy expended on their behalf seems to help them. When their background is investigated, one or more unresolved traumatic events gradually surface. Many times, the people have buried the memory of these events so deeply that they are unaware of them and the impact they are having on their present-day health.

■ HEALING THE SPIRIT

Steps must be taken to correct the spiritual injury or issue. If the person can acknowledge and accept that there is a problem,

much can be done to heal the spirit, mind, and body. This is often more difficult than addressing the physical problems and taking steps to correct them. If the damage is severe, counseling with an understanding and knowledgeable counselor may be necessary for complete recovery.

■ ACCEPTANCE

Acceptance is not a one-time commitment leading to perfect health, but rather is a daily—sometimes hourly—dedication to working toward better health. The battle is not only with the physiology of your body but also with your psyche. Accepting yourself as you are involves recognizing the limitations of your illness, which allows the expansion to a new self with different coping skills.

At some stage in every illness, we have to assume a degree of responsibility for ourselves, whether it involves completely revamping our lifestyle, changing our diet, or remembering to take supplements and extracts. Understanding the underlying concepts of the disease process and the preventive measures that can help alleviate our distress is essential. This open attitude and acceptance will help you progress to the final stage of hope.

■ THE FOCUS OF HOPE

An environmentally sensitive person does not have to get stuck in depression or grief, nor does the person with a spiritual injury have to remain ill. We have been given the gift of an innate ability to maintain hope. Positive, constructive, energizing thoughts can aid recovery, and should be applied on a daily or hourly basis along with the other aspects of therapy. In *Love, Medicine, and*

436

Miracles, Dr. Bernie Siegel states that healing is a creative art, calling for all the hard work and dedication needed for other forms of creativity.

There are many health-supporting mechanisms that can be used to change the perception of environmental illness. Norman Vincent Peale proved that there is power in positive thinking. Norman Cousins' recovery from illness was a prime example of the curative powers of personal belief. He asks in his book, *Anatomy of an Illness*: "If negative emotions produce negative chemical changes in the body, wouldn't the positive emotions produce positive chemical changes? Is it possible that love, hope, faith, laughter, confidence, and will to live have therapeutic value?"

Taking Steps to Wellness

The following steps to wellness can have a profound effect on healing the body, mind, and spirit. Their simplicity can be deceptive, making some people feel that they are simply "busy work." However, if they are incorporated into a person's life and are faithfully utilized, an astonishing amount of healing will take place.

▌▌ CHANGES IN ATTITUDE AND FOCUS

- Take off the mask of adulthood and become a child again. The child in us loves to laugh. Aristotle described laughter as a "bodily exercise precious to health."
- Release feelings of anger, fear, guilt, or pain. Our emotions do not just happen to us—we choose them. Allow yourself to feel joy, hope, life, peace, and love.

- Adopt a positive, hopeful attitude toward recovery from your illness. Concentrate on the present, not the past.
- Use visual imagery—see yourself as a healthy person.
- Adopt a spirit of thankfulness for the inherent gifts, talents, and abilities you possess.
- Improve your self-esteem and gain confidence in your coping ability.
- Gradually restructure any faulty psychological defenses and work at seeing yourself as happy and healthy! You will begin to see the world differently.
- Learn to benefit each day from your experiences. Remember that you have choices and options as you learn how to create a new life.
- Focus on wellness rather than on illness; focus on changes rather than on problems. Remember that you are in control.
- Make an effort to face and accept the present moment and formulate an image of health that empowers you to take action.
- Seek a personal sense of purpose and meaning by looking at new dimensions and definitions for your life. As Siegel said, "You can create your own opportunities out of the same raw materials from which other people create their defeats."
- Forgive yourself and others for any wrongdoing. If you cannot forgive someone who has hurt you, consider turning over your feelings to your higher power. It can help to write the person's name on a piece of paper, ask your higher power to do the forgiving, then throw away or burn the paper. Over time, many people find that forgiveness has become possible without their

conscious awareness of the healing process.

- When a negative thought occurs, replace it with positive, constructive work that will absorb you and stop the negative pattern from becoming a habit. Dr. Jesse Stoff writes: "Transforming negative thoughts is not merely saying 'no' to a negative thought. It is a creative process of generating positive feelings from within."

▌▌ CHANGES IN ACTIVITIES

- Start each day by concentrating on a beautiful music or a scene, poem, or affirmation. An affirmation can be as simple as one word: determination, energy, strength, hope, courage. Be inventive and design a new affirmation each week.
- Nurture a sense of humor—read comedies, cartoons. Let laughter be your best medicine.
- Seek spiritual support and comfort through meditation and prayer.
- Strengthen your interpersonal relationships.
- Work on a hobby that is compatible with your illness.

▌▌ CHANGES IN LIFESTYLE

- Simplify your lifestyle and reduce stress in those areas over which you have control.
- Determine your limits by "testing the waters." Reconcile what you want from life with what you can do.
- Habits are hard to break; repetition is essential. Follow the adage, "Fake it until you make it."
- Live life to the fullest each day even though you may experience some limitations.

Stretch yourself a bit further in your endeavors each day.

- Look for new beginnings in your lifestyle or occupations.
- Network with others and extend your talents and personality into the community around you. That community may consist of other environmentally ill people elsewhere in the country.
- "Whatever you do, do it with a sense of joy, enthusiasm, and a purpose. This will gradually help with extending your powers of concentration, and strengthening your ability to make decisions" (Dr. Jesse Stoff, *Chronic Fatigue Syndrome*).

In *Love, Medicine, and Miracles*, Dr. Siegel tells of a quotation found on a wall in a bombed-out basement in Germany, after the close of World War II. "I believe in the sun—even when it does not shine. I believe in God—even when I do not hear him speak." As you begin taking a positive approach to your life, this attitude may last only for a fleeting moment each day. However, your approach will expand and become a large part of your recovery from environmental illness.

Set realistic goals by taking into consideration your strengths and weaknesses. Do not push yourself to the point of exhaustion; exercises of faith can be just as tiring as physical activity. It may be wise to set aside a few minutes each day to practice these positive concepts. By taking short breaks away from depressing thoughts, even physical symptoms of depression will begin to lift.

You have the innate ability—as well as the responsibility—to do something about your health. Working on a positive program

438

to improve your health will give you an increased sense of well-being. Take one small step at a time that will lead to conscious control of your illness. Dr. Siegel describes a person who exercises hope and control as "an exceptional patient." These people learn to take charge of their lives, and they work hard to achieve health and peace of mind.

Seek out every avenue of help and support from traditional medicine, as well as from alternative forms of healing. Use your symptoms as signposts for discovering treatments that are most effective, rather than as indicators of failure. Use your inner strength to overcome what may seem to be impossible, and allow the innate restorative powers of your body to work their miracles.

Glossary

Absorption: The process by which nutrients are taken up through the intestinal wall and passed into the bloodstream.

Acetaldehyde: An aldehyde found in cigarette smoke, vehicle exhaust, and smog. It is a metabolic product of *Candida albicans* and is synthesized from alcohol in the liver.

Acetylcholine: A neurotransmitter manufactured in the brain, used for memory and control of sensory input and muscular output signals.

Acid: Any compound capable of releasing a hydrogen ion; its pH is less than 7.

Acute: Extremely sharp or severe, as in pain; can also refer to an illness or reaction that is sudden and intense.

Adaptation: The ability of an organism to integrate new elements into its environment.

Addiction: A dependent state characterized by cravings for a particular substance if that substance is withdrawn. People can have emotional and psychological addictions, as well as physical ones.

Additive: A substance added in small amounts to foods to alter them in some way.

Adrenalin: Trademark for preparations of epinephrine, a hormone secreted by the adrenal gland. It is given sublingually and by injection to stop allergic reactions.

Aerobic: Organisms or metabolic processes that require oxygen.

Air cleaner: A filtering machine that, depending on the type of filter, can remove pollen, dust, mold, bacteria, viruses, and chemicals from the air.

Aldehydes: A class of organic compounds obtained by the oxidation of alcohols. Formaldehyde and acetaldehyde are members of this class.

Alkaline: Also called basic; any substance that accepts a hydrogen ion; its pH is greater than 7.

Allergenic: Causing or producing an allergic reaction.

Allergens: Substances that cause adverse symptoms, such as pollens. molds, animal danders, food and drink (often those most liked or disliked), or chemicals found in air, water, or food. Also called incitants.

Allergic reaction: Adverse, varied symptoms or a group of symptoms, unique to each person, resulting from the body's response to exposure to allergens.

Allergic shiners: Dark circles under the eyes, usually indicative of allergies.

Allergy: Attacks by the immune system on harmless or even useful substances entering the body; abnormal responses to substances well tolerated by most people.

Amino acid: An organic acid that contains an amino (ammonia-like) chemical group; the building blocks that make up all proteins.

Anabolism: A metabolic process involving the production of energy, by which simple substances are synthesized into complex substances; shifts the body pH toward alkalinity.

Anaerobic: Organisms or metabolic processes that do not require oxygen.

Anaphylactic shock: An infrequent, extreme and immediate allergic reaction that can cause difficulty in breathing or even death.

Antibody: A protein molecule produced to protect the body. It is made by B-lymphocytes or plasma cells in response to a perceived foreign or abnormal substance or organism.

Antigen: Any substance recognized by the immune system that causes the body to produce antibodies; also refers to a concentrated solution of an allergen.

Antihistamine: A chemical that blocks the action of histamine, released by the mast cells and basophils during an allergic reaction.

Antioxidant: A substance that slows oxidation. In nutrition, a substance that prevents damage from free radicals.

Artificial: Made by people, often in imitation of something natural.

Assimilate: To incorporate into a system of the body; to transform nutrients into living tissue.

Autoimmune: A condition resulting when the body makes antibodies against its own tissues or fluid. The immune system attacks the body it inhabits, causing damage or alteration of cell function.

Bacteria: Single celled microorganisms that occur as spheres (cocci), rods (bacilli), curved cells (vibrios), or spiral-shaped cells (spirochetes or spirilla). A special bacterial form, rickettsiae, are coccobacilli.

Basal temperature: A "resting" temperature often used to determine hypothyroidism. Also used as a marker to follow effects of treatments for hypothyroidism.

Basophils: A type of white blood cell that mediates inflammatory reactions. They are functionally similar to mast cells and are found in mucous membranes, skin, and bronchial tubes.

B-cell: A white blood cell that produces antibodies as directed by the T-cells.

Binder: A substance added to tablets to help hold them together.

Binding: The uniting of two substances, such as a mineral binding to an enzyme, or a neurotransmitter to a receptor site.

Bioaccumulation: Buildup of chemicals or substances in cells and tissues.

Biochemical individuality: A distinct cellular makeup, basic and unique to each person, which determines cellular needs, responses, and metabolism.

Blood-brain barrier: A cellular barrier that prevents certain chemicals from passing from the blood to the brain.

Buffer: A substance that minimizes changes in pH.

Candida albicans: A type of yeast normally found in the body. It can multiply and cause infections, allergic responses, or toxicity.

Candidiasis: An overgrowth of Candida organisms, which are part of the normal flora of the mouth, skin, intestines, and vagina.

Carbohydrate, complex: A large molecule consisting of simple sugars linked together, found in whole grains, vegetables, and fruits. Metabolizes more slowly to glucose (a body nutrient) than refined carbohydrates.

Carbohydrate, refined: A molecule of sugar, found in such foods as white flour, sugar, and white rice, that metabolizes quickly to glucose (a body nutrient).

Cascade: A succession of metabolic events that accelerate an allergic reaction or immune response.

Catabolism: A metabolic process involving the release of energy, in which complex substances are broken down into simpler substances; shifts the body pH toward acidity.

Catalyst: A chemical that speeds up a chemical reaction without being consumed or permanently affected in the process.

Cerebral allergy: Mental dysfunction caused by sensitivity to foods, chemicals, inhalants, or toxins in the environment.

Cerebral symptoms: Symptoms that affect the brain, cognitive functions, and emotions.

Chelation: In nutrition, a process whereby an amino acid is combined with another substance to increase its absorption and ease its assimilation into the body.

Chemical: A substance produced by chemical processes. Chemicals are classified according to their structure.

Chronic: Of long duration; refers to constant pain, or a condition or illness that has been present for a long time.

Chronic fatigue syndrome: Also known as chronic fatigue immune dysfunction syndrome. Characterized by extreme fatigue, muscle pain, and cognitive dysfunction. Recurrent fevers and swollen lymph glands may also be present.

Clinical ecology: The original term for a branch of medicine that treats allergies and sensitivities through diet, environmental control, and immunotherapy techniques. Now known as environmental medicine. *See also* Environmental medicine physician.

Coenzyme: Organic molecules that enhance or are necessary for enzyme function. Vitamins are among the compounds that serve as coenzymes.

Cofactor: In nutrition, a substance necessary to cause a given process to take place. Minerals serve as cofactors.

Complement: Over 20 proteins in the fluid of the blood, which constitute a system in partnership with antibodies that contributes to the destruction of disease-causing organisms.

Contact dermatitis: Skin rash resulting from exposure to an irritating substance.

Cross-reactivity: The reaction of an antigen with antibodies formed against another antigen. Cross-reactivity occurs, for example, between some foods and pollens.

Cumulative reaction: A type of reaction caused by an accumulation of allergens in the body.

Cyclic allergy: A type of allergy which, with abstinence and/or nonexposure, will disappear and will not reappear unless overexposure to the substance occurs.

Cytokine: A chemical produced by the T-cells during an infection. Examples of cytokines are interleukin 2 and gamma interferon.

Dander: The skin scales that are produced and shed by animals that have fur or feathers.

Desensitization: The process of building up body tolerance to allergens through the use of extracts of the allergenic substance.

Detoxification: A variety of methods used to reduce toxic materials accumulated in body tissues.

Detoxification pathways: The series of chemical reactions in the body by which it cleanses itself of toxic materials accumulated in tissues. Detoxification reactions are grouped into Phase I and Phase II reactions.

Die-off: Uncomfortable symptoms caused when cells of organisms rupture and release toxic metabolic products in the body.

Digestive system: Includes the mouth, esophagus, stomach, small and large intestine, salivary glands, and portions of the liver and pancreas. Its function is to digest food and transfer nutrients and water from the external environment to the body's internal environment.

Disorder: A disturbance of regular or normal functions.

Eczema: Dry, itchy, noncontagious skin rash frequently caused by allergy.

Edema: Excess fluid accumulation in tissue spaces. May be local or generalized.

Electromagnetic: A type of energy involving emissions and interactions of both electric and magnetic components. Magnetism arises from an electrical field.

Elimination diet: A diet in which common allergenic foods and those suspected of causing allergic symptoms are temporarily eliminated.

Endocrine: Refers to ductless glands that manufacture and secrete hormones into the bloodstream or extracellular fluids. The hormones released exert specific effects on other organs.

Endocrine system: Includes the thyroid, parathyroid, pituitary, hypothalamus, adrenal glands, pineal glands, and the gonads. The intestinal tract, kidneys, liver, and placenta may also be included.

Endogenous: Originating from or due to internal causes.

Endpoint: The treatment dose as determined by serial dilution titration.

Environment: The total of circumstances and/or surroundings in which an organism exists. May be a combination of internal or external influences that can affect an individual.

Environmental illness: A complex and extensive set of symptoms caused by adverse reactions of the body to external and internal environments and toxins.

Environmental medicine physician: A physician who specializes in the diagnosis, management, and prevention of the disruption of body homeostasis that results from toxic environmental exposures (foods, inhalants, and chemicals). Treatment may include a combination of environmental control, immunotherapy, nutritional supplements, and rotation diet, with minimal use of drugs.

Enzyme: A substance, usually a protein and formed in living cells, that starts or stops biochemical reactions.

Eosinophil: A type of white blood cell. Eosinophil levels may be high in some cases of allergy or parasitic infection.

Erythrocyte: Red blood cell.

Essential: Refers to nutrients needed for building and repair of the body that cannot be manufactured in the body and must be supplied in the diet.

Excipient: An inert substance added to a prescription or vitamin to give a certain consistency or form to the preparation.

Exocrine: Refers to substances released through ducts that lead to a body compartment or surface, such as sweat or salivary glands.

Exogenous: Originating from or due to external causes.

Extracellular: Situated or occurring outside a cell or cells.

Extract: Treatment dilution of an antigen (allergen) used in immunotherapy, such as a food, chemical, or pollen extract.

Fatty acids: Organic acids from which fats and oils are made.

"Fight or flight": The activation of the sympathetic branch of the autonomic nervous system, preparing the body to meet a threat or challenge.

Fixed allergy: See Permanent allergy.

Food addiction: Similar to drug addiction; the person becomes "hooked" on a particular allergenic food and must keep eating it regularly in order to prevent withdrawal symptoms.

Food family: A grouping of foods according to their botanical or biological characteristics.

Free radical: A substance with unpaired electrons, which is attracted to cell membranes and enzymes where it binds and causes damage.

Fungi: Organisms from the plant world that do not contain chlorophyll and cannot synthesize food from water and carbon dioxide; include mushrooms, toadstools, puffballs, and various yeasts and molds.

Gastrointestinal: Relating to both the stomach and intestines.

Glucose: The sugar that is the principal source of energy for the cells of the body.

Heparin: A body chemical released during allergic reactions. Preparations of heparin, in the proper concentrations and administered sublingually, have an anti-inflammatory action.

Herb: Any plant part that has medicinal, nutritional, or cleansing value.

Histamine: A body chemical released by mast cells and basophils during allergic reactions.

Holistic: Refers to the view that health and wellness depend on a balance between mind, body, emotions, and spirit.

Homeopathic: A branch of medicine in which patients take minute amounts of plant and other substances that in larger doses would produce effects similar to the condition being treated.

Homeostasis: The balance of functions and chemical composition within an organism that is maintained by the actions of regulatory systems.

Hormone: A chemical substance that is produced in the body and secreted into body fluids, then transported to other organs, where it produces a specific effect on metabolism.

Hydrocarbon: A chemical compound that contains only hydrogen and carbon.

Hyperinsulinemia: An excess of insulin caused by the resistance of insulin receptor sites or a deficit of receptor sites, and accompanied by a serotonin deficiency.

Hypersensitivity: An acquired reactivity to an antigen that produces bodily damage upon subsequent exposure to that particular antigen.

Hyperthyroidism: A condition resulting from overfunction of the thyroid gland.

Hypoallergenic: Refers to products formulated to contain the fewest possible allergens. Such products are not necessarily safe for everyone.

Hypothyroidism: A condition resulting from underfunction of the thyroid gland.

IgA: Immunoglobulin A, an antibody found in secretions associated with mucous membranes.

IgD: Immunoglobulin D, an antibody found on the surface of B-cells.

IgE: Immunoglobulin E, an antibody responsible for immediate hypersensitivity and skin whealing.

IgG: Immunoglobulin G (known as gamma globulin), the major antibody in the blood that protects against bacteria and viruses.

IgM: Immunoglobulin M, the first antibody to appear during an immune response.

Immune system: The body's defense system, composed of specialized cells, organs, and body fluids. It has the ability to locate, neutralize, metabolize, and eliminate unwanted or foreign substances.

Immunity: Inherited, acquired, or induced state of being able to resist a particular antigen by producing antibodies to counteract it.

Immunocompromised: A person whose immune system has been damaged or stressed and is not functioning properly; the condition may or may not be reversible, depending on the extent of the damage.

Immunoglobulin: A specific antibody. *See* IgA; IgD; IgE; IgG; IgM.

Immunotherapy: Treatment with allergy extracts over a period of time, with extract doses based on individual test results.

Incitant: See Allergens.

Inflammation: The reaction of tissues to injury from trauma, infection, or irritating substances. Affected tissue can be hot, reddened, swollen, and/or tender. Oxygen availability may be reduced in these tissues.

Inhalant: Any airborne substance small enough to be inhaled into the lungs, such as pollen, dust, mold, and animal danders.

Intolerance: Inability of an organism to endure a substance.

Intracellular: Situated or occurring within a cell or cells.

Intradermal: Between skin layers; a method of testing in which a measured amount of antigen is injected between the top layers of the skin.

Ion: An atom that has lost or gained an electron and thus carries an electrical charge.

Kinins: A peptide formed in the tissues that causes blood vessels to dilate and smooth muscle to contract.

Latent: Concealed or inactive.

Leaky gut: A digestive problem that occurs when abnormal intestinal permeability allows larger food molecules to be absorbed through the intestinal wall. This condition heightens food allergy.

Leukocytes: White blood cells.

Lipids: Fats and oils that are insoluble in water. Oils are liquid at room temperature and fats are solid.

Lymph: A clear, watery, alkaline body fluid found in the lymph vessels and tissue spaces. Contains predominantly white blood cells.

Lymphocyte: A type of white blood cell, usually classified as T- or B-cells, and with many subsets.

Macrophage: A white blood cell that kills and ingests microorganisms and other body cells.

Maladaption: An alternative term to describe sensitivity.

Masking: Suppression of symptoms due to frequent exposure to a substance to which a person is sensitive.

Mast cells: Large cells containing histamine, found in mucous membranes and skin cells. The histamine in these cells is released during certain allergic reactions.

Mediated: Serving as the vehicle to bring about a phenomenon. An IgE-mediated reaction is one in which IgE changes cause the symptoms and the reaction to proceed.

Membrane: A thin sheet or layer of pliable tissue that lines a cavity, connects two structures, or provides a structural, selective barrier (e.g., cell membranes).

Metabolism: Complex chemical and electrical processes in living cells by which energy is produced and life is maintained. New material is assimilated for growth, repair, and replacement of tissues; waste products are excreted.

Metabolite: Any product of metabolism.

Metal: A chemical element characterized by properties of luster, malleability, ductility, and ability to conduct electricity. Also called a mineral when referring to nutrition.

Migraine: A condition marked by recurrent severe headaches, frequently on one side of the head, often accompanied by nausea, vomiting, and a light aura. These headaches are frequently attributed to food allergy.

Mineral: An inorganic substance that must be present in trace amounts to maintain normal metabolic processes; insufficient amounts result in deficiency states. The major minerals

in the body are calcium, phosphorus, potassium, sulfur, sodium, chloride, and magnesium.

Modulator: A molecule attached to a protein, which adapts the properties of other binding sites and regulates the functional activity of the protein.

Mold: A type of fungus that is composed of tubular structures called hyphae, which grow by branching and longitudinal extension. Molds produce spores, which are very allergenic.

Monocyte: A type of white blood cell.

Mucous membranes: Moist tissues forming the lining of body cavities that have an external opening, such as the respiratory, digestive, and urinary tracts.

Nervous system: A network made up of nerve cells, the brain, and the spinal cord, which regulates and coordinates body activities.

Neurotransmitter: A molecule that transmits electrical and/or chemical messages from nerve cell (neuron) to nerve cell or from nerve cells to muscle, secretory, or organ cells.

Neutralize: To render an allergic reaction inactive. In chemistry, to make a substance neither acidic nor alkaline, with a pH of 7.

Neutralizing dose: The dilution of a particular antigen that gives relief from or prevents allergic symptoms. This treatment dose is determined by provocative-neutralization testing.

Nutrients: Vitamins, minerals, amino acids, fatty acids, and glucose, which are the raw materials needed by the body to provide energy, effect repairs, and maintain functions.

Optimal dose: Dose that gives the most complete relief for the longest period of time.

Organic foods: Foods grown in soil free of chemical fertilizers, and without pesticides, fungicides, or herbicides.

Orthomolecular: Pertaining to the "right" molecule: treating disease by supplying the proper balance and concentration of substances found in the body, such as vitamins, minerals, trace elements, amino acids, enzymes, and hormones.

Outgasing: The releasing of volatile chemicals that evaporate slowly and constantly from seemingly stable materials such as plastics, synthetic fibers, or building materials.

Overload: The overpowering of the immune system due either to massive, concurrent exposure or to low-level continuous exposure caused by many stresses, including allergens.

Oxidation: The chemical process by which a substance combines with oxygen and changes to another form. In chemistry, refers to that portion of a chemical reaction in which an electron is lost by an atom or group of atoms.

Parasite: An organism that depends on another organism (host) for food and shelter, contributing nothing to the survival of the host.

Pathogenic: Capable of causing disease.

Pathway: The metabolic route used by body systems to facilitate biochemical functions.

Permanent allergy: An allergy to a substance that always provokes symptoms, even after prolonged abstinence.

Petrochemical: A chemical derived from petroleum or natural gas.

pH: A scale from 1 to 14 used to measure acidity and alkalinity of solutions. A pH of 1–6 is acidic; a pH of 7 is neutral; a pH of 8–14 is alkaline or basic.

Phagocyte: White blood cells possessing the ability to ingest bacteria, foreign particles, and other cells.

Phagocytosis: The process of ingestion and digestion by cells (e.g., lymphocytes ingest bacteria).

Phenolic food compounds: Aromatic food compounds that occur naturally in all foods, and which become antigenic after entering the bodies of susceptible people.

Pollen: Part of the reproductive system of a plant; analogous to human sperm. Windborne pollen is the allergenic pollen.

Postnasal drip: The leakage of nasal fluids and mucus into the back of the throat.

Precursor: A substance from which another sub-

stance is made, such as a substance that is converted into an active enzyme, vitamin, neurotransmitter, or hormone.

Prostaglandins: A group of unsaturated, modified fatty acids with a regulatory function.

Provocative-neutralization: An allergy test that uses an antigen to provoke a reaction and then neutralizes the reaction with a lower or higher dose of the same antigen.

Radiation: The process of emission, transmission, and absorption of any type of waves or particles of energy, such as light, radio, ultraviolet, or X-rays.

Receptor: Special protein structures on cells where hormones, neurotransmitters, and enzymes attach to the cell surface.

Reduction: The chemical process by which oxygen is removed from a substance, changing it to another form. In chemistry, refers to that portion of a chemical reaction in which an electron is gained by an atom or group of atoms.

Respiratory system: Includes the nostrils, nasal passages, throat, larynx, and lungs.

Rotation diet: A diet in which a particular food and other foods in the same "family" are eaten only once every four or seven days.

Sensitivity: A state in which a person develops a group of adverse symptoms to the internal or external environment. Generally refers to non–IgE-mediated "allergic" reactions.

Sensitization: The process that leads to the development of allergic symptoms to a specific substance.

Serotonin: A constituent of blood platelets and other organs that is released during allergic reactions. It also functions as a neurotransmitter.

Steroid: A subclass of naturally occurring lipid molecules such as hormones, bile acids, precursors for vitamins, and certain natural drugs; in pharmacology, a synthetic compound used to suppress the action of the immune system.

Stress: The responses of a person that place undue strain upon normal body functions. Stress may be internal in origin (such as disease, malnutrition, dysfunction of a system, or allergic reaction) or external (such as environmental factors).

Sublingual: Under the tongue; a method of testing or treatment in which a measured amount of an antigen or extract is administered under the tongue. The absorption of material is rapid.

Supplement: Nutrient material taken in addition to food in order to satisfy extra demands, effect repair, and prevent degeneration of body systems.

Susceptibility: An alternative term to describe sensitivity.

Symptoms: A recognizable change in a person's physical or mental state, representing a departure from normal function, sensation, or appearance, which may indicate a disorder or disease.

Synapse: A specialized junction between two nerve cells where the electrical and chemical activity in one cell affects the action of the second.

Syndrome: A group of symptoms or signs that, occurring together, produce a pattern typical of a particular disorder.

Synthesis: The combining of separate elements and substances to make a new, coherent whole.

Synthetic: Made in a laboratory; not normally produced in nature, or may be a copy of a substance made in nature.

Systemic: Affecting the entire body.

Target organ: The particular organ or system in an individual that will be affected most often by allergic reactions to varying substances.

T-cell: A white blood cell that instructs B-cells to produce antibodies in an allergic or immune reaction.

Terpene: A type of chemical that occurs naturally in plants and animals. Widely distributed in plants, terpenes are responsible for a plant's odor and taste.

Tolerance: The capacity of the body to withstand repeated exposures without symptoms.

Total load: The total body burden, consisting of physical, environmental, emotional, and spiritual toxins and stresses.

Toxicity: A poisonous, irritating, or injurious effect resulting when a person ingests or produces a substance in excess of his or her tolerance level.

Toxin: A poisonous, irritating, or injurious substance.

Trace mineral: An inorganic substance found in minute quantities in the body. The major trace minerals are chromium, cobalt, copper, iodine, iron, zinc, manganese, molybdenum, selenium, and vanadium.

Transmission: The conveyance or spread of an infectious disease from one person to another.

Universal reactor: A person who is allergic to or has symptoms from numerous materials.

Urticaria: Allergic hives or welts.

Vascular: Pertaining to blood vessels.

Virus: A microorganism that consists of a nucleic acid (DNA or RNA) core and a protein coat, which reproduces within a living cell by infecting and taking over the host cell.

Vitamin: A complex organic molecule that must be present in trace amounts to maintain normal metabolic processes; insufficient amounts result in deficiency states. Occurs naturally in plants and animals.

Volatile: Readily vaporizes.

Wheal: A raised bump on the skin surface caused by injection of an antigen between the top layers of skin.

Withdrawal: Short-term, adverse symptoms experienced when a person avoids a substance to which he or she is allergic or addicted.

Xenobiotic: A chemical that is foreign to the body, such as drugs, fertilizers, insecticides, herbicides, or fungicides.

Yeast: A form of fungus that is typically oval or round and usually reproduces by budding. *Candida albicans* is a common body yeast.

Suggested Reading

You may want to read some of these books to further your understanding of your total health picture. Most of them are available at health stores and bookstores.

A Consumer's Dictionary of Cosmetic Ingredients, Ruth Winter. New York: Three Rivers Press, 1999.

Excellent resource for unraveling the mystery of cosmetic labeling. The material is understandable for people with no scientific training.

A Consumer's Dictionary of Food Additives, Ruth Winter. New York: Three Rivers Press, 1999.

Helps consumers to understand food labeling and make informed food choices.

A Consumer's Dictionary of Household, Yard, and Office Chemicals. New York: Crown Publishers, 1992.

Allows consumers to learn about harmful and desirable chemicals found in everyday home products, yard poisons, and office pollutants.

An Alternative Approach to Allergies, Theron G. Randolph and Ralph W. Moss. New York: Harper and Row, 1980.

This classic book describes a new approach to allergy and chronic illness. The authors explain that many illnesses, both physical and mental, are caused by our contaminated indoor and outdoor environments.

Biomagnetic Handbook, William Philpott and Sharon Taplin. Choctaw, OK: Envirotech Products, 1999.

A guide to the use of magnetic energy in diagnosing and treating health problems.

Brain Allergies, William H. Philpott and Dwight Kalita. New Canaan,CT: Keats Publishing, 2000.

Presents an overview of depression, schizophrenia, and degenerative disease as they relate to food allergy/addiction and to other substances to which our bodies are exposed.

Chemical Sensitivity, volumes 1–4, William J. Rea. Boca Raton, FL: Lewis Publishers, 1992–1997.

Four volumes on chemical sensitivity that are very detailed and well referenced; a scientific background would be helpful for readers. These books emphasize the effects of environmental pollution on detoxification systems and the importance of maintaining a balance between body systems and nutrient levels.

The Complete Food Allergy Cookbook, Marilyn Gioannini. Rocklin, CA: Prima Publishing, 1996.

This substitutions cookbook contains more than 150 recipes that are free of wheat, corn, dairy, eggs, and sugar.

Cross Currents, Robert O. Becker. Los Angeles: Jeremy P. Tarcher, 1991.

Dr. Becker discusses the application and promise of electricity in medicine and the perils of electropollution.

Earl Mindell's Vitamin Bible for the 21st Century, Earl Mindell. New York: Warner Books, 1999.

A full description of vitamins, minerals, and nutrition is presented in this book. The easy-to-read presentation allows the reader to assess nutrient needs and to select quality vitamins.

Finding the Right Treatment. Jacqueline Krohn and Frances A. Taylor. Point Roberts, WA: Hartley & Marks, 1999.

This comprehensive book discusses the strengths and weaknesses of modern and alternative medicine, as well as presenting what each has to offer for over 70 common health problems.

Guess What Came to Dinner, Ann Louise Gittleman. Garden City Park, NY: Avery Publishing Group, 1993.

A thorough discussion of parasites and parasitic infections and their effects on health. Prevention techniques and treatments are also included.

Healthy by Design, David Rousseau and James Wasley. Point Roberts, WA: Hartley & Marks, 1997.

An in-depth guide for creating a living and working space that is free from toxic chemicals. Indoor health hazards, building materials, air quality products, water and electrical systems, and heating and cooling systems are all reviewed in careful detail.

Healthy for Life, Richard Heller and Rachael Heller. New York: Plume/Penguin, 1995.

Written in a more scientific manner than their first book, the Hellers tell how to reduce obesity and the risk of serious illness and early death by controlling hyperinsulinemia. A diet plan, menus, and recipes are included.

The Healthy School Handbook, Norma L. Miller, editor. NEA Professional Library, 1995.

A comprehensive overview of the school environment and its effects on students. Corrective actions for problems are discussed.

Human Ecology and Susceptibility to the Chemical Environment, Theron Randolph. Springfield, IL: Charles C. Thomas, 1962.

This classic book on clinical ecology, written by a pioneer in this emerging field of medicine, describes chemical susceptibility problems and a working model of the stages of allergy/addiction.

Is This Your Child? Doris Rapp. New York: William Morrow, 1991.

An excellent guide for identifying allergies related to health problems in children. All aspects of treatment are presented, and practical advice on diet and home environment is provided.

It's All in Your Head, Hal. A. Huggins. Garden City, NY: Avery Publishing Group, 1993.

Discusses the relationship between chronic illness and mercury toxicity from amalgam dental fillings. It includes evidence of toxicity and its effect on the immune system, as well as considering alternative restoration materials.

Natural Detoxification, Jacqueline Krohn and Frances A.Taylor. Point Roberts, WA: Hartley & Marks, 2000.

An encyclopedic coverage of detoxification and cleansing, balancing, and preventive methods. Nutritional, homeopathic, and herbal methods of detoxification are discussed in detail.

The Natural Pharmacy, Skye Lininger, Jonathan Wright, Steve Austin, Donald Brown, and Alan Gary. Rocklin, CA: Prima Health, 1998.

This excellent book discusses all major ailments and conditions, and includes sections on herbs, nutritional supplements, and homeopathy.

Nontoxic, Natural, and Earthwise, Debra Lynn Dadd. Los Angeles: Jeremy P. Tarcher, 1990.

A presentation of how to protect yourself from harmful products and live in harmony with the earth. It includes more than 400 do-it-yourself formulas.

Prescription for Nutritional Healing. James F. Balch and Phyllis A. Balch. Garden Park, NY: Avery Publishing Group, 1997.

This book is an A–Z reference to drug-free remedies using vitamins, minerals, herbs, and quality supplements. It is a comprehensive and up-to-date self-help approach to good health.

Root Canal Cover-Up, George E. Meining. Bion Publishing, Ojai, CA, 1994.

A reading must if you have a root canal or think you need one. Discusses side effects of root canals caused by migration of bacteria and toxins from root canal teeth.

Rotation Isn't Just For Tires, Frances Taylor, Deborah Brandt, and Jacqueline Krohn. Los Alamos, NM: Krohn, 1996.

A how-to rotation diet cookbook that takes the reader step by step through using a rotation diet. Several variations of rotation diets are included, complete with suggested menus and accompanying recipes for appetizers, main dishes, salads, dips, sauces, snacks, desserts, and vegetable/vegetarian dishes.

Wellness Against All Odds, Sherry A. Rogers. Syracuse, NY: Prestige Publishing, 1994.

Dr. Rogers discusses treating and helping to defend against toxic insults from the environment. She also includes dietary and nutritional information.

The Yeast Connection and the Woman, Jackson, TN: William G. Cook Professional Books, 1995.

A comprehensive book on yeast problems and health for all family members. This book discusses yeast-related problems that affect people of all ages and both sexes. It also covers nutrition, diet, and yeast control agents, both nonprescription and prescription.

Recommended Sources
and Organizations

The following sources and organizations are those mentioned in the text of this book. They represent only the products and companies with which we are familiar. Certainly there are other sources and other products that would be of benefit in treating allergy and restoring and maintaining health.

Organizations

PATIENT AND VOLUNTEER ORGANIZATIONS

H.E.A.L. (Human Ecology Action League)
2250 N. Druid Hills Rd. NE #236
Atlanta, GA 30329-3118
(404) 248-1898

PROFESSIONAL ORGANIZATIONS

AAEM
American Academy of Environmental
  Medicine
c/o American Finance Center
7701 East Kellog, Suite 625
Wichita, KS 67207
(316) 684-5500
Fax: (316) 684-5709

AAOA
American Academy of Otolaryngic Allergy
1990 M St. NW
Washington, DC 20036
(202) 955-5010
Fax: (202) 955-5016

American Association of Naturopathic
  Physicians
601 Valley St. Suite 105
Seattle, WA 98109
(206) 298-0126
Fax: (206) 298-0129

ACAM
American College for Advancement in
  Medicine
23121 Verdugo Drive, Suite 204
Laguna Hills, CA 92653
(714) 583-7666
(800) 532-2680

International Society for Orthomolecular
  Medicine
16 Florence Ave.

Toronto, ON M2N 1E9
Canada
(416) 733-2117
Fax: (416) 733-2352

National Center for Homeopathy
801 N. Fairfax Street, Suite 306
Alexandria, VA 22314
(703) 548-7790
Fax: (703) 548-7792

Hands-On Techniques

BioSET™
Dr. Ellen Cutler
P.O. Box 5356
Larkspur, CA 94977
(877) 927-0741
Fax: (415) 945-0465

NAET
Nambudripad's Allergy Elimination
   Technique
Dr. Devi Nambudripad
6714 Beach Blvd.
Buena Park, CA 90621
(714) 523-8900
Fax: (714) 523-3068

NET
NeuroEmotional Technique
Dr. Scott Walker
524 Second Street
Encinitas, CA 92024
(619) 944-1030
(800) 888-4638
Fax: (619) 753-7191

TBM
Total Body Modification

Dr. Victor Frank
1907 E. Foxmoor Circle
Sandy, UT 84092
(801) 571-2411
(800) 243-4TBM
Fax: (801) 567-0806

Detoxification Centers

Center for Environmental Medicine
Dr. Allan Lieberman
7510 Northforest Drive
N. Charleston, SC 29420
(803) 572-1600
Fax: (843) 572-1792

Environmental Health Center
Dr. Bill Rea
8345 Walnut Hill Lane, Suite 220
Dallas, TX 75231
(214) 368-4132
Fax: (214) 691-8432

Healing Naturally
Dr. Walter Crinnion
11811 NE 128th St., Suite 202
Kirkland, WA 98034
(425) 821-8118
Fax: (425) 821-4353

Robbins Environmental Medicine Clinic
Dr. Albert Robbins
400 S. Dixie Highway, Building 2, Suite 210
Boca Raton, FL 33432
(561) 395-3282
Fax: (561) 395-3304

Housing Consultants

Archemy Consulting Ltd.
David Rousseau

1662 West 75th Ave.
Vancouver, BC Canada
V6P 6G2
(250) 935-6878
drouss@oberon.ark.com

Environment Education and Health
   Services, Inc.
Mary Oetzel
P. O. Box 92004
Austin, TX 78709-2004
(830) 238-4589

Green Eclipse
Bruce M. Small, P. Eng.
2269 Conc. 4
R.R. #1
Goodwood, ON L0C 1A0
(905) 642-3082
Fax: (905) 649-1314

Healthy House Institute
John Bower
430 N. Sewell Rd.
Bloomington, IN 47408
Phone and Fax (812) 332-5073

Supplies

AIR CLEANERS

AllerMed Corporation
31 Steel Road
Wylie, TX 75098
(972) 442-4898
Fax: (972) 442-4897

Foust Air Purifiers
E.L. Foust Co.
Box 105
Elmhurst, IL 60126

www.foustco.com
(312) 834-4952
(800) 225-9549
Fax: (708) 834-5341

AIR SAMPLERS

Practical Allergy Research Foundation
1421 Colvin Blvd.
Buffalo, NY 14223
(716) 875-0398
Fax: (716) 875-5399
(Air samplers, charcoal masks, books, water
purifiers, videos, audio tapes, peak flow meters)

COTTON AND NATURAL
FIBER PRODUCTS

Janice Corporation
198 US Hwy 46
Budd Lake, NJ 07828
(800) J-A-N-I-C-E-S
Fax: (973) 691-5459
JSWACK@worldnet.att.net
(Natural-fiber bedding, clothes, shoes, fabric,
household accessories, and bath products)

Voice of the Mountain
Vermont Country Store
P. O. Box 3300
Manchester Center, VT 05255-3000
Mail Order (802) 362-2400
Customer Service (802) 362-4647
www.vermontcountrystore.com
vos@sover.net
(Wool and cotton clothing and other products)

Winter Silks
11711 Marco Beach Dr.
Jacksonville, FL 32224
(800) 648–7455

Fax: (800) 648-0411
www.wintersilks.com
*(Silk garments, underwear, loungewear, hats,
and scarves for men and women)*

ELECTROMAGNETIC

ELF Teslar
State Route 1, Box 21
St. Francisville, IL 62460
(618) 948-2393
Fax: (618) 948-2650
(Watches)

Ener-G Polari-T
P.O. Box 2449
Prescott, AZ 86302-2449
(520) 778-5039
Fax: (520) 771-0611
(Diodes)

Enviro-Tech Products
17171 S.E. 29th Street
Choctaw, OK 73020
(405) 390-3499
(800) 445-1962
Fax: (405) 390-2968
(Magnets)

Essentia
100 Bronson, Suite 1001
Ottawa, ON K1R 6G8
(613) 238-4437
Fax: (613) 235-5876
(EMF meters, full-spectrum lights, air systems)

Radon Environmental Monitoring, Inc.
3334 Commercial Ave.
Northbrook, IL 60062
(847) 205-0110

Fax: (847) 205-0114
(Radon monitoring equipment)

Tachyon Energy Research, Inc.
4400 186th Street
Redondo Beach, CA 90278
(310) 542-3035
(800) 888-2509 (orders only)
Fax: (310) 542-3685
(Tachyon beads)

ENVIRONMENTALLY SAFE PRODUCTS

The following companies carry a large variety of environmentally safe products, including personal care products, cleaning supplies, supplements, water and air filters, household products, paints, books, bedding, and many other items. Most of them produce catalogs.

Allergy Relief Shop, Inc.
3360 Andersonville Hwy.
Andersonville, TN 37705
Housing and Environmental Consulting
   (865) 494-4100
Sales and Catalog Orders (800) 626-2810
Allergya@IX.net

Allergy Resources, Inc.
301 E. 57th Ave.
Denver, CO 80216
(719) 689-2969
(800) USE-FLAX

Karen's Non-Toxic Products
110 N. Washington St.
Havre de Grace, MD 21078
(800) 527-3674

The Living Source
P. O. Box 20155
Waco, TX 76702
(254) 776-4878
(800) 662-8787 (orders)
Fax: (254) 776-9329
www.livingsource.com

N.E.E.D.S.
National Ecological and Environmental Delivery System
527 Charles Avenue, Suite 12A
Syracuse, NY 13209
(800) 634-1380
Fax: (315) 488-6336 or (800) 295-NEED
www.needs.com

HERBS AND HERBAL PRODUCTS

Eclectic Institute
14385 S.E. Lusted Rd.
Sandy, OR 97055
(503) 668-4120
(800) 332-4372
Fax: (503) 668-3227

Gaia Herbs
108 Island Ford Rd.
Bervard, NC 28712
(828) 884-4242
(800) 831-7780
Fax: (828) 883-5960

MacroPharma International
1857 N. 105 East Ave.
Tulsa, OK 74116
(918) 833-5060
Fax: (918) 833-5061

HOMEOPATHIC REMEDIES AND SUPPLIES

APEX Energetics, Inc.
1701 E. Edinger Ave., Suite A-4
Santa Ana, CA 92705
(714) 973-7733
(800) 736-4381 (orders)
Fax: (714) 973-2238
Fax: (888) 286-1676 (orders)
(Complex remedies)

BHI Homeopathic Products
11600 Cochiti, S.E.
Albuquerque, NM 87123
(505) 293-3843
(800) 621-7644
Fax: (505) 275-1642
(Classical and complex remedies)

Boiron
East coast: Campus Boulevard Building A
Newtown Square, PA 19073
West coast: 98C W. Cochran St.
Simi Valley, CA 93065
(800) BLU-TUBE
(Classical remedies)

Dolisos America, Inc.
3014 Rigel Ave.
Las Vegas, NV 89102
(702) 871-7153
(800) 365-4767
Fax: (702) 871-9670
(Classical remedies)

Homeopathic Educational Services
2124 Kittredge Street
Berkeley, CA 94704

(510) 649-0294
(800) 359-9051 (orders)
(Homeopathic books and educational materials)

HVS Laboratories
HomeoViticS
3427 Exchange Avenue
Naples, FL 34104
(800) 521-7722
Fax: (941) 643-7370
(Adaptosode RR, complex homeopathic remedies)

PHP Professional Health Products
211 Overlook Dr. Suite 5
Sewickley, PA 15143
(800) 929-4133
Fax: (412) 741-6372
(Complex remedies)

Vibrant Health
150 des Grands Couteau
St-Mathieu-de-Beloeil, PQ J36 2C9
Canada
(450) 536-1295
(888) 337-8427 (orders)
Fax: (450) 536-1294
(Complex remedies)

HOME SAUNAS

Heavenly Heat
1106 Second Street
Encinitas, CA 92024
(760) 942-0478
(800) MY SAUNA
Fax: (760) 634-1268

MASKS

American Environmental Health
Foundation
8345 Walnut Hill Lane, Suite 225
Dallas, TX 75231-4262
(214) 361-9515
(800) 428-2343
Fax: (214) 362-2534
(Ceramic oxygen masks, Tygon tubing)

Diane Anderson
53760 Avenida Mendoza
La Quinta, CA 92253
(619) 564-1709
(Cotton surgical-style flat charcoal masks)

Sandra Den Braber, RN
114 Ray Street
Arlington, TX 76010
(817) 469-9626
(Cotton and silk fitted charcoal masks)

Foust Air Purifiers
E.L. Foust Co.
Box 105
Elmhurst, IL 60126
www.foustco.com
(312) 834-4952
(800) 225-9549
Fax: (708) 834-5341
(Impregnated fiber charcoal face masks)

MISCELLANEOUS

Advanced Health Products
24000 Mercantile Rd., Ste. 7
Beachwood, OH 44122
(888)262-5700
Fax: (216) 514-5700
(High Performance Hygiene Systems)

NEOLIFE PRODUCTS

Neolife
GNLD Distributor Services
3500 Gateway Blvd.
Fremont, CA 94538
(510) 651-0405
(800) 432-5848
Fax: (510) 440-2818
(NeoLife Green)

NUTRITIONAL, ANTIPARASITIC, AND ANTIVIRAL MATERIALS

AMNI
Advanced Medical Nutrition, Inc.
700 Trumbull Dr.
Pittsburgh, PA 15205
(800) 437-8888
Fax: (888) 245-4440
(Organic germanium, hypoallergenic nutrients)

Ecological Formulas
(Cardiovascular Research/Arteria)
1061-B Shary Circle
Concord, CA 94518
(800) 351-9429
(Tapioca vitamin C, Tri-Salts, antiparasitic and antiviral preparations, and hypoallergenic nutritional materials)

Nutricology, Inc./Allergy Research Group
P. O. Box 489
San Leandro, CA 94577
(800) 545-9960 (information)
(800) 782-4274 (orders)
(570) 639-4572 (international orders)
Fax: (570) 635-6730
(Beet vitamin C, antiparasitic preparations, FOS, grape pips, hypoallergenic nutrients, Bottoms Up rectal nutrients, organic germanium)

Pain and Stress Therapy Center
Dr. Billie Sahley
5282 Medical Drive, Suite 160
San Antonio, TX 78229-6023
(800) 669-2256 (orders)
(210) 614-7256 (consultations)
Fax: (210) 614-4336
(Specialty nutrients, Balanced Neurotransmitter Complex, Anxiety Control)

Thorne Research
P. O. Box 25
Dover, Idaho 83825
(208) 263-1337
Fax: (208) 265-2488
info@thorne.com
(Formula SF 722 and other pure supplements—not available at health food stores. Order from company with physician's signature.)

Twin Labs
150 Motor Parkway, Suite 210
Hauppauge, NY 11788
(631) 467-3140
(800) 645-5626
Fax: (631) 630-3484
(Vitamin C, amino acids, CoQ10, hypoallergenic nutrients)

Uni Key Health Systems
P. O. Box 7168
Bozeman, MT 59771
(800) 888-4353
(406) 586-9424 (customer service)
Fax: (406) 585-9892

www.unikey.com
(Paratox 11 and Paratox 22)

Vital Life (Klaire Laboratories)
140 Marine View Rd., Suite 110
Solana Beach, CA   92075
(619) 744-9680
(800) 533-7255
Fax: (858) 350-7883
(Bi-Carb Formula, powdered ascorbic acid,
*   ProBiotics (FOS), grape seed extract, and*
*   other hypoallergenic nutrients)*

RESPIRATORS AND SUPPLIES

Sanderson Safety
1101 SE 3rd Ave.
Portland, OR 97214
(503) 238-5700
(Wilson half-mask and other respirators and
*   supplies)*

SHOWER FILTERS

American Environmental Health
   Foundation
8345 Walnut Hill Lane, Suite 225
Dallas, TX 75231-4262
(214) 361-9515
(800) 428-2343
Fax: (214) 361-2534

STABILIZED OXYGEN

Aerobic Life Industries
2916 N. 35th Ave., Suite 8
Phoenix, AZ 87017
(602) 455-6380
(800) 798-0707
(Aerobic 07)

American Biologics
1180 Walnut Ave.
Chula Vista, CA 91911
(619) 429-8200
(800) 227-4473
Fax: (619) 429-8004
(Dioxychlor)

Good For You Canada Corporation
295 Midpark Way S.E., Suite 210
Calgary, AB T2X 2A8
(403) 296-2816
(800) 661-8364
Fax: (403) 254-8744
(Aerobic Oxygen)

Laboratories and Services

COMPREHENSIVE STOOL AND DIGESTIVE ANALYSIS

Great Smokies Diagnostic Labs
63 Zillicoa St.
Ashville, NC   28801-1074
(828) 253-6621
(800) 522-4762
Fax: (828) 253-1127

Meridian Valley Clinical Laboratory
515 West Harrison, Suite 9
Kent, WA 98032
(253) 859-8700
(800) 234-6825
Fax: (253) 859-1135

DETOXIFICATION TESTS FOR LIVER FUNCTIONS

Diagnos-Techs, Inc.
6620 S. 192nd Place, Suite J-104
Kent, WA 98032

(800) 878-3787
Fax: (425) 251-0637
(Caffeine metabolism test)

Doctor's Data Laboratories, Inc.
170 W. Roosevelt Rd.
P. O. Box 111
West Chicago, IL 60185-9986
(630) 231-9190
(800) 323-2784
Fax: (630) 587-7860
www.doctorsdata.com
(D-glucaric acid and mercapturic acid)

Great Smokies Diagnostic Labs
63 Zillicoa Street
Ashville, NC 28801-1074
(828) 253-6621
(800) 522-4762
Fax: (828) 253-1127
(Detoxification Profile)

DUST/DUST MITE COLLECTOR

Vespa Laboratories
1095 Upper Georgia's Valley Rd.
Spring Mills, PA 16875
(814) 422-8165
Fax: (814) 422-8424

FORMALDEHYDE MONITOR

Occupational and Environmental Safety
  Division of 3M
(800) 328-1667 for referral to local
  distributor

HEIDELBERG GASTROGRAM
PH SYSTEM

Heidelberg International, Inc.
933 Beasley St.

Blairsville Industrial Park
Blairsville, GA 30512
(800) 241-7517
(706) 781-6229

IMMUNOGLOBULIN E TEST KIT

MAST Immunosystems
630 Clyde Court
Mountain View, CA 94043
(650) 961-5501

MOLD TESTING (MOLD PLATES)

American Environmental Health
  Foundation
8345 Walnut Hill Lane, Suite 225
Dallas, TX 75231-4262
(214) 361-9515
(800) 428-2343
Fax: (214) 361-2534

Mold Survey Service
Dr. Sherry A. Rogers
P.O. Box 2716
Syracuse, NY 13220
(315) 488-2856

NUTRIENT TESTING

SpectraCell Laboratories, Inc.
7051 Port West 100
Houston, TX 77024
(713) 621-3101
(800) 227-5227
Fax: (713) 621-3234

PARASITE TESTING

Great Smokies Diagnostic Labs
63 Zillicoa Street
Ashville, NC 28801-1074
(828) 253-6621

(800) 522-4762
Fax (828) 253-1127
(Parasite test kits and laboratory testing)

**SPECIMEN TESTING FOR
PESTICIDES, SOLVENTS,
HERBICIDES, AND HEAVY METALS**

AccuChem Laboratories
990 North Bowser, Suite 800
Richardson, TX 75081
(800) 451-0116
Fax: (972) 234-6095

Bibliography

Books

Abrahamson, E. M., and A. W. Pezet. *Body, Mind, and Sugar*. New York: Avon, 1951.

Altman, Philip L., and Dorothy S. Dittmar. *Metabolism*. Bethesda, MD: Federation of American Societies for Experimental Biology, 1968.

Asai, Kazukiko. *Miracle Cure: Organic Germanium*. Tokyo: Japan Publications, 1980.

Atkins, Robert C. *Dr. Atkins' Vita-Nutrient Solution*. New York: Simon and Schuster, 1998.

Balch, James F., and Phyllis A. Balch. *Prescription for Nutritional Healing – A-to-Z Guide to Supplements*. Garden City Park, NY: Avery Publishing Group, 1998.

Balch, James F., and Phyllis A. Balch. *Prescription for Nutritional Healing*. Garden City Park, NY: Avery Publishing Group, 1997.

Barnes, Broda O., and Lawrence Galton. *Hypothyroidism: The Unsuspected Illness*. New York: Harper and Row, 1976.

Bartholomew, Mel. *Square Foot Gardening*. Emmaus, PA: Rodale Press, 1981.

Beaver, P. C.; Rodney C. Jung; and Eddie W. Cupp. *Clinical Parasitology*. Philadelphia: Lea and Febiger, 1984.

Becker, Robert O. *Cross Currents*. Los Angeles: Jeremy P. Tarcher, 1990.

Becker, R. O., and G. Selden. *The Body Electric*. New York: William Morrow, 1985.

Bell, Iris. *Clinical Ecology*. Bolinas, CA: Common Knowledge Press, 1982.

Bellanti, Joseph A. *Immunology III*. Philadelphia: W. B. Saunders, 1985.

Bender, Arnold E. *Dictionary of Nutrition and Food Technology*. Stoneham, MD: Butterworth, 1982.

Bland, Jeffrey. *Your Health Under Siege*. Brattleboro, VT: Stephen Greene Press, 1982.

Bland, Jeffrey, ed. *Medical Applications of Clinical Nutrition*. New Canaan, CT: Keats Publishing, 1985.

Bland, Jeffrey, ed. *The 1984–1985 Yearbook of Nutrition Medicine*. New Canaan, CT: Keats Publishing, 1985.

Bliznakov, Emile, and Gerald Hunt. *The Miracle Nutrient Coenzyme Q10*. Toronto: Bantam Books, 1987.

Bradshaw, John. *Homecoming: Reclaiming and Championing Your Inner Child*. New York: Bantam Books, 1990.

Braverman, Eric R., with Carl Pfeiffer. *The Healing Nutrients Within*. New Canaan, CT: Keats Publishing, 1987.

Breneman, James C. *Basics of Food Allergy*. Springfield, IL: Charles C. Thomas, 1984.

Bricklin, Mark, and Sharon Claessens. *The Natural Healing Cookbook*. Emmaus, PA: Rodale Press, 1981.

Brodeur, Paul. *Currents of Death*. New York: Simon and Schuster, 1989.

Brody, Jane. *Jane Brody's Nutrition Book*. New York: W. W. Norton & Company, 1981.

Brostaff, Jonathan, and Stephen J. Challacombe. *Food Allergy and Intolerance*. London: Bailliere Tindall, 1987.

Bucholz, Ilene K.; Karen S. Cook; and Theron G. Randolph. *An Alternative Measure*. Chicago: Human Ecology Research Foundation, 1982.

Budoff, Penny Wise. *No More Menstrual Cramps and Other Good News*. New York: Penguin Books, 1980.

Buist, Robert. *Food, Chemical Hypersensitivity*. Garden City Park, NY: Avery Publishing Group, 1988.

Calabrese, Edward J., and Michael W. Dorsey. *Healthy Living in an Unhealthy World*. New York: Simon and Schuster, 1985.

Cameron, Evan, and Linus Pauling. *Cancer and Vitamin C*. Palo Alto, CA: The Linus Pauling Institute, 1979.

Chaitow, Leon. *Amino Acids in Therapy*. Rochester, VT: Healing Arts Press, 1988.

Challem, Jack Joseph. *Vitamin C Updated*. New Canaan, CT: Keats Publishing, 1983.

Cheraskin, E.; W. M. Ringsdorf; and E. L. Sisley. *The Vitamin C Connection*. New York: Harper and Row, 1983.

Cheraskin, E.; M. W. Ringsdorf; and J. W. Clark. *Diet and Disease*. New Canaan, CT: Keats Publishing, 1977.

Clendening, Logan. *Source Book of Medical History*. New York: Dover Publications, 1942.

Colgan, Michael. *Your Personal Vitamin Profile*. New York: William Morrow, 1982.

Colgrove, Melba; Harold Bloomfield; and Peter A. McWilliams. *How to Survive the Loss of a Love*. New York: Bantam Books, 1976.

Cousins, Norman. *Head First: The Biology of Hope*. New York: E. P. Hutton, 1989.

Cousins, Norman. *Healing Heart*. New York: Avon Books, 1984.

Cousins, Norman. *Anatomy of an Illness*. New York: Norton, 1979.

Cousteau, Jacques-Yves. *The Cousteau Almanac*. New York: Doubleday,1981.

Crook, William G. *The Yeast Connection and the Woman*. Jackson, TN: Professional Books, 1995.

Crook, William G. *The Yeast Connection*. Jackson, TN: Professional Books, 1983.

Crook, William G. *Tracking Down Hidden Food Allergy*. Jackson, TN: Professional Books, 1980.

Crook, William G., and Cynthia Crook. *Chronic Fatigue Syndrome and the Yeast Connection*. Jackson, TN: Professional Books, 1992.

Cummings, Stephen, and Dana Ullman. *Everybody's Guide to Homeopathic Medicines.* Los Angeles, CA: Jeremy P. Tarcher, 1991.

Cutler, Ellen. *Winning the War Against Asthma and Allergies*. New York: Delmar Publishers, 1998.

Cutler, Ellen. *Winning the War Against Immune Disorders and Allergies*. New York: Delmar Publishers, 1998.

Dadd, Debra Lynn. *Nontoxic, Natural, and Earthwise*. Los Angeles, CA: Jeremy P. Tarcher, 1990.

Dadd, Debra Lynn. *The Nontoxic Home*. Los Angeles: Jeremy P. Tarcher, 1986.

Dadd, Debra Lynn. *Nontoxic and Natural*. Los Angeles: Jeremy P. Tarcher, 1984.

Dadd, Debra Lynn, and Alan S. Levin. *A Consumer Guide for the Chemically Sensitive*. San Francisco: Nontoxic Lifestyles, 1982.

Davis, Roy, and Walter Rawls. *Magnetism and Its Effect on the Living System*. Kansas City, MO: Acres USA, 1988.

Dickey, Lawrence D., ed. *Clinical Ecology*. Springfield, IL: Charles C. Thomas, 1976.

Dickey, Lawrence D., and John G. Maclennan. *Clinical Ecology Office Procedures Manual*, 6th ed. Society for Clinical Ecology:1981.

Eagle, Robert. *Eating and Allergy*. Garden City, NY: Doubleday, 1979.

Editors of *Prevention* Magazine. *Everyday Health Hints*. Emmaus, PA: Rodale Press, 1985.

Faelten, Sharon, and editors of *Prevention* Magazine. *The Allergy Self-Help Book*. Emmaus, PA: Rodale Press, 1983.

Fasciana, Guy S. *Are Your Dental Fillings Hurting You?* Springfield, MA: Health Challenge Press, 1986.

Feingold, Ben F. *Why Your Child Is Hyperactive*. New York: Random House, 1975.

Foreman, Robert. *How to Control Your Allergies*. New York: Larchmont Books, 1979.

Franz, Marion. *Fast Food Facts*. Wayzato, MN: Diabetes Center, 1987.

Frazier, Claude. *Coping and Living with Allergies*. Englewood Cliffs, NJ: Prentice-Hall, 1980.

Frazier, Claude. *Coping with Food Allergy*. New York: Quadrangle Press, 1974.

Frazier, Claude, and F. K. Brown. *Insects and Allergy*. Norman, OK: University of Oklahoma Press, 1980.

Fuchs, Kathryn. *The Nutrition Detective*. New York: St. Martin's Press, 1985.

Gaby, Alan. *The Doctor's Guide to Vitamin B6*. Emmaus, PA: Rodale Press, 1984.

Galland, Leo. *The Four Pillars of Healing*. New York: Random House, 1997.

Galland, Leo, with Dian Dincin Buchman. *Superimmunity for Kids*. New York: C. P. Dutton, 1988.

Garcia, Lynne S., and David A. Bruckner. *Diagnostic Medical Parasitology*. Washington, D.C.: AMS Press, 1997.

Garrison, Robert Jr. *Lysine, Tryptophan and Other Amino Acids*. New Canaan, CT: Keats Publishing, 1982.

Gioannini, Marilyn. *The Complete Food Allergy Book*. Rockland, CA: Prima Publishing, 1996.

Gittleman, Ann Louise. *Guess What Came to Dinner?* Garden City Park, NY: Avery Publishing Group, 1993.

Golos, N.; and F. Golbitz. *If This is Tuesday, It Must Be Chicken*. New Canaan, CT: Keats Publishing Inc., 1983.

Golos, N.; F. Golbitz; and F. Leighton. *Coping with Your Allergies*. New York: Simon and Schuster, 1979.

Golos, Natalie; James F. O'Shea; and Francis J.

Waickman; with Frances Golos Golbitz. *Environmental Medicine*. New Canaan, CT: Keats Publishing, 1987.

Hagglund, Howard E., and Marsha Ferrier. *Help! I Feel Awful!* Norman, OK: HEH Medical Publications, 1985.

Hallenbeck, W. H., and K. M. Cummingham-Burns. *Pesticides and Human Health*. New York: Springer-Verlag, 1985.

Heller, Richard F., and Rachael F. Heller. *Healthy for Life*. New York: Plume/Penguin, 1995.

Heller, Rachael F., and Richard F. Heller. *The Carbohydrate Addict's Diet*. New York: Signet, 1993.

Hoffer, Abram, and Morton Walker. *Orthomolecular Nutrition*. New Canaan, CT: Keats Publishing, 1978.

Huggins, Hal. *It's All in Your Head*. Garden City, NY: Avery Publishing Group, 1993.

Hunter, Beatrice Trum. *The Sugar Trap*. Boston: Houghton Mifflin, 1982.

Hunter, Beatrice Trum. *How Safe is the Food in Your Kitchen?* New York: Charles Scribner's Sons, 1981.

Hunter, Beatrice Trum. *The Additives Book*. New Canaan, CT: Keats Publishing, 1980.

Hunter, Beatrice Trum. *The Great Nutrition Robbery*. New York: Charles Scribner's Sons, 1978.

Hunter, Beatrice Trum. *Consumer Beware*. New York: Simon and Schuster, 1971.

Inlander, Charles B., and Ed Weiner. *Take This Book to the Hospital With You*. Emmaus, PA: Rodale Press, 1985.

Jacobson, Michael F. *Eater's Digest: The Consumer's Factbook of Food Additives*. Garden City, NY: Anchor Books, 1972.

Jampolsky, Gerald. *Out of Darkness and into the Light*. New York: Bantam Books, 1989.

Jampolsky, Gerald. *Love is Letting Go of Fear*. Millbrae, CA: Celestial Arts, 1979.

Jelks, Mary. *Allergy Plants That Cause Sneezing and Wheezing*. Tampa, FL: World Wide Printing, n.d.

Johns, Stephanie Bernardo. *The Allergy Guide to*

Brand-Name Foods and Food Additives. New York: New American Library, 1988.

Joklik, Wolfgang K.; Hilda P. Willett; Bernard D. Amos; and Catherine M. Wilfert. *Zinsser Microbiology*. Norwalk, CT: Appleton and Lange, 1988.

Joneja, Janice Vickerstaff, and Leonard Bielory. *Understanding Allergy, Sensitivity and Immunity*. New Brunswick and London: Rutgers University Press, 1990.

Jones, M. H. *The Allergy Self-Help Cookbook*. Emmaus, PA: Rodale Press, 1984.

Justice, Blair. *Who Gets Sick: Thinking and Health*. Houston: Peak Press, 1987.

King, Jonathan. *Troubled Waters*. Emmaus, PA: Rodale Press, 1985.

Kirschman, John D. *Nutrition Almanac*. New York: McGraw-Hill, 1979.

Krohn, Jacqueline, and Frances A. Taylor. *Finding the Right Treatment*. Point Roberts, WA: Hartley & Marks, 1999.

Krohn, Jacqueline and Frances Taylor. *Natural Detoxification*. 2nd ed. Point Roberts, WA: Hartley & Marks, 2000.

Krohn, Jacqueline; Frances A. Taylor; Judy Storms; and Homer Woolf. *A Guide to the Identification and Treatment of Biocatalyst and Biochemical Intolerances*. Los Alamos, NM: Krohn, 1994.

Kubler-Ross, E. *On Death and Dying*. New York: Macmillan, 1969.

Lafavore, Michael. *Radon: The Invisible Threat*. Emmaus, PA: Rodale Press, 1987.

Langer, S., and J. Scheer. *Solved: The Riddle of Illness*. New Canaan, CT: Keats Publishing, 1984.

Larson, June, and Bonnie Nugent. *Very Basically Yours*. Chicago: The Board of the Human Ecology Study Group, 1967.

Lederberg, Joshua; Robert E. Shope; and Stanely C. Oaks, Jr. *Emerging Infections*. Washington, D.C.: National Academy Press, 1992.

Lesser, Michael. *Nutrition and Vitamin Therapy*. New York: Bantam Books, 1981.

Levin, Alan, and Merla Zellerbach. *The Type 1/ Type 2 Allergy Relief Program*. Los Angeles: Jeremy P. Tarcher, 1983.

Levine, Stephen, and Parris M. Kidd. *Antioxidant Adaptation*. San Leandro, CA: Biocurrents Division, Allergy Research Group, 1986.

Lifton, Bernice. *Bugbusters*. New York: McGraw-Hill, 1985.

Lininger, Skye; Jonathan Wright; Steve Austin; Donald Brown; and Alan Gaby. *The Natural Pharmacy*. Rocklin, CA: Pima Health, 1998.

Lippman, Morton, and Richard B. Schlesinger. *Chemical Contaminations in the Human Environment*. New York: Oxford University Press, 1979.

Mackarness, R. *Chemical Victims*. London: Pan Books, 1980.

Mackarness, R. *Living Safely in a Polluted World*. New York: Stein and Day, 1980.

Mackarness, R. *Not All in the Mind*. London: Pan Books, 1976.

Male, David. *Immunology*. St. Louis, MO: The C. V. Mosby Company, 1986.

Mandell, Gerald L.; R. Gordon Douglas, Jr.; and John E. Bennett. *Principles and Practice of Infectious Diseases*. New York: Churchill Livingstone, 1990.

Mandell, Marshall, and Lynne Scanlon. *Dr. Mandell's 5–Day Allergy Relief System*. Denver: The Nutri-Books Corporation, 1979.

McElroy, William D. *Cell Physiology and Biochemistry*. Englewood Cliffs, NJ: Prentice-Hall, 1971.

McGilvery, Robert W., and Gerald W. Goldstein. *Biochemistry—A Functional Approach*. Philadelphia: W. B. Saunders, 1983.

McKelway, Ben, ed. *Guess What's Coming to Dinner?* Washington: CPSI, 1987.

Meinig, George E. *Root Canal Cover-Up*. Ojai, CA: Bion Publishing, 1994.

Miller, Joseph B. *Food Allergy Provocative Testing and Injection Therapy*. Springfield, IL: Charles C. Thomas, 1972.

Miller, Norma, ed. *The Healthy School Handbook*. Washington, D.C.: NEA Professional Library, 1995.

Mindell, Earl. *Earl Mindell's Vitamin Bible for the 21st Century*. New York: WarnerBooks, 1999.

Mindell, Earl. *Earl Mindell's Herb Bible*. New York: Simon and Schuster, 1992.

Moore, Raymond, and Dorothy Moore. *Home-Made Health*. Waco, TX: World Books Publisher, 1986.

Morrison, Roger. *Desktop Companion to Physical Pathology*. Nevada City, CA: Hahnemann Clinic Publishing, 1998.

Morrison, Roger. *Desktop Guide to Keynotes and Confirmatory Symptoms*. Albany, CA: Hahnemann Clinic Publishing, 1993.

Murphy, Robin. *Homeopathic Medical Repertory*. Durango, CO: Hahnemann Academy of North America, 1996.

Murphy, Robin. *Lotus Materia Medica*. Pagosa Springs, CO: Lotus Star Academy, 1995.

Nambudripad, Devi S. *Say Goodbye to ADD and ADHD*. Buena Park, CA: Delta Publishing, 1999.

Nambudripad, Devi S. *Say Goodbye to Allergy-related Autism*. Buena Park, CA: Delta Publishing, 1999.

Nambudripad, Devi S. *Say Goodbye to Illness*. Buena Park, CA: Delta Publishing, 1999.

Nelson, Ray. *Pollen Guide for Allergy*. Spokane, WA: Hollister-Stier/Miles Laboratories, 1990.

Newbold, H. L. *Mega Nutrients for Your Nerves*. New York: Berkley Publishing, 1978.

Nugent, Nancy, and editors of *Prevention* Magazine. *Food and Nutrition*. Emmaus, PA: Rodale Press, 1983.

Null, Gary, and Steven Null. *How to Get Rid of the Poisons in Your Body*. New York: Arco Publishing, 1978.

Ogle, Irving. *The Healing Mind*. Berkeley, CA: Celestial Arts, 1974.

Ory, Robert L. *Anti-Nutrients and Natural Toxicants in Foods*. Westport, CT: Food and Nutritional Press, 1981.

Oski, Frank A. *Don't Drink Your Milk*. Syracuse, NY: Mollica Press, 1983.

Packard, Vernal S. *Processed Foods and the Consumer: Additives, Labeling, Standards, and Nutrition*. Minneapolis: University of Minnesota Press, 1976.

Passwater, Richard A. *Supernutrition for Healthy Hearts*. New York: The Dial Press, 1977.

Passwater, Richard A. *Super Nutrition*. New York: Pocket Books, 1975.

Pauling, Linus. *How to Live Longer and Feel Better*. New York: Avon Books, 1987.

Pauling, Linus. *Vitamin C and the Common Cold*. San Francisco: W. H. Freeman, 1976.

Pearson, Durk, and Sandy Shaw. *The Life Extension Companion*. New York: Warner Books, 1984.

Pfeiffer, Carl C. *Mental and Elemental Nutrients*. New Canaan, CT: Keats Publishing, 1975.

Philpott, William H., and Dwight K. Kalita. *Brain Allergies*. New Canaan, CT: Keats Publishing, 2000.

Philpott, William H., and Dwight K. Kalita. *Victory Over Diabetes*. New Canaan, CT: Keats Publishing, 1983.

Philpott, William H., and S. Taplin. *Biomagnetic Handbook*. Chocktaw, OK: Envirotech Products, 1999.

Randolph, Theron. *Environmental Medicine—Beginnings and Biographies of Clinical Ecology*. Fort Collins, CO: Clinical Ecology Publications, 1987.

Randolph, Theron. *Human Ecology and Susceptibility to the Chemical Environment*. Springfield, IL: Charles C. Thomas, 1962.

Randolph, Theron G., and Ralph W. Moss. *Allergies, Your Hidden Enemy*. Wellingborough, England: Thorsons Publishers, 1981.

Randolph, Theron G., and Ralph W. Moss. *An Alternative Approach to Allergies*. New York: Harper and Row, 1980.

Rapp, Doris J. *Is This Your Child?* New York: William Morrow, 1991.

Rapp, Doris J. *Allergies and Your Family*. New York: Sterling Publishing, 1984.

Rapp, Doris J. *Allergies and the Hyperactive Child*. New York: Simon and Schuster, 1979.

Rapp, Doris, J., and Dorothy Bamberg. *The Im-*

possible Child. Buffalo, NY: Practical Allergy Research Foundation, 1986.

Rea, William J. *Chemical Sensitivity, Volumes 1–4.* Boca Raton, FL: Lewis Publishers, 1992–97.

Rea, W. "Inter-Relationships between the Environment and Premenstrual Syndrome" in *Functional Disorders of the Menstrual Cycle,* 135–37. New York: John Wiley and Sons, 1988.

Remington, Dennis, and Barbara Higa. *The Bitter Truth About Artificial Sweeteners.* Provo, UT: Vitality House International, 1987.

Remington, Dennis, and Barbara Higa. *Back to Health.* Provo, UT: Vitality House International, 1986.

Rinkel, H.; T. Randolph; and M. Zeller. *Food Allergy.* Springfield, IL: Charles C. Thomas, 1951.

Rippon, John W. *Medical Mycology.* Philadelphia: W. B. Saunders, 1982.

Robinson, Trevor. *The Organic Constituents of Higher Plants.* North Amherst, MA: Cordus Press, 1983.

Rogers, Sherry. *Wellness Against All Odds.* Syracuse, NY: Prestige Publishing, 1994.

Rogers, Sherry A. *Tired or Toxic?* Syracuse, NY: Prestige Publishing, 1990.

Rogers, Sherry A. *The E.I. Syndrome, An Rx for Environmental Illness.* Syracuse, NY: Prestige Publishing, 1986.

Roitt, Ivan; Jonathan Brostoff; and David Male. *Immunology.* St Louis, MO: The C. V. Mosley Company, 1985.

Rousseau, David, and James Wasley. *Healthy by Design.* Point Roberts, WA: Hartley & Marks, 1997.

Rousseau, David; W. J. Rea; and Jean Enwright. *Your Home, Your Health, and Well-Being.* Point Roberts, WA: Hartley and Marks/Ten Speed Press, 1987.

Saifer, Phyllis, and Merla Zellerbach. *Detox.* Los Angeles: Jeremy P. Tarcher, 1984.

Satir, Virginia. *Making Contact.* Berkeley, CA: Celestial Arts, 1976.

Schauss, Alexander. *Diet, Crime, and Delinquency.* Berkeley, CA: Parker House, 1987.

Schroeder, Henry A. *The Trace Elements and Man.* Old Greenwich, CT: The Devin-Adair Company, 1973.

Schutte, Karl H., and John A. Myers. *Metabolic Aspects of Health—Nutritional Elements in Health and Disease.* Kentfield, CA: Discovery Press, 1979.

Selye, Hans. *The Stress of Life.* New York: McGraw-Hill, 1978.

Selye, Hans. *Stress Without Distress.* New York: New American Library—Dutton, 1975.

Sheinkin, C.; M. Schachter; and R. Hutton. *Food, Mind and Mood.* New York: Warner Books, 1979.

Sherris, John C., ed. *Medical Microbiology.* New York: Elsevier Science Publishing, 1984.

Siegel, Bernie S. *Love, Medicine, and Miracles.* New York: Harper and Row, 1986.

Simonton, Carl O. *Getting Well Again.* New York: Bantam Books, 1982.

Small, Bruce M. *The Susceptibility Report.* Longueuil, PQ, Canada: Deco Books, 1982.

Smith, Cyril, and Simon Best. *Electromagnetic Man.* New York: St. Martin's Press, 1989.

Smith, Lendon. *Feed Yourself Right.* New York: McGraw-Hill, 1983.

Smith, Lendon. *Feed Your Kids Right.* New York: Dell Publishing, 1979.

Spohn, Richard B. *Clean Your Room: A Compendium on Indoor Pollution.* State of California: Department of Consumer Affairs, 1982.

Stanier, Roger Y.; Michael Duodoroff; and Edward A. Adelberg. *The Microbial World.* Englewood Cliffs, NJ: Prentice-Hall, 1970.

Stecher, Paul G., ed. *The Merck Index.* 7th ed. Rahway, NJ: Merck and Company, 1960.

Stevens, Laura J. *The Complete Book of Allergy Control.* New York: Macmillan Company, 1983.

Stoff, Jessie, and Charles Pellegrino. *Chronic Fatigue Syndrome: The Hidden Epidemic.* Westminster, Maryland: Random House, 1988.

Stone, Irwin. *The Healing Factor: Vitamin C Against Disease.* New York: Grosset and Dunlap, 1972.

Stortebecker, Patrick. *Mercury Poisoning from Dental Amalgam—A Hazard to the Human Brain*. Orlando, FL: Bio-Probe, 1985.

Streltwieser, Andrew Jr., and Clayton Heathcock. *Introduction to Organic Chemistry*. New York: Macmillan, 1976.

Stryer, Lubert. *Biochemistry*. New York: W. H. Freeman, 1988.

Taylor, Frances; Deborah Brandt; and Jacqueline Krohn. *Rotation Isn't Just for Tires*. Los Alamos, NM: Krohn, 1996.

Trowbridge, John Parks. *The Yeast Syndrome*. New York: Bantam Books, 1986.

Truss, C. Orian. *The Missing Diagnosis*. Birmingham, AL: C. Orian Truss, 1983.

Ullman, Dana. *Homeopathic Medicine for Children and Infants*. Los Angeles, CA: Jeremy P. Tarcher, 1992.

Vander, Arthur J.; James H. Sherman; and Dorothy S. Luciano. *Human Physiology: The Mechanisms of Body Function*. New York: McGraw-Hill, 1998.

Walczak, Michael, ed. *Nutrition—Applied Personally*. La Habra, CA: International College of Applied Nutrition, 1979.

Weiss, Linda. *The Kitchen Magician*. Milford, MI: Prosperity Publishing, 1986.

Weiss, Linda, and Milton Weiss. *How to Live with the New 20th Century Illness*. Milford, MI: Weiss, and X-Press Publishing, 1983.

Wheeler, Margaret F., and Wesley A. Volk. *Basic Microbiology*. Philadelphia: J. B. Lippincott, 1969.

Whitney, Eleanor, and Eva Hamilton. *Understanding Nutrition*. New York: West Publishing, 1984.

Williams, Robert Hardin, ed. *Textbook of Endocrinology*. Philadelphia: W. B. Saunders, 1974.

Williams, Roger J. *Advancement of Nutrition*. Austin, TX: Clayton Foundation, Biochemical Institute of the University of Texas at Austin, 1982.

Williams, Roger J. *Nutrition Against Disease*. New York: Bantam Books, 1973.

Williams, Roger J. *Biochemical Individuality*. Austin, TX: University of Texas Press, 1956.

Williams, Roger J., and Dwight Kalita. *A Physician's Handbook on Orthomolecular Medicine*. New Canaan, CT: Keats Publishing, 1977.

Wilson, E. Denis. *Wilson's Syndrome*. Orlando, FL: Cornerstone Publishing, 1991.

Windholz, Martha, ed. *The Merck Index*. 10th ed., Rahway, NJ: Merck, 1983.

Winter, Ruth. *A Consumer's Dictionary of Cosmetic Ingredients*. New York: Three Rivers Press, 1999.

Winter, Ruth. *A Consumer's Dictionary of Food Additives*. New York: Three Rivers Press, 1999.

Winter, Ruth. *A Consumer's Dictionary of Household, Yard, and Office Chemicals*. New York: Crown Publishers, 1992.

Wright, Jonathan V. *Dr. Wright's Guide to Healing With Nutrition*. Emmaus, PA: Rodale Press, 1984.

Wright, Jonathan V. *Dr. Wright's Book of Nutritional Therapy*. Emmaus, PA: Rodale Press, 1979.

Yepsen, Roger B., Jr. *The Encyclopedia of Natural Insect and Disease Control*. Emmaus, PA: Rodale Press, 1984.

Zamm, Alfred V. *Why Your House May Endanger Your Health*. New York: Simon and Schuster, 1980.

Journals and Periodicals

Baines, T.; J. H. Somers; and K. H. Hellman. "EPA Motor Vehicle Emissions Characterization Projects on Light and Heavy Duty Diesels." *Journal of the Air Pollution Control Association* 32(7): 725–28 (1982).

Barbul, A., and E. Seifter. "Wound Healing and Thymotropic Effects of Arginine: A Pituitary Mechanism of Action." *American Journal of Clinical Nutrition* 37: 786 (1983).

Barnes, R.M.; Allan S. Taylor-Robinson; R. Finn; and P.M. Johnson. "Serum antibodies reactive with *Saccharomyces cerevisiae* in inflammatory bowel disease: Is IgA antibody a marker for Crohn's disease?" *International*

Archives of Allergy & Applied Immunology 92(1): 9–15 (1990).

Bell, Iris R. "White Paper: Neuropsychiatric Aspects of Sensitivity to Low-Level Chemicals: A Neural Sensitization Model." *Toxicology and Industrial Health*, 10 (4/5): 277–312 (1994).

Bell, Iris. "Environmental Illness and Health: The Controversy and Challenge of Clinical Ecology for Mind–Body Health." *Advances* IV(3): 45–55 (1987).

Bionic Products. "Components of Sidestream Smoke." *Manual for Eleventh Clinical Ecology Instructional Course, Part I—Primary.* Aurora, CO: 15 (April 18–20, 1986).

Bou-Holaigah, I.; P.C. Rowe; J. Kan; and H. Calkins. "The relationship between neurally mediated hypotension and the chronic fatigue syndrome." *Journal of the American Medical Association.* 271(12): September 27, 1995.

Branch, David R. "Fetus's Nicotine Exposure Equals Smoking Adult's." *Pediatric News.* May 1997: 8.

Brault, Heather P. "More research says RSV infection increases a child's asthma risk." *Infectious Diseases in Children.* August 2000: 81–82.

Brault, Heather P. "Pollution decrease causes decline in respiratory illnesses in Germany." *Infectious Diseases in Children.* August 2000: 85-88.

Brostaff, Jonathan. "The Brain–Allergy Axis." *American Academy of Environmental Medicine Newsletter* 20(3): 1 (Summer 1985).

Brown, Norman. "10 Foods to Keep Your Immune System Fit." *Let's Live.* (August 1986): 32–34.

Buist, Robert. "New Light on Chronic Fatigue Syndrome." *Journal of Orthomolecular Medicine* III(3): 186–89 (1988).

Burks, A.; S. Mallory; L. Williams; and M. Shirrell. "Atopic Dermatitis: Clinical Rebalance of Food Hypersensitivity Reactions." *Journal of Pediatrics* 113(3): 447–51 (1988).

Cathcart, Robert F. "The Vitamin C Treatment of Allergy and the Normally Unprimed State of Antibodies." *Medical Hypothesis* 21(3): 307–21 (1986).

Cathcart, Robert F. "Vitamin C: The Nontoxic Nonratelimited, Antioxidant Free Radical Scavenger." *Medical Hypothesis* 18: 61–77 (1985).

Cathcart, Robert F. "The Method for Determining Proper Doses of Vitamin by Titrating to Bowel Tolerance." *Journal of Orthomolecular Psychiatry* X(2): 125–32 (1981).

Cernansky, Nicholas P. "Diesel Exhaust Odor and Irritants: A Review." *Journal of the Air Pollution Control Association* 33(2): 97–104 (1983).

Challem, Jack Joseph, and Renate Lewin. "War in the Wards: A Guide for Surviving Surgery and the Hospital." *Let's Live.* May 1987: 10–14.

Challem, Jack Joseph, and Renate Lewin. "Turn Off Your Allergies with Neutralization Therapy." *Let's Live.* March 1987: 34–36.

Choy, Ray; Jean Monro; and Cyril Smith. "Electrical Sensitivities in Allergy Patients." *Clinical Ecology* IV(3): 93–101 (November 1986).

Clark, Linda. "More Help for Your Allergies, Part II." *Let's Live.* February 1981: 89–99.

Committee on Substance Abuse. "Tobacco-Free Environment: An Imperative for the Health of Children and Adolescents." *Pediatrics* 93 (5): 866–68 (May 1994).

Curtis, Luke. "Latex Sensitivities." *The Human Ecologist.* Number 80: 10–12 (1998).

Drews. Carolyn; Catherine C. Murphy; Marshalyn Yeargin-Allsop; and Pierre Decouflé. "The Relationship Between Idiopathic Mental Retardation and Maternal Smoking During Pregnancy." *Pediatrics* 97 (4): 547–52. (April 1996).

Editors. "Do Superfoods Deliver Less?" *Health.* November/December 1999: 34.

Eurman, Nina. "The Immunity Arsenal vs. the Attackers." *Let's Live.* August 1986: 16–19.

Fackelmann, K. A. "Mother's smoking linked to child's IQ drop." *Science News.* February 12, 1994, 101.

Fasciana, Guy S. "The E.I. Dentist—Dental

Materials Part I." *The Human Ecologist* (25): 9–11 (Spring 1984).

Fasciana, Guy S. "The E.I. Dentist—Dental Materials Part II." *The Human Ecologist* (26): 11–12 (Summer 1984).

Fields, Debra. "Toss That Toothbrush." *Let's Live*. February 1988: 6.

Finn, R., et al. "Hydrocarbon Exposure and Glomerulonephritis." *Clinical Nephrology* 14(4): 173–75 (1980).

Fox, Arnold. "The B Complex." *Let's Live*. February 1984: 18–22.

Fox, Arnold, and Barry Fox. "Immunity." *Let's Live*. October 1987:10–17.

Fox, Arnold, and Barry Fox. "Supplementing Your Immune System." *Let's Live*. July 1987:14–18.

Fox, Arnold, and Barry Fox. "Super Foods and Your Immune System." *Let's Live*. October 1986: 10–14.

Fox, Arnold, and Barry Fox. "Take Care of Your Immune System." *Let's Live*. August 1986: 10–14.

Frank, Ellen Perley. "Rosacea: A Reaction, Not a Disease." *Cosmetic Dermatology*. February 1991, 27–28.

Gaul, John W. "The Immune System." *Let's Live*. October 1981: 117–21.

Grant, Alexander, ed. "Aspartame Headache." *Healthwise* XI(6): 1 (June 1988).

Hahn, L. J.; R. Kloiber; M. J. Vimy; Y. Takahashi; and F. L. Lorscheider. "Dental Silver Tooth Fillings: A Source of Mercury Exposure Revealed by Whole-body Image Scan and Tissue Analysis." *The FASEB Journal*. III: 2641 (1980).

Halloran, Jean, and Michael Hansen. "Unlabeled Genetically Engineered Food Is a Recipe for Danger." *Sully's Living Without*. Winter 1999/2000: 26–29.

Huggins, Hal A. "Root Canals." *Let's Live*. November 1990: 71.

Hunter, Beatrice Trum. "Gluten Intolerance." *Clinical Ecology* IV(3): 120–26 (Fall 1986).

IOM Report. "Exposure to indoor substances can lead to or worsen asthma, study says." *Pediatric Asthma*. February 2000: 17–19.

Jemmott, J.B., and D. C. McClelland. "Secretory IgA as a measure of resistance to infectious disease: Comments on Stone, Cox, Valdimarsdottir, and Neale. *Behavioral Medicine*. 15 (2): 63–71 (Summer 1989).

Jones, M. H. "Superfood #4–Teff." *Mastering Food Allergies* IV(7): 1–2 (July–August 1989).

Jones, M. H. "Amaranth and Quinoa." *Mastering Food Allergies* I(3): 1–2, 4 (March 1986).

Kalsner, S., and R. Richards. "Coronary Arteries of Cardiac Patients are Hyperreactive and Contain Stores of Amines: A Mechanism for Coronary Vasospasm." *Science* 223: 1435–37 (1984).

Kebbekus, Barbara; Arthur Greenberg; Liam Horgan; Joseph Bozzelli; Faye Darack; and Carol Eveleens. "Concentration of Selected Vapor and Particulate-Phase Substances in the Lincoln and Holland Tunnels." *Journal of the Air Pollution Control Association* 33(4): 328–30 (1983).

Kellerman, R. W., and Richard C. Graham, Jr. "Kinins—Possible Physiologic and Pathologic Roles in Man." *New England Journal of Medicine* 279(16): 859–64 (1968).

Kordash, Terance R. "Environmental Control of Molds." *Allergy Forum* II(3): 1–7 (November 1990).

Krassner, Michael B. "Brain Chemistry." *Chemical and Engineering News* 61(35): 22–33 (August 29, 1983).

LaMarte, F. P.; J.A. Merchant; and T.B. Casale. "Acute systemic reactions to carbonless copy paper associated with histamine release." *Journal of the American Medical Association*. 260 (2): 242–43 (July 8, 1988).

Langone, John. "Emerging Viruses." *Discover*. December 1990: 63–68.

Levine, Stephen, and Jeffrey H Reinhardt. "Biochemical Pathology Initiated by Free Radicals, Oxidant Chemicals and Therapeutic Drugs." *Journal of Orthomolecular Psychiatry* XII(3): 166–83 (1983).

Lindsey, Bill. "Off, Off Ye Mildew!" *Sports Afield.* June–July 1999: 67.

Lorenzani, "Symptoms by Allergy Management Procedures." *Obstetrics and Gynecology* 50(5): 560–64 (1982).

MacKenzie, William R., et al. "Massive Outbreak of Waterborne Cryptosporidium Infection in Milwaukee, Wisconsin: Recurrence of Illness and Risk of Secondary Infection." *Communicable Infectious Disease.* 21: 57–62 (1995).

MacKenzie, William R., et al. "A Massive Outbreak in Milwaukee of Cryptosporidium Infection Transmitted through the Public Water Supply." *New England Journal of Medicine.* 331 (3): 161–67 (July 21, 1994).

McGrath, Mike, ed. "Do In Your Dust Mites Now!" *Rodale's Allergy Relief* 1I(8): 1, 4–5 (1987).

McGrath, Mike, ed. "Dust Mites: A Microscopic Monster You Can Tame." *Rodale's Allergy Relief* I(9): 1, 3 (1986).

Miller, Claudia. "Chemical Susceptibilities' Many Guises." *The Human Ecologist* (3): 3–8 (June 1979).

Miller, Dana. "Electromagnetic Bodies, Electromagnetic Pollution." *The Human Ecologist* 34: 7–11 (Spring 1987).

Mitchell, E. A., et al. "Smoking and the Sudden Infant Death Syndrome." *Pediatrics.* 91 (5): 893–96 (May 1993).

Monro, J.; J. Brostoff; C. Carini; and K. Zilkha. "Food allergy in migraine: Study of dietary exclusion and RAST." *Lancet.* 2(8184): 1–2 (July 5, 1980).

Morales, Betty Lee. "Immunity: What Is it?" *Let's Live.* August 1986. 56–57.

Morgan, Joseph T. "The Water Problem." *The Human Ecologist.* June 1980: 3–4.

Moser, Penny Ward. "All the Real Dirt on Dust." *Discover.* November 1986: 106–15.

Nelson, P. F. "Evaporative Hydrocarbon Emissions from a Large Vehicle Population." *Journal of the Air Pollution Control Association.* 31(11): 1191–93 (1981).

Nennella, Julie A., and Gary K. Beauchamp. "Smoking and the Flavor of Breast Milk." *New England Journal of Medicine.* 339: 1559–60 (1998).

Okamoto, W. K.; Robert A. Gorse; and W. R. Pierson. "Nitric Acid in Diesel Exhaust." *Journal of the Air Pollution Control Association.* 33(11): 1098–1100 (1983).

Olds, David L.; Charles R. Henderson Jr.; and Robert Tatelbaum. "Intellectual Impairment in Children of Women Who Smoke Cigarettes During Pregnancy." *Pediatrics.* 93 (2): 221–27 (February 1994).

Olds, David L.; Charles R. Henderson, Jr.; and Robert Tatelbaum. "Prevention of Intellectual Impairment in Children of women Who Smoke Cigarettes During Pregnancy." *Pediatrics.* 93 (2): 228–33. (February 1994).

Oldstone, Michael B. A. "Viral Persistence and Immune Dysfunction." *Hospital Practice.* 81–98 (May 15, 1990).

Oldstone, Michael B. A. "Viral Alteration of Cell Function." *Scientific American.* August 1989: 42–48.

Orfan, Nicholas, et al. "Systemic cold urticaria in a five-year-old boy." *Annals of Allergy.* 67: 143–46 (August 1991).

Pfeiffer, Carl C., and Audette, Lianne. "Pyroluria—Zinc and B6 Deficiency." *International Chemical Nutrition Review.* VIII(3): 107–10 (July 1988).

Pike, Arnold. "Feeding Your Immune System." *Let's Live* (October 1987):34–38.

Rennie, John. "The Body Against Itself." *Scientific American.* December 1990: 107–15.

Ringsdorf, M. W., and E. Cheraskin. "Nutritional Aspects of Urolithiasis." *Journal of Orthomolecular Psychiatry.* XII(2): 142–46 (1983).

Rogers, Sherry A., and William Rea. "Surgery and the E.I. Patient." *The Human Ecologist.* (30): 10–11 (Fall 1985).

Rothschild, Jonathan. "The Thymus—Your Master Gland of Immunity." *Let's Live.* April 1982: 43–47.

Rowe, A. "Chronic Ulcerative Colitis—An Allergic Disease." *Annals of Allergy.* VII(6): 727–819 (1949).

Rowe, P.C., and H. Calkins. "Neurally mediated hypotension and chronic fatigue syndrome. *American Journal of Medicine.* 105(3A): 15S-21S (September 28, 1998).

Saifer, Mark, and Phyllis Saifer. "A Guide to Drinking Water." *The Human Ecologist* IX (June 1980).

Saifer, Phyllis, "Universal Reactivity—Some Underlying Causes." *The Human Ecologist.* (20): 4–5 (Winter 1982–83).

Schultzle, Dennis, and Joseph M. Perez. "Factors Influencing the Emissions of Nitrated-Polynuclear Aromatic Hydrocarbons (Nitro-PAH) from Diesel Engines." *Journal of the Air Pollution Control Association.* 33(8): 751–53 (1983).

Scinto, J., et al. "In Vitro Leukocyte Histamine Release (LHR) to Progesterone (PG) and Pregnandediol (PD) in a Patient With Recurrent Anaphylaxis Associated with Exogenous Administration of Progesterone." *Immunology and Allergy Practice.* 12(11): 29/430 (November 1990).

Siegel, J. "Inflammatory bowel disease: Another possible effect of the allergic diathesis." *Annals of Allergy.* 47 (2): 92–94 (August 1981).

Sigsby, John E.; Silvestre Tejada; William Ray; John Lang; and John Duncan. "Volatile Organic Compound Emissions from 46 In-Use Passenger Cars." *Environmental Service and Technology.* XXI(5): 466–75 (1987).

Strauss, S. E., and J. K. Dale. "Allergy and the Chronic Fatigue Syndrome." *Journal of Allergy Clinical Immunology.* 81: 791–95 (1988).

Tabor, Robert N. "A Unified Theory of Chemical Hypersensitivity." *Journal of Orthomolecular Psychiatry.* XIII(1): 6–14 (1984).

Vimy, M.J.; Y. Takahashi; and F. L. Lorscheider. "Maternal-fetal distribution of mercury (203-Hg) released from dental amalgam fillings." *American Journal of Physiology* 258: R939-R945 (1990).

Wallis, Claudia. "Viruses." Reported by Chestine Gorman; Madeline Nash; and Dick Thompson. *Time.* November 3, 1986: 66–78.

Weitzman, Michael; Steven Gortmaker; and Arthur Sobol. "Maternal Smoking and Behavior Problems of Children." *Pediatrics* 90 (3): 342–48 (September 1992).

Witkin, Steven S.; Ing Ru Yu; and William J. Ledger. "Inhibition of *Candida albicans*-induced lymphocyte proliferation by lymphocytes and sera from women with recurrent vaginitis." *American Journal of Obstetrics and Gynecology.* 147 (7): 809–11 (December 1, 1983).

Yacenda, John. "Your Immune System and Addictions—Any Link?" *Let's Live.* October 1987: 20–23.

Zoler, Mitchel L. "Immune complexes initiate RSV pathology." *Journal of the American Medical Association.* 249 (4): 447–52 (January 28, 1983).

Other

American Cancer Society. "General Facts on Smoking and Health." Pamplet. November 1985.

American Cancer Society. "Women and Smoking." Pamphlet. November 1985.

American Lung Association. "Emphysema." August 30, 2000. *http://www.lungusa.org/diseases/lungemphysem.html*

Ashford, Nicholas, and Claudia Miller. "Chemical Sensitivity." A Report to the New Jersey State Department of Health. December 1989.

Associated Press. "Irradiated Beef Makes Its Way to the Marketplace." The Salt Lake Tribune. February 23, 2000. *http://www.sltrib.com/02232000/business/28664.htm*

Baker, Sidney, and Leo Galland. "Case Presentations: Magnesium, Histamine, Allergic Reactions." Presented at Evaluating and Treating the Environmentally Sensitive/Complex Patient. San Diego, CA. January 18, 1987.

Bland, Jeffrey. "Introductory Nutrition." Audio Training Series. Torrance, CA: 1985.

Bland, Jeffrey. "Therapeutic Uses of Nutrition: Vitamins A to Zinc." Presented at Denver, CO, December 8–9, 1984.

Cardiovascular Research. "Clinical Uses of Coenzyme Q10." Pamphlet. Concord, CA: Cardiovascular Research, 1985.

Colburn, Don. "Allergens Travel Well, Even to the south Pole." The Cutting Edge. June 22, 1999.

Duncan, Bruce. "Chronic Fatigue Syndrome." Pre-publication manuscript. Palmerston, North New Zealand (1989).

Ecological Formulas. "Free Radical Quenchers." Pamphlet. Ecological Formulas. Concord, CA: n.d.

Editor. "More Foods Implicated in Latex Allergies." Allergy Hotline newsletter. March: 2, 2000.

Epidemiologic Notes and Reports. "Plague— South Carolina." Morbidity and Mortality Weekly Report, Centers for Disease Control. 32 (32): 1258 (1983).

Garfinkle, Ellen. "The Role of Psychotherapy in the Treatment of Environmental Illness." Source unknown.

GY&N—Nutrient Pharmacology. "L-Carnitine." Pamphlet. GY&N—Nutrient Pharmacology. Carlsbad, CA: n.d.

Harper, Tara K. "Virus: Hantavirus." Science and Literary Links for Writers, Science and Technical References for Writers. 2000. *http://www.teleport.com/~until/v_hanta.htm*

Hoechst, Marion Rousel. "Interesting Facts About Those Annoying Allergies." Asthma Magazine newsletter. n.d.: 16.

Lieberman, Allan D., and Ellis Kline. "Microbiological Flora: An Antigenic Source of Ecological Illness." Presented at the 19th Advanced Seminar of the American Academy of Environmental Medicine. Phoenix, AZ, November 3, 1985.

Marx, Andreas. "Why Use Drainage Remedies?" Professional Information, n.d.

Myers, John A. "Biological Medicine." Presented at Tacoma, WA, January 1976.

National Center for Infectious Diseases. "All About Hanta Virus." Centers for Disease Control and Prevention. September 9, 2000. *http://www.cdc.gov/ncidod/diseases/hanta/hps /noframes/at risk.htm*

National Center for Infectious Diseases. "Tracking a Mystery Disease: The Detailed Story of Hantavirus Pulmonary Syndrome. Centers for Disease Control and Prevention. September 9, 2000. *http://www.cdc.gov/ncidod/ diseases/hanta/hps/noframes/outbreak.htm*

National Center for Infectious Diseases, "Tracking a Mystery Disease: Highlights of the Discovery of Hantavirus Pulmonary Syndrome." Centers for Disease Control and Prevention. September 9, 2000. *http://www.cdc.gov/ ncidod/diseases/hanta/hps/noframes/ history.htm*

National Institutes of Health. "21st Century Management of Upper Respiratory Allergic Diseases." Highlights from a Conference. 1-8, 1998.

NIOSH Alert. "Preventing Allergic Reaction to Natural Rubber Latex in the Workplace." DHHS Publication No. 97-135, June 1997. *http://www.cdc.gov/niosh/latexalt.html*

Office of Communications and Public Liaison. "Post Polio Syndrome Resources." National Institutes of Health, Bethesda, MD. July 1996. *http://ppsr.com/ppsfactsheets.html*

Pangborn, J. B. "Functions of Important Amino Acids." Lisle, IL: Technical Memorandum #2, Bionostics, Inc., February 1983.

Randolph, Theron G., and R. Michael Wisner. Detoxification: Personal Survival in a Chemical World. Pamphlet. Heathmed, Inc., 1988.

Squires, Sally. "Designer Foods Take Off." Washington Post. May 18, 1999, H15. *http://washingtonpost.com/wp-srv/health/digest/may99/ foods0518.htm*

U.S. Department of Health and Human Services. "The Health Consequences of Involuntary Smoking: A Report of the Surgeon General." Public Health Service, Office on Smoking and Health, 1986.

U.S. Department of Health and Human Services. "The Health Consequences of Smoking-Chronic Obstructive Lung Disease: A

Report of the Surgeon General." Public Health Service, Office on Smoking and Health, 1984.

U.S. Food and Drug Administration. The Regulations Restricting the Sale and Distribution of Cigarettes and Smokeless Tobacco to Protect Children and Adolescents. September 7, 2000. *http://www.lawpublish.com/fdarule.html*

Answers

1. Pollen allergies will cause the eye to itch, but if the eye only itches on the inner corner you may have a food allergy.

2. In his book on Chronic Fatigue, Dr. Jesse Stoss implicated allergies. In environmental clinical practices Chronic Fatigue Syndrome is a common complaint.

3. An allergy to milk can result in bed-wetting (or nocturnal enuresis).

4. All allergic people should be tested for sensitivities to wheat, yeast, corn, soy, eggs, milk and sugar.

5. Proper digestion is a key factor in recovering from food sensitivities and understanding your digestive system will help you to make informed food choices.

Index